Leonid Hanin

Modeling Cancer Progression and the Effects of Treatment

De Gruyter Series in Mathematics and Life Sciences

Volume 15

Leonid Hanin

Modeling Cancer Progression and the Effects of Treatment

Mathematical, Statistical and Computational Methodologies with Clinical Perspectives

DE GRUYTER

Author
Leonid Hanin
Professor Emeritus
Department of Mathematics and Statistics
Idaho State University
USA
hanin@isu.edu

ISSN 2195-5530
ISBN 978-3-11-133332-8
ISBN 978-3-11-133403-5 (PDF)
ISBN 978-3-11-133425-7 (E-PUB)
DOI https://doi.org/10.1515/9783111334035

Library of Congress Control Number: 2026932582

Bibliographic information published by the Deutsche Nationalbibliothek
The Deutsche Nationalbibliothek lists this publication in the Deutsche Nationalbibliografie; detailed bibliographic data are available on the Internet at https://dnb.dnb.de.

De Gruyter and Walter de Gruyter GmbH are part of De Gruyter Brill.
www.degruyterbrill.com

Questions about General Product Safety Regulation: productsafety@degruyterbrill.com

Printing: CPI books GmbH, Leck

FSC www.fsc.org MIX Papier | Fördert gute Waldnutzung FSC® C083411

Contents

1 Introduction: A message to cancer patients

Hundreds of books and many millions of articles have been published on the subject of cancer. Apart from just a handful of exceptions, they deal with very specific questions and due to their technical nature are inaccessible to the vast majority of cancer patients and other nonspecialists. This book is very different. It is patient-centered in that its primary focus is on a number of basic questions that are of vital personal interest and importance to cancer patients and those around them—including family, friends and caregivers who help them go through the existential crisis of cancer.

I made every effort to make the exposition in the book as accessible as possible. However, I expect that from time to time the reader will have to look up the definitions of concepts and pieces of biomedical, mathematical or statistical terminology. In some chapters of the book, the arguments made for the purpose of understanding cancer and the effects of its treatment or evaluating the existing methodologies are mathematical in nature. Comprehending these arguments would require only the standard calculus (or analysis) sequence or its equivalent and a first course in probability. On a few occasions, results presented in the book have more intricate proofs. In these instances, I provided references to my articles containing detailed rigorous arguments. Since Poisson processes are critical for the formulation in Chapters 8–10 of mathematical models and model-based results leading to significant biomedical insights, I collected everything the reader would need to know about Poisson processes in a fairly self-contained appendix. Those not familiar with the mathematical methods employed in the book may gloss over the technical parts and focus on their biomedical essence. Such readers will be aided by nontechnical explanations and summaries that appear with some regularity throughout the book.

The subject of cancer, including its biology, epidemiology, treatment and mathematical modeling, is enormous, and this book is by no means an attempt to do any justice to it all. Rather, biological and clinical aspects of cancer as well as mathematical models and solutions are only discussed to the extent necessitated by cogent exposition of the ideas, principles, results and methodological analyses presented in the book.

Two biomedical caveats are in order. First, this book discusses in detail only solid cancers, which constitute more than 90 % of all cancer cases. More rarely occurring disseminated cancers of blood and bone marrow cells such as leukemias, lymphomas and myelomas diverge from solid cancers in clinical symptoms, mechanisms of disease progression, and methods of treatment. Second, the greatest emphasis is placed on metastasizing solid cancers because metastasis accounts for about 90 % of all cancer-related deaths. A notable example of non-metastasizing solid cancers is the majority of brain tumors, which spread through cancer-cell migration and invasion within the brain.

https://doi.org/10.1515/9783111334035-001

Finally, mathematical notation, if any, is consistent within each chapter of the book but not necessarily across the chapters.

1.1 A common cancer treatment scenario that should not be

Having observed firsthand many cases of cancer among relatives, friends and colleagues, as well as strangers who had read my publications and wrote to me seeking advice, I became convinced that something is amiss at a very basic level in the methodology and practice of oncological care.

Here is a scenario all too familiar to patients afflicted with a malignant solid tumor and to their families. Shortly after a patient receives a diagnosis of cancer and goes through tests and diagnostic imaging procedures that determine cancer type, stage, size of the primary tumor, and various histological and molecular characteristics of the disease, the treating physician enthusiastically offers the patient a treatment plan. If cancer was detected at an early or intermediate stage, the proposed treatment usually consists of surgery and/or radiation therapy, often combined with systemic therapies such as cytotoxic chemotherapy, hormonal therapy or immunotherapy. The patient may naturally find it hard to resist such a definitive offer of hope for a cure and goes along with the plan. All these treatments are designed to eliminate cancer cells or at least thwart or restrict their proliferation. Quite often, as a result of administered therapies, the primary tumor shrinks below the detection threshold. The patient is then triumphantly declared cancer-free and assigned a schedule of periodic check-ups and perhaps a recommendation to take some maintenance medications. Unfortunately, in a large percentage of such patients, within a few years or even months, their cancer returns with a vengeance, either as a recurrence of the primary tumor or, even worse, as metastatic relapse. At that point, more radiation and/or potent second-line chemotherapy or other drugs are deployed. As a result, the patient often beats cancer back for a while to only see it come back again, which triggers a new round of treatment.

Radiation, chemotherapy and other anticancer drugs produce numerous harmful and debilitating side effects. Perhaps the most consequential among them is damage to the immune system, which serves as the best natural defense against immunogenic cancers (i. e., those eliciting an immune response). Weakening of the immune system, in turn, may lead to recurrent infections, which are dangerous in themselves and whose treatment can bring about new side effects. Also, radiation therapy is well-known to cause secondary cancers. Additionally, cancer patients often go through health crises caused by cancer treatment-induced damage to hematopoietic (blood cell generating) system, kidneys, the liver and other vital organs. They may also suffer from fatigue, depression and anxiety, and feel that their mind is beclouded.

After a number of treatment cycles with diverse, and increasingly more potent and toxic, drugs and an uphill battle against snowballing side effects, the time comes for the treating oncologist to tell the patient that progressing metastasis is unstoppable and that medicine has exhausted its options. The patient is then sent home with pain management and other symptom-relief medications or admitted to a hospice for comfort and palliative care.

The described pattern of aggressive cancer treatment is based on a broad consensus of multiple panels of experts, approved by the medical establishment and is viewed as the best standard of care. Ultimately, aggressive cancer therapy is predicated on an intuitively appealing and almost self-evident idea that cancer cells should be eliminated as soon as possible, lest they proliferate and make a delayed treatment increasingly less likely to succeed. This idea has three important implications: (a) frequent use of surgery and radiation as radical first-line treatments for early- and intermediate-stage cancer; (b) starting treatment as soon as possible; and (c) administering the largest dose of radiation, chemotherapy or other agent a patient can tolerate, which is termed the *maximum tolerated dose* (MTD) principle. In this book, I present a number of biomedical and mathematical arguments to explain why tenets (a)–(c) are dubious and why aggressive cancer treatment may actually worsen survival in a fraction of cancer patients, compared to more conservative options.

Poor outcomes of conventional cancer treatments, doubts about their scientific rationale raised in Chapter 4, methodological problems that plague biomedical sciences and their capture by academic orthodoxy and vested interests uncovered in Chapters 12 and 13 are among the many reasons why I urge cancer patients and those who share their journey through cancer to try and develop their own understanding of the basic principles of cancer biology and cancer treatment. The principal aim of the book is to assist them in reaching such an understanding. And to cancer researchers and oncologists, this book is an invitation to take a critical look at the conventional wisdom on cancer and its management.

1.2 The gist and novelty of this book

A combination of the following features constitutes the conceptual essence of the book and distinguishes it from countless other publications related to cancer.

Focus on individual patients

Patients' demographic and clinical attributes, the course of their disease and responses to treatment display great heterogeneity. As a result, population-based descriptions of the natural history of cancer and assessment of the effectiveness of anticancer interventions essentially deal with a nonexistent average patient and may prove grossly inapplicable to a given individual case. The book, therefore, systematically eschews the population approach to cancer and its treatment unless it is indispensable to the subject of inquiry, as is the case, for example, in parts of Chapter 13. Thus, in this book, the discussion of the biology of cancer, responses to cancer therapies and related mathematical models and solutions is tailored to an individual patient. This approach has recently gained popularity under the name of *personalized medicine* [1].

Importance of clinical case studies
Among the most precious sources of knowledge about cancer are detailed, well-documented clinical case studies. Each of them represents a raw manifestation of natural processes operating in an individual patient and thus a nugget of biomedical truth. Unlike cohort and population studies, clinical case studies are unadulterated with inter-patient variation. Taken collectively, individual case studies of patients with the same type of cancer map out the range of possible trajectories of the disease and treatment outcomes. They also provide valuable hints on cause-and-effect relationships associated with cancer and its treatment. Many individual cases will be presented in this book to illustrate general principles.

Generality
Solid cancers number more than 150 types with many subtypes differing in the clinical course of the disease and methods of treatment. Despite such diversity, this book is mostly concerned with general principles encapsulating cancer progression and the effects of treatment that are applicable to all, or many, solid cancers.

Phenomenological approach
What does it mean to know cancer? The knowledge of cancer is almost universally pursued by uncovering detailed molecular mechanisms of cancer origination, progression and treatment-induced response. This approach involves thousands of genes, proteins and other classes of molecules, their proximal and long-distance interactions and associated intricate molecular pathways. Some of the latter are so complex that comprehending their operation in detail is not humanly possible. Following this mechanistic, reductionist way of knowing cancer, scientists have uncovered layers upon layers of complexity in the molecular organization and regulation of life and disease with no end in sight. Although such knowledge is important for drug development, it has not brought about so far a decisive breakthrough in the "War on Cancer." The reason is very simple: Cancer is a living, dynamically evolving and largely unpredictable entity irreducible to the sum of its ultramicroscopic components and their interactions.

Due to its sheer volume and complexity, the research literature on cancer is mostly out of reach for nonspecialists, including a vast majority of cancer patients. What's more, even experts can master only a small fraction of the collectively accumulated knowledge. Finally, and equally importantly, many cancer-driving mechanisms, and perhaps significant ones, have not even been discovered! Thus, the mechanistic and reductionist understanding of cancer has fundamental limitations.

In this book, knowing cancer is viewed in a different light in that it is predominantly *phenomenological*. This means that, instead of focusing on intricate mechanisms of cancer, the book zeros in on timing, rates and other quantitative characteristics of clinically relevant cancer-related processes. In other words, rather than dealing with *whys* and *hows* of cancer, the book asks questions such as *when?*, *where?*, *how many?*, *for how long?* and *at what rate?*

From the perspective of this book, knowing the natural history of metastatic cancer in an individual patient means being able to answer the following basic questions, and many similar ones:

(1) What was the patient's age at the emergence of the first malignant cancer cell?
(2) What was the rate of growth of the primary tumor?
(3) When and at which site was it detected and what was its size at detection?
(4) What was the patient's age when the first viable metastasis was seeded?
(5) How many viable metastases were disseminated by a given time and in which organs or tissues did they take root?
(6) What were the rates of growth of these metastases?
(7) What were the effects of treatment on the growth rates of the primary tumor and metastases?

Of note is that these questions make no reference to molecular mechanisms, whether known or unknown. The very basic, quantitative nature of this phenomenological approach to cancer has two implications. First, it makes the book accessible to a broader readership, including cancer patients and their families, compared to the vast specialized literature that views cancer and its treatment through the lens of molecular biology, genomics and pharmacology. Second, it lends centrality to mathematical modeling, discussed next.

The paramount role of mathematical modeling

Among the seven questions, the third one deals with observable quantities, the first and fourth involve strictly unobservable events, while the remaining questions address partially observable clinical variables and processes. The tool of choice for making inference about the unobservable or partially observable biological processes in an individual subject is mathematical modeling.

Mathematical models depend on unknown parameters whose estimation by statistical or other means requires data. Within the phenomenological, single-patient paradigm adopted in this book, a natural example of such data would be the volume of the primary tumor and the volumes of metastases detected in a certain organ or tissue such as the lungs, liver, bones or the brain.

Importantly, detection of primary tumor or metastases in an individual patient is separated from the occurrence of critical microevents that propel cancer progression (see questions 1 and 4) by years or even decades. This is another compelling reason that makes mathematical models indispensable. As one example, I introduce in Chapter 8 a very general phenomenological model that, surprisingly, leads to the formulation of a general principle regarding the effects of the primary tumor and its ablation by surgery or radiation on metastases—treated in Chapter 9. Although extensive empirical foundation for this principle has been built over the last 120 years, its clear-cut formulation proved refractory to experimental, clinical and epidemiological methods. How specific parametric versions of the general model enable reconstruction of clinically significant unobservable aspects of individual natural history of cancer is demonstrated in Chapters 9 and 10.

Emphasis on methodology
Combining rigorous mathematical analysis of the natural history of cancer and the effects of treatment with statistical inference from data and inputs from biology requires great care about the methods being used. Therefore, methodology of mathematical modeling and statistical analysis constitutes a centerpiece of this book and is discussed at length in Chapters 6, 12 and 13.

Careful formulation of assumptions
Many biomedical articles read like revelations of absolute truth from "the source." The problem, however, is that the "truth" varies among the articles and often fails replication. One reason for this gaping uncertainty is that the authors of such articles never spell out their assumptions. If they did, they would occasionally find that some of the assumptions are not as general as they are believed to be, some restrict the scope of the claims being made, while others are empirically untestable. That is why in this book I strive to carefully formulate all the assumptions, both mathematical and biological, to the best of my ability. For a very brief discussion of the role of assumptions and hypotheses in science, see Section 6.1; great insights into this subject can be found in the classic book [2].

1.3 Should cancer patients unconditionally trust the experts?

A legitimate question cancer patients may, should and frequently do ask is: *Why not just trust the experts and the science they represent?*

As a preamble to a more detailed answer to this question in the next section, let me quote two notable authorities. The first is Linus Pauling (1901–1994), one of the greatest chemists of all time and the winner of the Nobel Prize in Chemistry (1954). In a letter dated 24 October, 1979 and addressed to Dr. Ralph Moss, an American science writer, Linus Pauling stated:

> Everyone should know that the "war on cancer" is largely a fraud, and that the National Cancer Institute and American Cancer Society are derelict in their duties to the people who support them.

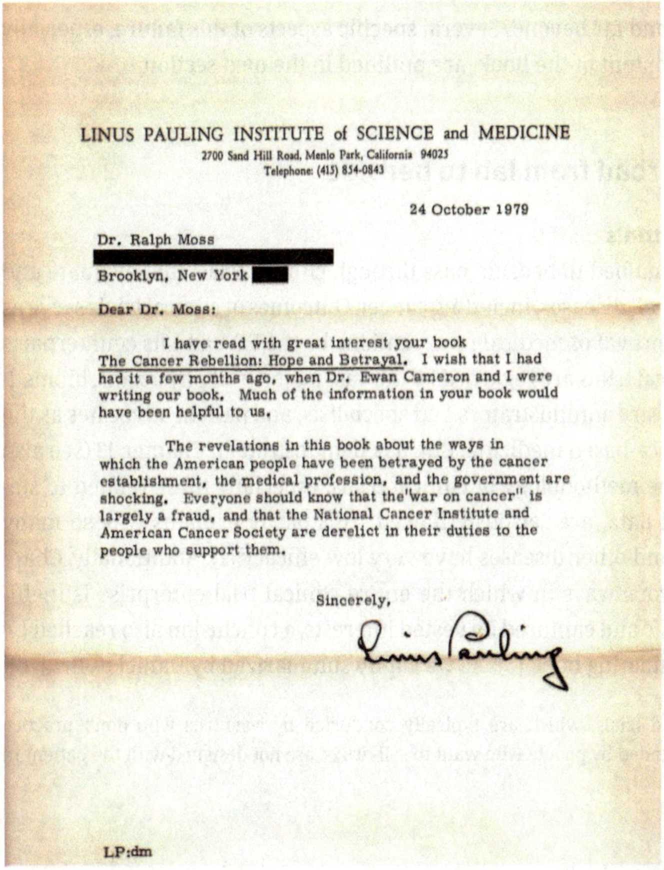

LINUS PAULING INSTITUTE of SCIENCE and MEDICINE
2700 Sand Hill Road, Menlo Park, California 94025
Telephone: (415) 854-0843

24 October 1979

Dr. Ralph Moss
[redacted]
Brooklyn, New York [redacted]

Dear Dr. Moss:

I have read with great interest your book The Cancer Rebellion: Hope and Betrayal. I wish that I had had it a few months ago, when Dr. Ewan Cameron and I were writing our book. Much of the information in your book would have been helpful to us.

The revelations in this book about the ways in which the American people have been betrayed by the cancer establishment, the medical profession, and the government are shocking. Everyone should know that the "war on cancer" is largely a fraud, and that the National Cancer Institute and American Cancer Society are derelict in their duties to the people who support them.

Sincerely,

Linus Pauling

LP:dm

Figure 1.1: Photocopy of Linus Pauling's letter of 24 October, 1979 to Ralph Moss. For context and provenance, see Section 1.3.

A photocopy of the letter is shown in Figure 1.1 and displayed on the website [3].

And here is what Marcia Angell, an acclaimed medical doctor and medical ethicist, and a former Executive Editor and interim editor-in-chief of *The New England Journal of Medicine*, one of the world's most prestigious medical journals, wrote in 2009 [4]:

> It is simply no longer possible to believe much of the clinical research that is published, or to rely on the judgment of trusted physicians or authoritative medical guidelines. I take no pleasure in this conclusion, which I reached slowly and reluctantly over my two decades as an editor of The New England Journal of Medicine.

But one need not take the word of these renowned scientists for granted—their opinions are backed up by a large body of evidence, some of which is presented in this book and a lot of it elsewhere; see, for example, [5–8]. A systemic failure of science, medicine, healthcare and the biomedical industry has occurred in many areas of cancer-related research and practice, and far beyond. Several specific aspects of this failure, especially those previewing the content of the book, are outlined in the next section.

1.4 Blocks on the road from lab to bedside

Problems with clinical trials

Nowadays, all roads from bed to bedside pass through clinical trials that evaluate and compare treatments for all diseases, including cancer. Outcomes of clinical trials serve as a principal basis for approval of medical interventions by the FDA and its counterparts around the world. Clinical trials are regarded by the vast majority of physicians, biomedical researchers, healthcare administrators and specialists, and patient advocates as the gold standard of evidence-based medicine. But, as I demonstrate in Chapter 13 (see also [9]), many aspects of the methodology of clinical trials, especially those related to statistical analysis of trial data, are seriously flawed. This partly explains why so many treatments for cancer and other diseases have very low efficacy [1]. Additionally, Chapter 13 describes numerous ways in which the entire clinical trial enterprise is inefficient, wasteful, ritualistic and captured by vested interests, a conclusion also reached by Clifton Leaf in his illuminating book [5]. As was aptly summarized by Daniel Kolitz [10],

> Randomized controlled trials, which are typically conducted by scientists who don't practice medicine, and often funded by people who want to sell drugs, are not designed with the patient in mind.

The use of questionable endpoints

The most informative criterion for the assessment and comparison of anticancer agents in clinical trials is overall survival, i. e., which treatment leads to a longer average duration of the residual lifetime of cancer patients. Waiting for this endpoint to manifest in a particular patient may take years or even decades. That is why similar but less definitive shorter-term criteria, such as the length of disease-free, progression-free or recurrence-free survival, are widely used. Under pressure from pharmaceutical companies, who want to expedite clinical trial completion even further in order to cash in on their drugs before their exclusive licenses and patent protections expire, a surrogate criterion—the extent of treatment-induced tumor shrinkage, somewhat elusively called *tumor response to treatment*—is ubiquitously employed. However, as I show in Chapter 11, contrary to almost universal belief, extensive tumor shrinkage at the end of treatment is a poor substitute for longer overall survival and, in fact, may actually be a predictor of *shorter* overall survival in a fraction of cancer patients. This paradoxical effect of tumor shrinkage, studied in Chapter 11 through a combination of biological and mathematical perspectives, explains why a "fast and furious" cancer comeback often occurs after an ostensibly successful treatment.

The folly of indiscriminate averaging

If you ask an oncologist about the most important lesson he or she has learned from treating cancer patients, there is a good chance that the answer would be that there are as many cancers as there are patients. It is just an undeniable empirical fact that the natural course of the same type of malignancy, its clinical manifestations and response to identical treatments in different patients are highly idiosyncratic.

A key feature of themethodology of clinical trials is the comparison of treatment outcomes by averaging individual responses within each arm of the trial. As I argue in Chapter 12, averaging distributionally heterogeneous variables, while mathematically feasible, is biologically meaningless and akin to computing, say, the average weight or height for the entire global human population. Yet, comparatively favorable values of arm-specific averages of individual responses in clinical trials serve as the single most important measure required for the approval of treatments for cancer and other medical conditions. Since time immemorial, physicians have been treating patients individually, one at a time. The idea of averaging responses of various patients to a given treatment would have come across to them as absurd and antithetical to the tenets and practice of medicine.

Abuse of statistics

Indiscriminate averaging is but one example of misuse and abuse of statistical methods in biomedical and other sciences scrutinized in Chapter 12. I demonstrate there how and why cavalier use of statistical inference in empirical sciences has led to massive accumulation of false knowledge and irreplicable results (see also [11]). This is one important reason that has caused the trust in science and scientists to plummet in the court of American public opinion [12].

In the world of contemporary medicine, a promising treatment may be doomed just because some purely statistical measures (such as statistical significance, *p*-value or statistical power), only loosely related to the treatment's efficacy, fail to fall within arbitrarily chosen limits. Conversely, meeting these criteria due to chance or expedient selection of study design and/or methods of data analysis may give a green light to poor treatments. As a result, many findings in biomedical sciences including cancer research are "statistically but not clinically significant" [13]. Such are some of the consequences of the statistical diktat increasingly imposed on medicine, health care, epidemiology and biological sciences starting in the 1930s [8].

Reductionism of modern medicine

As a science and practice, contemporary medicine embraces a reductionist view of the patient as essentially a genetically programmed biological machine. In this conception of human being, a patient's consciousness—including one's emotions, beliefs, intentions and personal views on life and death, health and disease as well as qualities of character—are deemed irrelevant to the outcomes of treatment for cancer and other somatic diseases. Among several thousands of articles on clinical aspects of cancer I have read, merely a couple have mentioned the harrowing emotional state of cancer patients vacillating between hope and despair, passionate desire to live and fear of death, as if this is some immaterial anecdotal detail. Just the opposite, the diagnosis of cancer often has a devastating effect on the patient's mental health and can cause adverse and even catastrophic cardiovascular events [14]. Furthermore, the psychological state of cancer patients can negatively affect in many essential ways their immune, endocrine and gastrointestinal systems. Finally, it has significant implications for compliance with prescribed treatment and patient drop-out rate in clinical trials.

One particularly troubling aspect of the reductionist philosophy of medicine is the notion that physicians should treat the disease rather than the patient by following objective measures of the state of disease and its progression, such as test results, diagnostic images, and mutation profiles obtained by sequencing the DNA of cancer cells. As a crude comparison, this is much like how a car mechanic or electrician would approach repair of a broken car or an electrical device. Such a dehumanizing attitude is another major cause of the growing public distrust of medicine. This alienates and repels a lot of patients, for elsewhere in real life—in the family and in relationships, at work, in school and postsecondary education, research institutions, business, politics and sports, and in the military—intention, belief, determination, courage, perseverance and other qualities of mind and character are praised, encouraged and produce great results.

Unsurprisingly, mainstream medicine disdains alternative countermeasures against cancer such as vigorous exercise, radical change of diet, interaction with other cancer patients, attending group therapy sessions, and many others. These measures, however, are known to not only amplify the placebo effect but can also have specific beneficial effects of their own, including extending a patient's life and improving its quality, and ameliorating side effects of toxic drugs. For an inspiring discussion of such non-clinical options of cancer management, see the book by Dr. David Servan-Schreiber [6]. An outline of a holistic, integrative, patient-centric approach to treating cancer is provided in a remarkable book by Jeremy Geffen [15].

It should be stated emphatically that many brave medical doctors make it their professional credo to treat the whole patient and not just the patient's disease. Such was Judah Folkman (1933–2008), one of the greatest and most innovative American surgeons and oncologists, who was the first to discover the fundamental role of angiogenesis, the process by which solid tumors induce the development of new blood vessels that enable their unbridled growth. Dr. Folkman's signature way of treating his patients was to develop a relationship of trust and compassion with them and their families and to gain an intimate knowledge of their individual and family medical history as well as their personal circumstances and preferences. This is one reason why he was relentlessly ridiculed, and his work deprecated and sabotaged, his position at the pinnacle of the Harvard medical world notwithstanding, by the snobbish biomedical establishment engrossed in molecular biology and genetics [16].

Ethics concerns

A universal recommendation of putting cancer patients on an aggressive course of treatment may not only be wrong scientifically but also questionable from an ethical standpoint, for at least two reasons.

Firstly, cancer patients are often not given the full information about their treatment options, associated side effects and overall chances of cure. To quote from the title of the book by Clifton Leaf [5], they are given "the truth in small doses." Cancer patients should know that in spite of considerable progress in treating several types of cancer, such as some childhood leukemias, Hodgkin's lymphoma, most types of thyroid cancer, testicular cancer and a few others, the most common invasive solid cancers that claim the greatest toll of human life, including lung, breast, prostate, colorectal, liver, gastric, renal, pancreatic, esophageal, ovarian, head and neck , and brain cancers, currently remain largely incurable. They should also know that if treated creatively and in an individualized and adaptive manner, many of these deadly cancers can be controlled by medications for an extended period of time with tolerable side effects.

Secondly, the choice between an aggressive treatment and a more conservative one is often, albeit by far not always, the choice between the length and quality of a patient's residual life. The latter choice is deeply personal and rooted in the patient's philosophy of life and death, religious beliefs and what has the greatest meaning and purpose for the patient like seeing children graduate or get married, or grandchildren to be born. Such choice should be an informed one, but eventually entirely up to the patient. Yet quite frequently, instead of providing the patient with expert medical advice in making difficult treatment, and at times life-and-death, decisions and rendering medical services implementing them, physicians railroad cancer patients into standard therapies approved by the medical establishment and considered by experts, rightly or wrongly, the best practice of patient care.

Playing it safe and following the officially approved guidelines regardless of the patient's best interest has deep roots in the contemporary academic and medical culture permeated with an overcautious ethos, fear of reprisals, conformity, self-censoring, rampant groupthink and tight administrative control, all on full display during the Covid-19 pandemic [17]. This environment encourages academic orthodoxy and enables unchallenged transmission and propagation of unproven theories, debatable claims and misconceptions from one generation of biomedical scientists and clinical practitioners to the next (for a wider and more detailed picture, see Chapters 4, 12 and 13). In such an academic milieu, broad swaths of cancer research were allowed to exist largely for their own sake and lose sight of their primary purpose—treatment of cancer patients and alleviation of their suffering.

1.5 My scientific and personal journey

I am a rigorously trained Ph.D. mathematician and as such I have a keen interest in things that are abstract and very general as well as in all sorts of rigorous arguments. On the other hand, I have always been attracted to the workings of the universe and especially of living beings. Although I don't have formal medical education, I have used every opportunity since my middle school years to study medicine, and I was elated by the glimpses into the hidden wisdom of life and the human body that this study has occasionally revealed.

The confluence of these two currents within my academic life occurred in 1986 when I met Dr. Andrei Yakovlev (1944–2008), a visionary scientist who straddled the four sciences, cultures and intellectual worlds of medicine, biology, mathematics and statistics [18]. We quickly discovered the great affinity between our philosophies of science and the complementarity of our knowledge and expertise. Our friendship and collaboration lasted 22 years until his untimely death and produced one book and 22 research articles. Some of his unique views on the synthesis between mathematics and biology and his deep methodological ideas about mathematical modeling are laid out in my article [19].

Over the last 35 years, an overarching goal of my work was to bring rigorous, top-down mathematical thinking and methodology into biomedical sciences, mostly in the fields of cancer research and radiation biology, to the best of my knowledge and ability. I have found that developing mathematical models of cancer and its treatment is worthwhile only if the models are firmly rooted in the core principles of cancer biology and the practice of oncology. That is why I have devoted considerable time and effort to studying these subjects.

Diagnosis and treatment of cancer in a given patient is based on its *observable* clinical features. However, the accuracy of the diagnosis and prognosis of treatment outcomes are often determined by the critical aspects of the disease, such as the presence of subclinical metastases, that are *unobservable* at the time of the diagnosis or the start of treatment. Uncovering and quantifying these invisible attributes of the disease is the sole domain of mathematics, aided by statistical analysis of observables. Thus, the subject of cancer is a perfect ground for synthesis between biomedicine, mathematics and statistics.

I currently work as an independent researcher not beholden to any medical organization, biomedical or pharmaceutical company, or other private interest. I am not supported by any private or public foundation and am thus unencumbered by their views, expectations and policies.

* * *

I hope this book will help cancer patients and their families to successfully navigate the maze of dilemmas and treatment options they will encounter on their road through cancer and to forge a more effective and equitable partnership with their physicians.

Part I: **Cancer and its treatment**

2 The global cancer threat

If I were asked to name the two greatest threats currently facing humanity, I would say it is World War III, followed by the global scourge of cancer. In this chapter, I review very briefly a few well-known facts attesting to the frightening magnitude of the cancer prevalence and associated mortality using global data as well as statistics for the US and Western Europe as illustration. I will also outline trends in cancer incidence and mortality in the US population over a few recent decades. The data provided in this chapter pertain to all types of cancer combined, traditionally with the exclusion of mostly curable non-melanoma skin cancers. All population incidence and mortality counts are reported as *rates*, i. e., the number of cases per 100,000 individuals.

In 1971 President Richard Nixon declared an all-out War on Cancer with an ambitious goal of curing cancer, drastically reducing cancer mortality, and making a rapid progress in cancer prevention. The declaration was buttressed by the National Cancer Act passed by the US Congress and signed by President Nixon into law. This legislative package increased funding for basic research in cancer biology and more than doubled the budget of the National Cancer Institute (NCI) between the years 1970 and 1972. To monitor progress in the war on cancer, the Surveillance Epidemiology and End Results (SEER) database was created under the NCI and became operational in 1973. The SEER database contains detailed information on cancer cases, vital status of cancer patients and the cause of death.

Unfortunately, the grandiose War on Cancer was by and large a "more of the same" type of endeavor [5, Chapters 8, 9]. A cancer cure is still almost as elusive today as it was in 1971. Cancer prevention proved effective only for a very few types of cancer, most notably for lung and cervical cancer, and to a certain degree for melanoma. While cancer mortality in the US and globally is slowly declining for many types of cancer, for other types such as pancreatic cancer it continues to rise. But the SEER program proved to be an extremely valuable aid to cancer epidemiology.

US cancer statistics presented in the next section serves as a report card of sorts for the War on Cancer.

2.1 A few basic statistics

Cancer is the second leading cause of death after cardiovascular diseases globally, in the US and in Western Europe [20]. In the US, cancer had claimed this title for the first time in 1938 and has kept it ever since [5, Chapter 1]. The absolute cancer incidence in the US in 2024 was slightly over 2 million new cases, while mortality stood at about 612 thousand cancer-related deaths. Perhaps even more importantly, in the plurality of countries including the US, Canada, Argentina, Western European countries, Turkey, China and Australia, cancer is the leading cause of death for people under 70, i. e., in their most productive age [21].

https://doi.org/10.1515/9783111334035-003

Extrapolation of recent trends in the US cancer incidence and mortality has led to the following ominous predictions: American men currently have a 40 % probability to develop cancer during their lifetime and over a 17 % probability to die of it [22]. For American women, the respective probabilities are 39 % and 16 % [22]. Thus, the probability to die of cancer for US residents who have or will have developed it is 43 % for males and 41 % for females.

The lifetime probabilities to develop cancer and to die of it display significant geographic variation. For example, in Western Europe, the lifetime cancer occurrence probability is 48 % for males and 40.5 % for females [23], while the probability to die of cancer by the age of 75 is roughly 13 % for males and a little under 9 % for females [24]. It is worth comparing the US and Western European statistics with their global counterparts. The global sex-specific probabilities to develop cancer are over 26 % for males and about 24 % for females [23]. However, global data for the lifetime risk to die of cancer is less reliable due to great disparity in the quality of healthcare, longevity and data collection/reporting practices among different countries and regions of the world. Nevertheless, it is generally believed that 1 in 9 men and 1 in 12 women globally will die of cancer [25].

One of the more troubling signs of the persistence of cancer threat is the rising cancer incidence among children. For example, it was estimated in [26] that the overall cancer incidence in US children aged 0–19 was growing at an average annual rate of 0.73 % between 1975 and 2019. Extrapolating this trend leads to a conclusion that the increase in childhood cancer incidence over the 50-year period 1975–2025 is about 33 %. This is largely due to the growing number of cases of childhood leukemias, lymphomas and cancers of the central nervous system (CNS) [26]. The good news, however, is that the combined mortality for childhood cancers over the same period was steadily declining. For example, the overall 5-year childhood cancer survival rate between 1975 and 2019 increased from 63 % to 85 % [26]. This improvement was especially marked for leukemias and lymphomas. But on the negative side, for cancers of the CNS as well as bone and soft tissue tumors, the 5-year survival rate remained low, hovering at around 60 % [26].

Another concerning recent global trend is a sharp rise in early-onset cancer incidence and associated mortality. Early-onset cancer is defined as cancer diagnosed in patients younger than 50 years of age. For example, it was reported in [27] that the global incidence of early-onset cancer increased by almost 79 % between 1990 and 2019, while mortality caused by such cancers rose by about 27 %. Juxtaposing these figures with an overall global decline in the incidence and mortality for childhood cancers during this time period leads to a conclusion that the aforementioned trend in early-onset cancer is mostly due to an uptick in cancer incidence and the ensuing mortality among people aged 20–49.

The overall trends in cancer incidence and mortality in the US for the period 1975–2021 are displayed in Figure 2.1. It clearly shows that a period of continuous growth of mortality for both sexes was followed, since around 1991, by a tendency of steady decline. By contrast, the pattern of cancer incidence dynamics is sex-specific. The long-term pattern of cancer incidence in males was a slight increase with significant

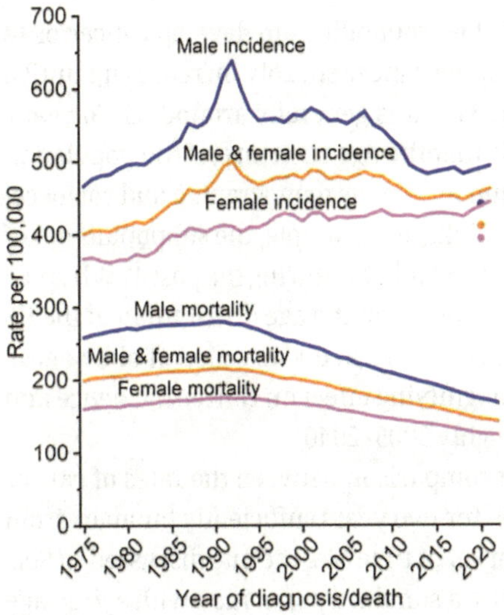

Figure 2.1: Trends in the US cancer incidence (1975–2021) and mortality (1975–2022) rates by sex. Rates are age adjusted to the 2000 US standard population, and incidence rates are adjusted for delays in case reporting. Due to the impact of Covid-19 pandemic, incidence data for 2020 do not fit the trend lines and are shown separately.
The figure was reproduced with permission from Siegel RL, Kratzer TB, Giaquinto AN, Sung H, Jemal A. Cancer statistics, 2025. CA Cancer J Clin 2025, 75, 10–45.

fluctuations including a sharp peak around 1992. This pattern closely follows a similar trend in the incidence of prostate cancer, the most common cancer in American men, with the peak attributable to the introduction of mass PSA screening of the male population around that time. In 2025 prostate cancer accounted for about 30 % of all new cases in US men and was the second leading cause of cancer-related deaths after lung cancer [28]. Cancer incidence in women was growing more steadily with only minor fluctuations. The growth pattern for women was greatly influenced by a considerable increase in the incidence of breast cancer, which is the most prevalent cancer in US women. In 2025 it accounted for about 32 % of new cases and was the second leading cause of cancer-related mortality among US women following lung cancer [28].

2.2 A word of caution

For any particular year, cancer incidence or mortality in a given population can be reported as a raw number representing new cases or deaths due to cancer, or as a relevant population rate per 100,000 people. An important source of such raw information in the US is the SEER database. However, such straightforward reporting is inadequate when cancer incidence and mortality are computed for, or compared across, a long span of years, or for the purpose of their prognostication. The two main reasons at play are as follows. The first is the drastic dependence of the probabilities to develop cancer or to die of it on age. For example, the risk of developing cancer sharply increases up until a certain age, which depends on the type of cancer but is generally around 65–70 years, and decreases thereafter. The second reason is that the age structure of the population of interest changes with the passage of time due to various demographic and socioeconomic processes as well as increased longevity. Take, for example, the subpopulation of baby boomers, i. e., US residents born between 1946 and 1964 during the post-WWII spike in birth rates. Baby boomers form a conspicuous bulge on the age distribution of the US population. As they age, the bulge moves to the right (i. e., in the direction of older ages), which had, has and will have a considerable magnifying effect on cancer incidence and mortality over an extended period of time, roughly 2005–2040.

A conventional statistical device enabling comparison between the rates of cancer incidence and mortality in the same population for two years sufficiently far apart from each other or charting a trend over a long interval of time like the one discussed in Section 2.1 is called *age adjustment*. The idea is to use a standard population with a *fixed* age distribution. In practice, such a standard population is extracted from a US census, typically the most recent one taken in 2000 and occasionally from one of the two previous censuses conducted in 1970 and 1940. Replacing the actual age distribution for a given year with a standard one, which for the year 2025 is 25, 55 or even 85 years older, can bring about considerable errors in the computation of cancer rates, most likely resulting in their underestimation (see [5, Chapter 2]).

I would be remiss without mentioning that cancer rates and other measures reported in various literature sources for the same year and population often display significant variation. This is due to many factors: (1) divergent criteria for what qualifies as cancer; (2) the source of raw data used for analysis; (3) differences in the methods of data processing; (4) selection of a particular standard population for the purpose of age adjustment; and (5) the size of age intervals (bins) chosen to represent the standard age distribution (e. g., 5-year vs. 10-year bins).

Thus, published data on cancer incidence and mortality and other epidemiological measures should be taken with a grain of salt.

I cannot emphasize strongly enough that cancers accounted for by the aforementioned statistics on incidence represent only the visible tip of the iceberg. A lot of cancers are microscopic and dormant and thereby undetectable by conventional means. Such cancers are discovered in great abundance on autopsies of people who died of causes unrelated to cancer. For a detailed treatment of cancer dormancy, the reader is referred to Section 3.6. The danger of such subclinical cancers lies in the fact that they can awaken either spontaneously or a result of medical interventions and other health-related events, see Sections 3.8, 5.2–5.4 and 14.4.

Finally, deaths caused by cancer can be due to either natural progression of the disease or cancer treatment. What is the contribution of the latter? This book shines some light on this fundamental question in Chapters 4, 5, 9 and 11.

3 Biology of cancer: the main principles

In line with the phenomenological approach of this book, the principal universal features of a clinically significant cancer considered here are uncontrolled proliferation of cancer cells and their invasion of surrounding normal tissue. Additionally, the majority of invasive cancers, including the most deadly ones, have the ability to colonize distant sites, i. e., to form metastases.

Among major diseases afflicting humans, cancer is perhaps the most baffling and poorly understood [29]. As Francis Peyton Rous (1879–1970), who was awarded in 1966 a Nobel Prize in Physiology or Medicine for his discovery of cancer-causing viruses, stated in his Nobel lecture [30],

> ... neoplastic cells neither give off any tell-tale substance indicative of their presence nor elicit any specific reaction from the body, whereby it can be certainly discerned; nor do they form any injurious substance characteristic of themselves even while flourishing in great number or undergoing necrosis. True, the body often reacts against them while they are small, as it does against grafts of incompatible normal tissue, destroying these; yet so rarely do established tumors disappear that such happenings seem miraculous. The generality of them, while growing, do away so completely with the initial resistance the body offers to strange cells that even grafts from animals of alien species may succeed.

3.1 The origins of cancer

The scientific field of carcinogenesis is dominated by the mutational theory of cancer. Here are, in a nutshell, the principal tenets of this theory, which can be found in every textbook in biology or medicine. Cancer arises from a single cell that has acquired one or, more likely, several mutations in critical genes. The accumulation of multiple mutations typically occurs sequentially. If a particular type of cancer is caused by, say, two mutations, then the second mutation occurs in one of the cells within the clone generated by the progenitor cell that had acquired the first mutation. Since unrepaired mutations are inherited by the progeny, the first fully malignant cell generates, under favorable conditions, a cancerous clone, the precursor of a malignant tumor. Depending on the affected genes, the mutations can disrupt or dysregulate such vital interrelated cellular processes as growth, proliferation, cell cycle, cell division and apoptosis (programmed cell death). As a result, cancer cells carrying such mutations and their offspring become less susceptible to regulatory signals emanating from the neighboring cells, the microenvironment (see the next section) and the organism at large. In particular, cancer cells can develop the ability to block or evade apoptotic signals, which gradually leads to uncontrollable and largely autonomous cell proliferation, one of the hallmarks of cancer. Despite this, cancer cells maintain, although often gradually lose, many traits and functions of their normal tissue of origin.

https://doi.org/10.1515/9783111334035-004

Carcinogenic mutations emerge either spontaneously or due to the action of chemical carcinogens, radiation or viruses. Mutations occurring in gametes (i. e., sperm in males and eggs in females) or in germ cells very early during embryonic development are carried by all cells in the body and are passed on to the progeny, which creates an inherited predisposition to certain types of cancer. A much more common scenario, however, is that carcinogenic mutations occur in somatic stem cells or differentiated functional cells, in which case they are not inherited by the next generation.

Some of the mutations can occur in genes controlling the fidelity of DNA replication or the molecular machinery of DNA damage repair. This leads to accelerated accumulation of additional mutations, which results in *genomic instability* of cancer cells. In advanced tumors, cancer cells are routinely found to harbor gross chromosomal abnormalities such as translocations (swapping of genetic material between sites on the same or different chromosomes or attachment of a broken piece of a chromosome to another chromosome), loss of fragments of a chromosome or even its entire arm, and a change in the number of chromosomes carried by a cell, called *aneuploidy*.

Some cancer cell lines are exceedingly resilient in that they can be transferred from one animal host to another without loss of malignant potency for decades, which makes them effectively immortal [30]. By contrast, the number of divisions a normal somatic differentiated cell can go through is bounded by the so-called *Hayflick limit*, typically around 40–60 [31].

The mutational theory of cancer implies that malignancy is an irreversible state of cancer cells or, as a popular dictum has it, *"once a cancer cell, always a cancer cell."* This notion has momentous consequences for cancer treatment, for it suggests that cancer cure can only be achieved by killing all cancer cells.

Over recent decades, the uniformity of scientific views on the genesis of cancer has been challenged by a few dissenters who proposed alternative theories, largely ignored and disdained by the mainstream biology. One of the most appealing among these heretical theories propounds that cancer originates at the tissue level and is rooted in deterioration of the tissue's morphology, function and signaling interactions [32–35]. This can be caused by many factors including hereditary disease, exposure to carcinogenic chemicals or radiation, bacterial or viral infection and wounding. According to this theory, mutations in cancer cells is a secondary phenomenon brought about by epigenetic mechanisms. In a dramatic departure from genetic determinism, the tissue paradigm posits that cancer is not a disease of individual cells but rather a malfunction of their collective organization and behavior. As Sir David Smithers, the British physician and radiologist, has aptly put it in 1962 [36], *"cancer is no more a disease of cells than a traffic jam is a disease of cars."*

A significant blow to the universality claim of the mutational theory of cancer was dealt in 1975 by a classic experimental study [37]. In the final stage of their meticulously conducted 8-year experiment, Beatrice Mintz and Karl Illmensee implanted cells of a highly malignant, metastasizing teratocarcinoma (a type of embryonal cancer) into mouse embryos at a very early stage of embryonic development. In spite of this, the embryos gave rise to viable perfectly normal mice carrying certain phenotypic traits of the lineage of mice from which cancer cells were derived. This demonstrates that under certain conditions cancer cells can be reprogrammed into normal ones. Thus, cancer is not always an immutable state but rather a reversible phenotype, a view that comports with the tissue theory of cancinogenesis. Reverting malignant phenotype by correction of signaling between cancer cells and their microenvironment has been extensively studied and successfully applied to the management of human acute promyelocytic leukemia (PML) [38].

There are many other systematic observations that favor the tissue theory of carcinogenesis over its mutational rival. One of them is *field cancerization*, i. e., that significant areas adjacent to malignant tumors consist of abnormal precancerous cells and have altered morphology and function. This is especially common in cancers caused by exposure to carcinogens such as lung cancer due to smoking, mouth cancer caused by chewing tobacco and skin cancer caused by exposure to UV light or polycyclic hydrocarbons. Remarkably, similar dysplastic changes are routinely observed in the contralateral breast of breast cancer patients without any evidence of the presence of cancer cells [35]. The field effect is often accompanied by the finding of multiple cancerous foci. For example, such multifocality is present in 40–54 % of breast cancers [35]. Finally, an indication that cancer can occur without initial changes in the genome is furnished by animal studies where insertion of tissue-separating, non-carcinogenic foreign objects such as glass or plastic film triggered malignant transformation [39].

Understanding carcinogenesis is important because it illuminates the entire phenomenon of cancer and is consequential for cancer prevention. However, for the purposes of this book, the question of whether mutations precede and cause tissue dysplasia or the other way around is largely irrelevant, for the book is mostly focused on the phenomenology of cancer progression and clinical effects of cancer treatment irrespective of how cancer came into being.

3.2 The role of tumor microenvironment

During embryonic development, a fertilized egg and its immediate offspring first undergo several mitotic divisions forming a clump of *totipotent* stem cells, i. e., those that can give rise to any organ or tissue in the body. Subsequently, under the action of precisely timed signals emanating from the mother's reproductive system, the incipient fetus starts to assume spatial orientation and form developmental axes. Concurrently, sequential divisions of stem cells produce increasingly more *differentiated* (specialized) cells that will eventually form all organs and systems of the emerging organism down to minute detail. Although the genomes of all cells in the body, including stem cells and differentiated cells of various degrees of "stemness" and differentiation, are identical, their geometric shapes, sizes, the physiological functions they perform and the morphology of the tissues they form are vastly different. This remarkable phenomenon is mostly the result of epigenetic control of selective gene expression effected by surrounding cells.

Under normal conditions, the process of embryonic development is characterized by perfect spatial and temporal order in sequence, structure, morphology and function. The same orderly operation and renewal is characteristic of normal tissues and organs. Exactly the opposite is happening in an inchoate tumor. It represents a chaotically growing cellular mass with deranged morphology, disordered behavior, blurry boundaries and altered physiological functions. A critical component of this disorganization is abnormal interactions with the *tumor microenvironment*.

The microenvironment of a normal or cancerous tissue consists of sparsely spaced cells of the connective tissue (also termed *stroma*) and noncellular material called *extracellular matrix* (ECM). The latter is comprised of a gel-like substance and fibrous proteins and is penetrated by blood vessels, lymph channels and nerves.

Modern methods of histopathology, including tissue staining and fluorescent labeling, which enable visualization of individual cells of various lineages, have demonstrated beyond reasonable doubt the presence of two phenomena: (1) that a growing tumor leads to progressive deterioration of both cellular and noncellular components of the microenvironment and (2) that malignant tumors depend critically on support by, and cooperation with, adjacent normal cells [40].

When cancer cells make direct contact with normal cells, the latter often die by apoptosis. However, if the normal cells adjacent to the tumor are refractory to stimulation by cancer cells, don't emit supporting signals and actively compete with them for space and vital chemicals, tumor growth is arrested or even reversed. Thus, a healthy normal microenvironment is a potent tumor suppressor [41].

The interaction between tumor and normal cells occurs on the interface between the tumor and the host, i. e., precisely in the tumor microenvironment. The latter is involved in many processes including engagement of membrane receptors of tumor cells by growth factors secreted by various cell types, bidirectional passage of signaling molecules and recruitment of normal cells into the expanding tumor. Additionally, immunogenic tumors often incorporate varied cells of the immune system.

3.3 Angiogenesis

Growing primary and secondary tumors encounter a hard barrier to their continued expansion. This is due to the fact that nutrients, oxygen and growth factors required for functioning and proliferation of tumor cells are supplied by the tumor microenvironment, mostly through diffusion at a rate proportional to tumor surface area or, in the special case of a spherical tumor, to the square of the tumor's diameter. At the same time, the demand for these resources is proportional to the number of tumor cells (in other words, to tumor volume or the cube of the diameter). Similarly, waste products of cellular metabolism accumulate at a rate proportional to the volume but are removed through the tumor surface at a rate proportional to the surface area. Therefore, when a tumor reaches sufficiently large size, the existing supply of material resources and waste removal capacity become inadequate to support further growth. As discovered experimentally by Judah Folkman [42], the limiting diameter of these stunted tumors in humans and animals is about 1–2 mm. Furthermore, lower estimates for the Folkman diameter found in the literature can even be as small as 0.5 mm [43].

In this book, the all-important phenomenon of size limitation for avascular tumors will be referred to as the *Folkman effect*.

As was mentioned in Section 3.1, cancer cells share many traits with normal cells from the tumor's organ or tissue of origin. One of them is the ability to produce and secrete special molecules that stimulate the growth of proximal capillaries in the direction of the gradient of the molecule's concentration, that is, toward the source. (The process of cell motion directed by a concentration field of a molecular agent is called *chemotaxis*.) Creation of a *de novo* capillary network is called *angiogenesis*, while the general term used for various stimulating molecules is *angiogenic factors*.

In normal organs and tissues, angiogenesis is critical for tissue regeneration after adverse events such as physical wound or infarction. It is also indispensable for embryonic growth and development, and for the enhancement of functional capacity in response to systematic increase in physical activity. For a cancerous tumor, angiogenesis is the principal mechanism enabling tumor growth beyond the Folkman's limit. It represents yet another manifestation of the critical role of tumor–host interactions mediated by the tumor microenvironment discussed in the previous section.

Following a general pattern of distortion of structure and function occurring within and around a malignant tumor, the new capillary network elicited by the tumor is defective in many respects. In particular, endothelium forming the walls of new capillaries is leaky and the geometry of the tumor's capillary network is irregular, compared to its normal counterparts.

Folkman began his systematic study of angiogenesis and realized its critical role in tumor growth in the early 1970s. His ideas had little to do with genes and molecular biology and, consequently, were out of sync with academic fashions of the day, still prevailing in our time. Rather, angiogenesis depends on much simpler phenomena such as chemical gradients, cell motility, chemotaxis, and fractal geometry of capillary networks. As a result, Folkman's ideas were kept out of the mainstream and rejected for about a quarter century. This challenged him to demonstrate the existence of angiogenic factors. An epic quest for their isolation and characterization took many years and is vividly described by Robert Cooke in his book [16]. This has led to the discovery of a family of signaling proteins called *vascular endothelial growth factors* (VEGFs) that stimulate growth and proliferation of endothelial cells. Subsequently, many other angiogenic factors have been discovered.

Normal physiological processes in living organisms are prevented from runaway snowballing by inhibitors of these processes. Angiogenesis is no exception. It was found by Folkman and others that tumors, their microenvironment, the liver and various types of cells in the body produce a number of angiogenesis inhibitors such as *angiostatin, endostatin* and *thrombospondin* [44, 45]. As a result, the outcome of angiogenesis is determined by the competition between pro- and anti-angiogenic factors and processes. If internal and external influences cause pro-angiogenic factors to prevail, an event termed *angiogenic switch* [46], the tumor enters a phase of active and potentially irreversible growth and may reach a lethal size. If, on the other hand, elicitation of new capillaries is thwarted by dominant locally and systemically produced angiogenesis inhibitors, the tumor will remain dormant due to a dynamic equilibrium between tumor cell proliferation, quiescence and death, or may even regress.

Many cancers, including certain kinds of breast, ovarian, uterine and prostate cancers, are hormone-dependent. When hormones bind to special receptors on the membrane of cancer cells, their growth and division are stimulated. Relevant hormones, such as estrogen and progesterone in the case of breast, ovarian and uterine cancers and testosterone and other androgens in the case of prostate cancer, are circulating in the blood. Thus, tumor angiogenesis enables more efficient delivery of hormones to cancer cells.

3.4 Tumor-cell heterogeneity

Heterogeneity of tumor cells represents one of the most formidable challenges to successful cancer treatment. In this section, I discuss a few principal aspects of this heterogeneity. As elsewhere in the book, I approach this phenomenologically, i. e., without going into molecular-biological and genomic attributes underlying distinctions between various classes and functional states of cancer cells.

Clonogenicity

Consider the following mental or actual experiment, termed *colony forming assay*. Pick a tumor cell and transfer it carefully to a petri dish containing a medium conducive to cell proliferation and kept under suitable experimental conditions such as appropriate temperature, humidity, and oxygen and CO_2 concentrations. Actual explantation assays of this kind have revealed that some cancer cells die, while others produce a small colony that peters out after a few generations. However, for some explanted cells, the scenario is very different—they produce a large colony, which continues to steadily expand until the growth is inhibited by overcrowding. Such cells are called *clonogenic* (or *tumorigenic*), and their characteristic property is that under favorable in vivo conditions they can regenerate the whole tumor.

From a clinical perspective, clonogenic cancer cells are the most harmful ones, and their elimination ought to be the primary goal of cancer treatment. Furthermore, it is commonly believed that only clonogenic cancer cells are capable of spawning metastases. It should be kept in mind, though, that the clonogenicity trait in a tumor-cell population in vivo is unobservable. Thus, although believed to be small, the size of the fraction of clonogenic cells in a tumor at a given time is unknown.

Quiescence

Under unfavorable conditions, both normal and cancer cells can become quiescent, i. e., enter G_0, the resting phase of the cell cycle, in which they can remain indefinitely. The reasons for quiescence are many. It can be a protective mechanism, whereby a cell is arrested at the first cell cycle checkpoint due to detection of damage to DNA in need of repair. Quiescence can also result from an insufficient supply of nutrients, oxygen or growth factors. Yet another reason for quiescence is overcrowding that triggers cell cycle arrest through signaling by neighboring cancer or normal cells. The same can be brought about by many other internal and external signals. Of note, quiescence of normal cells is often a natural physiological state, as is the case for stem cells and some terminally differentiated cells such as neurons and cells of the heart muscle.

The state of quiescence can be transient. In this case, a cell reenters the cell cycle, which leads to elongation of the latter.

Quiescent cancer cells are resistant to radiation and cytotoxic chemotherapy as well as many other treatment modalities that target actively proliferating cells. Under more favorable conditions, including post-treatment tumor regrowth following elimination of the majority of sensitive cancer cells, quiescent cancer cells can resume cycling and proliferation.

Hypoxy

When supply of oxygen is limited, tumor cells become *hypoxic*, which limits their ability to proliferate. Under conditions of severe hypoxia, such cells may become quiescent. Hypoxic cells are refractory to radiation and chemotherapy. In the post-treatment period, due to reduced competition for oxygen, hypoxic cancer cells within the residual tumor can become well-oxygenated. Such cells are a common source of cancer recurrence.

In mature tumors, hypoxic cells typically reside in the tumor core, away from the tumor surface perfused by the vasculature. Cancer cells in the inner core can become so hypoxic and undernourished that they undergo apoptosis or necrosis on a mass scale, forming a necrotic region.

Cancer stem cells

As was indicated in Section 3.2, every human, and more broadly mammalian, organism emerges through cell division and differentiation from a few totipotent embryonic stem cells, the offspring of a fertilized egg. All tissues in a body are generated, and replenished following cell loss due to apoptosis, injury or disease, from a pool of uni- or multipotent stem cells, which produce fully differentiated functional cells of one or several related tissues only. Thus, these stem cells serve as the organism's "golden reserve."

Because of their singular importance for tissue development, regeneration and homeostasis, stem cells have many special properties distinguishing them from differentiated cells:

(1) Depending on the needs of the organism, stem cells can either remain quiescent or divide either asymmetrically into one stem cell and one differentiated cell or symmetrically into two stem cells or two differentiated cells;
(2) Stem cells often occupy special protected anatomical niches;
(3) They have a strong efflux capability, i. e., can transport across the cell membrane various harmful substances that have entered the cell.

The concept of cancer stem cell (CSC) is not as clear-cut as that of normal stem cell and remains controversial [47]. While normal stem cells have been exhaustively characterized and can be identified with certainty (but a lot of effort, too), the notion of CSC is largely a matter of definition. Typically, CSCs are defined by postulating two properties: (1) tumorigenicity and (2) the capacity to self-renew through asymmetric division and thus produce differentiated nonstem cancer cells. Therefore, cancer stem cells form a subset of the subpopulation of clonogenic cells within a malignant tumor.

Definitive identification of cancer stem cells is an extraordinarily complex experimental procedure. That is why in practice CSCs are sought among cancer cells expressing certain combinations of membrane markers. These combinations are by no means specific to CSCs, which potentially leads to false-positive and false-negative identifications.

Originally CSCs were discovered for acute myeloid leukemia (AML) [48]. Later they were found for breast [49] and prostate [50] cancer, and subsequently for other common cancers such as lung, colon, pancreatic and some brain cancers as well as for melanoma, but not for all solid cancers.

The many faces of tumor cell heterogeneity can be summarized as follows. The principal dimensions of the heterogeneity are based on the classification of cancer cells into several functional states including: (1) clonogenic vs. nonclonogenic cancer cells; (2) actively proliferating vs. quiescent ones; and (3) cancer stem cells vs. differentiated cells in various stages of differentiation. Additionally, viability of cancer cells and their response to treatment depend on their oxygenation level mediated by their spatial position within the tumor, most notably proximity to tumor surface and blood vessels.

Finally, tumor cell heterogeneity is intertwined with evolutionary processes. Instability of the genomes of cancer cells leads to the emergence in these cells of a wide range of mutations, some of which may confer on these cells competitive advantage in proliferation, metabolic efficiency, motility, adaptation to the microenvironment and recruitment of noncancerous cells into the tumor. This causes lineages of fitter cells to gradually take over certain regions within the tumor.

3.5 Metastasis

Primary tumors are rarely lethal *per se*, unless they pose a threat to vital organs. It is distant metastases that account for about 90 % of all cancer-related deaths, and this is why every breakthrough in understanding metastasis could potentially go a long way in improving survival of cancer patients. However, despite enormous research effort on basic science, experimental, clinical, epidemiological and mathematical modeling fronts, metastasis still remains poorly understood, and genuine advances in therapy of the metastatic disease are few and far between. The unfortunate upshot is that once metastases start to aggressively grow, they almost invariably bring about a lethal outcome.

Metastasis is a process by which cancer cells from a primary tumor spread to other organs and tissues. This multi-stage process is extremely complex and highly selective [51]. A primary tumor may start shedding blood-borne cancer cells as soon as it becomes vascular. Therefore, angiogenesis and the resulting vascularization of the primary tumor has a particular significance for metastasis. Apart from the circulation, tumor cells can also spread via the lymphatic system, which can result in lymph-node metastases. Cancer cells disseminated via the lymphatic route that were not arrested or killed in the lymph channels and nodes eventually end up in the bloodstream because the lymphatic system merges with the systemic circulation through subclavian veins.

Metastasis is very often a fairly early event in the natural history of metastasizing solid cancers (see Section 4.1). For example, it was estimated in [52] that more than 75 % of malignant primary tumors have already metastasized by the time of their discovery; a more conservative estimate of 50 % was given in [53]. In the vast majority of cases, metastases surface within the first five years of primary tumor detection [52].

Disseminated cancer cells are frequently found in bone marrow. For example, it was reported in [54] that 25–43 % of breast cancer patients exhibit micrometastases including solitary cancer cells in bone marrow, following resection of their primary tumors.

One of the most influential discoveries related to metastasis was made by the British surgeon Stephen Paget (1855–1926). In a landmark study of 735 autopsy records of women with breast cancer published in 1889 [55], he uncovered a remarkable propensity of breast cancer cells to form metastases only in some specific distant organs, typically bones, lungs, liver and brain. He dubbed this phenomenon the "seed and soil hypothesis." A selective affinity for specific sites is also displayed by disseminated cancer cells originating from other organs [56]. This highlights a critical importance of the microenvironment ("soil") and cooperative interaction of seeded cancer cells with neighboring normal cells and noncellular tissue components for tumor growth (compare with Section 3.2).

The techniques of immunohistochemistry and fluorescent tagging enable labeling all cells of a given kind in a specimen. This was used in autopsy studies [40], experiments on animal models [40], and even in terminally ill cancer patients whose severe symptoms were relieved by an ingenuous system that enabled tracking disseminated cancer cells [57]. These investigations have uncovered a remarkable picture: While viable solitary cancer cells seeded by the primary tumor are present in all organs and tissues, they form micrometastases only in a few specific, predictable locations that can provide a hospitable microenvironmental niche.

The lungs hold a special significance for metastasis for a variety of reasons pertaining both to the anatomy of the circulatory system and to the biology of metastatic dissemination. The anatomic reasons are two-fold: (1) all closed blood-circulation routes pass through the lungs; and (2) the lungs' capillary bed is the first one encountered by *circulating tumor cells* (CTCs) (see Subsection 3.5.1) originating from all organs except for the gut (in the latter case, CTCs primarily pass through the liver, as shown in Figure 3.1). From the biological perspective, a special role of the lungs is due to the following factors: (1) They have an extensive capillary network, which favors CTC extravasation and makes angiogenesis limitation to metastatic growth less stringent; (2) oxygen-rich surface of blood vessels in the lungs is a favorable site for the migration of extravasated metastatic cells and colony formation. Taken collectively, these facts explain why the lungs is a frequent metastatic site for many types of solid cancer.

3.5.1 The metastatic cascade

To form a clinically detectable metastasis in a distant site (typically the lungs, liver, bones, brain, peritoneal cavity, skin, lymph nodes or soft tissue), a cancer cell from the primary tumor must go through numerous steps that collectively constitute the *metastatic cascade*. Specifically, a cancer cell has to (1) separate itself from the primary tumor, which requires the loss of cell adhesion; (2) degrade the basal membrane and extracellular matrix; (3) migrate to a blood vessel or lymph channel; (4) intravasate; (5) survive through the period of free circulation; (6) arrest in the capillary bed of a certain organ; (7) traverse the capillary wall (extravasate); (8) survive through the single-cell dormancy period; (9) start to proliferate; (10) induce angiogenesis and vascularize; and finally, (11) begin to actively grow and reach a clinically detectable size.

The metastatic cascade consists, therefore, of a sequence of critical microevents and processes. Each of them represents a barrier, which only a small proportion of cancer cells that have acquired relevant new attributes and gained additional functions can overcome. Thus, only a tiny fraction of cancer cells that are genotypically and phenotypically adapted to successful passage through all the stages of the metastatic cascade have a chance to give rise to clinically significant metastases.

3.5.2 Circulating tumor cells

The stages of the metastatic cascade are largely unobservable in clinical settings, with one exception—that of free circulation, where blood-borne CTCs can be detected in a

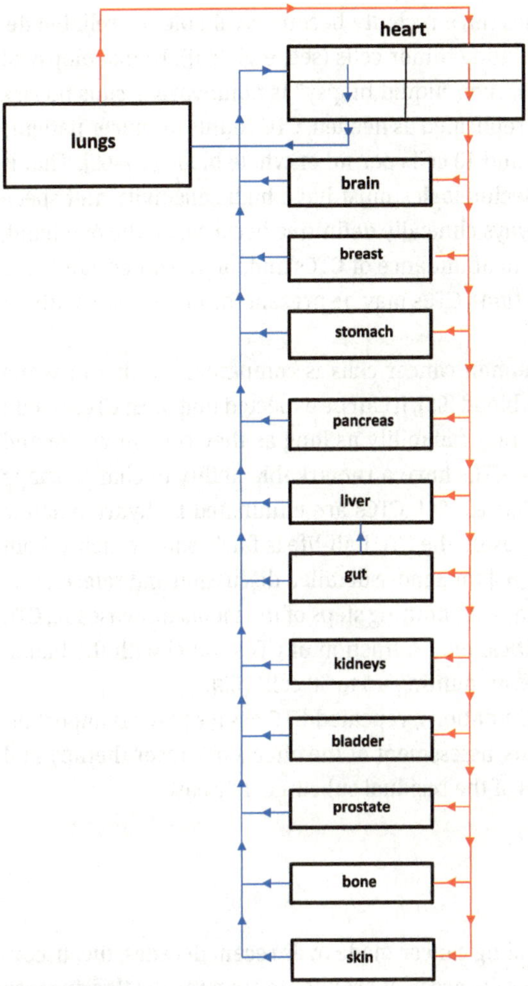

Figure 3.1: Schematic representation of the circulatory system. Red and blue lines represent arterial and venous blood, respectively. The direction of blood flow is indicated with arrows. Arterial blood flows from the heart's left ventricle through the aorta and reaches all the organs through a system of branching arteries supplying these organs with water, oxygen, ions, organic nutrients, hormones and blood cells. Deoxygenated blood carrying CO_2 and waste products flows from the organs through a reverse branching system of increasingly larger veins eventually forming the vena cava, a major vein that enters the heart's right atrium. The venous blood then exits the heart's right ventricle, goes through the bronchial artery to the lungs for oxygenation and finally flows back to the heart's left atrium and ventricle, thus completing one cycle of blood circulation.
The figure was reproduced with permission from Hanin LG. The circulation stage of the metastatic cascade: A mathematical description and its clinical implications. J Theor Biol 2023, 572, 111582.

blood sample, isolated and characterized. Therefore, CTCs provide a unique window into the metastatic cascade. The first report on CTCs was published by the Australian physician Thomas Ashworth in 1869 [58].

Numerous advanced technologies have recently become available for reliable detection and characterization of circulating tumor cells (see, e. g., [59]). Unlike biopsy of the primary tumor and lymph nodes, such "liquid biopsy" is noninvasive, runs no risk of spreading cancer cells and can be replicated as needed. CTC counts in cancer patients are typically low ranging between 1 and 10 cells per ml of whole blood [60–62]. That is why, to be effective, CTC detection technologies must have high sensitivity and specificity. However, CTC tests are not always clinically definitive because, on the one hand, some mature tumors don't produce an abundance of CTCs and, on the other hand, due to cancer dormancy (see the next section), CTCs may be present for many years without clinical evidence of cancer.

Since the size range for most human cancer cells is comparable to that of white blood cells that circulate freely in the blood [63], it can be expected that most CTCs would normally have the same free-circulation capability as long as they remain viable and don't extravasate. Additionally, some CTCs have a remarkable ability to change shape when passing through narrow capillaries [64]. CTCs are eliminated by hydrodynamic forces and the immune system. As a result, the CTC half-life is fairly short ranging from a few hours to perhaps 1–2 days (see [65] for a more detailed discussion and references). As was argued in [66], among the many rate-limiting steps of the metastatic cascade, CTC elimination is probably the most critical one. A fraction of CTCs travel with the bloodstream and extravasate in aggregates amounting up to 50 cells [63].

In spite of the aforementioned limitations, repeated CTC assays play an important role as a safe tool for cancer diagnosis, assessment of the effects of cancer therapy and monitoring post-treatment dynamics of the residual subclinical disease.

3.6 Cancer dormancy

Among major advances in understanding cancer made over recent decades, the discovery of cancer dormancy holds perhaps the greatest promise for turning the flagging war on cancer around. The phenomenon of cancer dormancy is heterogeneous and consists of at least two distinct forms—dormancy of solitary cancer cells and that of microscopic tumors. Apparently, the first publication on the subject of dormant cancer goes back to 1954 [67]. Since then, the interest in this phenomenon has seen a considerable acceleration. A wide ranging discussion of clinical aspects of breast cancer dormancy can be found in [68].

The biological basis of single-cell dormancy is cell quiescence, discussed in Section 3.4. It occurs when a cell exits the cell cycle and enters G_0 (the resting state), in which the cell is still metabolically active but cannot grow and divide. The most clinically significant examples of dormant solitary cancer cells (or small cell clumps) are: (1) circulating tumor cells (CTCs) (see Subsection 3.5.2); (2) viable metastatic cells that have extravasated into a foreign environment; and (3) residual cancer cells at a primary tumor site that have survived cancer treatment and can subsequently cause local recurrence.

Dormancy of microscopic tumors is a result of a dynamic equilibrium between tumor-cell proliferation, quiescence and death; a skillful experimental validation of this principle in a murine model of lung metastases was presented in [69]. The same homeostatic mechanism governs the maintenance of constant size of normal organs in an adult body over a lifetime.

The aforementioned equilibrium can be brought about by a number of nonmutually exclusive mechanisms:

(1) The tumor's failure to induce angiogenesis either due to lack of angiogenic phenotype or owing to the dominance of locally or systemically produced angiogenesis inhibitors (see Section 3.3);
(2) The tumor's presence in a hostile microenvironment and/or alongside noncooperative normal cells;
(3) Inhibition of tumor growth by the host's immune system. In particular, this can result from immunization to a tumor-associated antigen [60]; and
(4) Suppression of the growth of metastases by intact primary tumor (see Section 4.3).

The medical literature contains scores of case reports whose findings can in all likelihood be only explained by cancer dormancy. For example, the article [70] describes clinical cases of three women with biopsy-confirmed DCIS (ductal carcinoma *in situ*, a noninvasive form of breast cancer) who developed invasive breast cancer in the same location 23, 29 and 42 years after primary diagnosis. The study [71] describes a case of infiltrating ductal adenocarcinoma of the breast treated with radical mastectomy and radiation therapy that 39 years later produced pleural metastasis, which was again found to be an adenocarcinoma. As another example, the authors of [60] found that 36 % of breast cancer patients in their series had CTCs 7–22 years postmastectomy. Because the vast majority of local and distant recurrences of breast cancer happen within the first five years after treatment, such late occurrence of CTCs points to the existence of occult metastases that were continuously shedding cancer cells into the circulation.

Dormant cancer cells are also implicated in cancer transmission to the recipients of organ transplants. In one such case, metastatic prostate cancer cells were transferred through a heart transplant from a donor, whose autopsy confirmed prostate cancer, to a recipient, whose prostate was free of the disease but who developed prostate cancer metastases in the spine, sacrum and ribs 10 months after the transplantation [72]. Such precipitous adverse events are undoubtedly facilitated by the fact that recipients of organ transplants are put on immunosuppressants. This case highlights the ability of dormant cancer cells to persist in an inhospitable environment such as the heart, which only rarely harbors primary or secondary tumors. By contrast, normal cells typically cannot survive in an *ectopic* (foreign) environment for more than a few days [40]. For a systematic review of cancer transmission through organ transplants, see [52].

Dormant cancers are often viewed as an exotic state of the disease rarely observed in clinical practice. Contrary to this belief, it can be argued that this is a *natural stable state* for many types of cancer, while an aggressive form is a less common variant. In fact, dormancy is a universal phenomenon across all forms of life and represents a survival response to unfavorable conditions (such as insufficient supply of water, nutrients or oxygen, abnormal temperature, etc.) forged by evolution.

Chief among the sources of evidence for the ubiquity of tumor dormancy is autopsy studies. As an example demonstrating how large the pool of indolent breast cancers really is, it was reported in [73] that breast cancer *in situ* was discovered in more than one third of autopsied women who died of trauma between ages 40 and 50 and who never had a diagnosis of breast cancer. By comparison, invasive breast cancer is detected in only about 1 % of women in this age group [73]. Furthermore, an autopsy study [74] discovered *in situ* breast tumors in 16.9 % of Danish women who died from various causes unrelated to breast cancer and had never been diagnosed with it. For context, about 8.4 % of women in Denmark develop invasive breast cancer over their lifetime [74]. Likewise, indolent prostate cancer is very common in men. For example, prevalence of prostate cancer in men older than 79 years of age who died of causes unrelated to prostate cancer was found to be 59 % [75]. Even in much younger men in their twenties, the rate of prostate cancer discovery on autopsies was reported to be a staggering 8–11 % [76]! Finally, here is an even more striking example: Autopsies of virtually all people beyond the age of 50 have revealed the presence of *in situ* carcinomas of the thyroid gland, while only about 0.1 % of the population in this age group are diagnosed with clinical thyroid cancer [73].

3.7 Cancer, inflammation and the immune system

The main function of the immune system is to identify and eliminate foreign and abnormal cells (including cancer cells), toxins, viruses and fungi. This is achieved through the action of various kinds of leukocytes (white blood cells), the principal players of the immune system originating from the bone marrow. Leukocytes kill target cells by three mechanisms. First, macrophages, neutrophils, dendritic cells and eosinophils can directly eliminate target cells by phagocytosis. Second, some lymphocytes trigger apoptosis of target cells by binding to special receptors on their membrane, called *death receptors*. Third, antibodies produced by B lymphocytes bind to the corresponding antigens on the membrane of target cells, which creates antigen–antibody complexes and thereby marks such cells for elimination by macrophages and natural killer cells. Mounting a strong immune response is contingent on recognition of target cells by the immune system.

Thus, immunogenic tumors are engaged in complex interactions with the immune system, which manifests empirically as infiltration of such tumors by various cells of the immune system. Experimental evidence also suggests that the immune system can play a key role in suppressing cancer cell proliferation. For example, escape from dormancy of primary tumor and metastases and their subsequent aggressive growth in experimental animals can be triggered by immunosuppression through administration of cyclosporin

A or total body irradiation [77]. Likewise, inoculation of experimental mice with cancer cells works well only for special breeds of immunodeficient animals.

Unfortunately, the ability of the immune system to inhibit or eliminate malignant tumors can be severely hampered, or even reversed. The exact reasons are very complex and a subject of active research, but two of them can be stated with reasonable certainty:

(1) Many cancers are non-immunogenic ("cold"), which allows them to evade immune surveillance. In particular, membranes of such cancer cells have a low antigen footprint, which prevents an immune response mediated by B cells. Examples of non-immunogenic cancers include pancreatic cancer, glioblastoma (an aggressive brain cancer) and some types of breast, prostate and ovarian cancer. Alternatively, immunogenic cancers can reduce immunogenicity in the course of their evolution due to heritable variation and selection.

(2) Some cancers have, or can develop, the ability to co-opt certain cells and processes of the immune system. For example, macrophages, which are rich in growth factors, and several types of lymphocytes can be incorporated into the tumor microenvironment, which stimulates tumor growth and promotes local immunosuppression (see, e. g., [41, 78] for more details).

There exists a voluminous literature describing the role of local and systemic inflammation as boosters of tumor growth, invasion and metastasis. Elaborate molecular-biological narratives on this subject are exemplified by the article [79]. However, some of the conclusions reached in the literature are not supported by human autopsy studies or pathological examination of tumors surgically removed from cancer patients [40].

A universal mechanism both enabling and accompanying the immune response to infection, wound or irritation by a chemical agent is vasodilation, which makes capillaries more permeable. Vasodilation is brought about by a concerted action of molecular mediators of inflammation released by local cells of the immune system or derived from plasma proteins. Vasodilation creates conditions for massive trafficking of various cells of the immune system to the affected site. This results in local inflammation, which is a necessary initial stage of healing.

Vasodilation provides a crucial link among immunity, inflammation and cancer that is important to keep in mind for the rest of the book. Specifically, immunogenic tumors cause local inflammation and vasodilation, and the latter facilitates intravasation of disseminated cancer cells, thus feeding them into the metastatic pipeline.

3.8 Cancer and injury

This subject will be crucial for the discussion of various effects of cancer treatment in Chapter 5.

There is abundant experimental and clinical evidence that injury spurs the development of preexisting cancer at the site of injury and, although often to a lesser degree, at any other site in the body. We next discuss two seminal laboratory studies where the effects of injury on cancer progression were investigated in murine models. Then, to confirm translational value of these studies, I will review two relevant clinical cases.

The first study is an elaborate experiment where mice were subjected to surgical injury by electric cauterization or a laser and thereafter injected intravenously with various amounts of cancer cells of a specific mammary carcinoma cell line [80]. The injured organs were either a liver or kidney, the sites in which cancer cells in question never form actively growing spontaneous metastases. The main findings of this laboratory study are as follows:

(a) A large fraction of mice developed tumors at the injured organ, which demonstrates that injury creates conditions that override the "seed and soil" hypothesis (see Section 3.5).
(b) The fraction of injured mice that developed metastases in other organs increased compared to control (uninjured) mice, but not markedly so.
(c) The fraction of animals with metastases at the site of injury and the number of induced metastatic nodes increased with the extent of injury and the size of the inoculum.
(d) Delay in cancer cell inoculation relative to the timing of injury caused tapering of the effect on metastasis. Therefore, as healing progresses, wounds lose their ability to facilitate implantation and growth of metastases.

To explain their findings, the authors of [80] invoked formation of blood clots in response to wounding as an important factor causing entrapment of CTCs at the site of injury. The significance of blood coagulation and the formation of fibrin thrombi for tumor development and metastasis was also emphasized in [81].

The second experimental study represents a detailed investigation of the effects of skin injury on the growth of subcutaneous tumor grafts and lung metastases resulting from intravenous injection of cancer cells [82]. Tumor grafts comprised 16 different cancer cell lines of human or murine origin and were implanted in immunodeficient mice either at the site of injury or into the contralateral flank. For intravenous injections, a single melanoma cell line was used. The study resulted in the following conclusions:

(a) All human and murine tumors displayed a significantly, and often dramatically, increased rate of tumor growth in surgically traumatized animals compared to control (uninjured) mice.
(b) Although the increase in the rate of tumor growth was the highest when tumors were implanted at the site of injury, implantation at the distant site has also produced a substantially elevated tumor growth rate.
(c) Injured mice developed a significantly larger number of lung metastases than controls.
(d) Variation in the timing of tumor grafts relative to the time of injury revealed that the tumor growth-accelerating effect of injury is limited to 2–3 days.

A common theme of the two clinical cancer cases described next is that injury precipitates metastatic relapse. Although detailed mechanisms behind this phenomenon, as well as behind the findings uncovered in the two aforementioned experimental studies, are complex and poorly understood, the occurrence of the following two nonmutually exclusive effects involving two stages of the metastatic cascade seems fairly incontrovertible:

(1) Injury causes a surge in the local production of growth and angiogenic factors required for wound healing. They are captured by dormant metastases, which triggers their vascularization and aggressive growth.
(2) Inflammation response to injury causes local vasodilation, which, as was explained in Section 3.7, facilitates extravasation of CTCs shed by the primary tumor.

The following two clinical cases can be adduced in support of these two mechanisms. The first of them was presented in [83]:

> A 43 year-old male with a history of smoking was diagnosed with a non-small cell lung cancer (NSCLC) with no evidence of metastasis. He was treated with radiation and chemotherapy and responded positively to the treatment. About 16 month later, the patient suffered a minor injury to the right parietal bone on his skull with no bone fracture. In about a month, he developed a massive lump 7 cm in diameter at the site of injury. X-ray showed a bone lesion about 2 cm in diameter, while MRI imaging revealed a metastatic deposit in the right parietal bone with a considerable extracranial soft tissue and meningeal involvement. Radiotherapy reduced the size of the lesion, but 15 days after the end of treatment the patient died of profuse hemoptysis.

How could this clinical case be explained? Clearly, the site of injury contained a dormant or slowly growing subclinical metastasis. The injury altered its microenvironment, while the wound healing process brought about a spike in growth and angiogenic factors that were captured by the metastasis and triggered its explosive growth. To make sure this explanation is compatible with tumor growth kinetics, assume as an example that at the time of injury there was a single subclinical metastasis of spherical shape with a diameter of 5 mm, which grew exponentially over the period of 30 days into the observed metastatic lesion with the diameter of 20 mm. This implies (see Section 7.2 for mathematical details) that the metastasis' doubling time was 3.75 days. Although this doubling time falls into the very fast end of human tumor growth, it is still much longer than the duration of cell cycle in dividing somatic human cells (about 24 hrs) and is therefore within the range of biological possibilities.

The second clinical case was reported in [84] as follows:

> The case involves a 77-year-old male who presented with severe swelling of his right index finger that he had injured while gardening several months before seeking medical attention. Three years before visiting the doctor the patient underwent treatment for stage IIA melanoma on his left leg and had follow-up appointments every six months thereafter with no prior recurrence. A contrast-enhanced CT scan of his right hand revealed a solid tumor within the swollen region. The patient

was diagnosed with metastatic melanoma and four months later succumbed to the progression of the disease.

Just like the first clinical case, the second one can be explained by the growth of a preexisting micrometastasis at the site of injury accelerated by wounding and inflammation. However, the second case can alternatively be explained by aggressive proliferation of a clone spawned by a single melanoma CTC that was seeded by an occult primary or secondary tumor and extravasated at the site of the injury. To ascertain that this scenario is kinetically feasible, suppose that the CTC extravasated in a microenvironment with an abundance of growth and angiogenic factors and that the disseminated melanoma cell started an uninterrupted exponential growth four months prior to the detection of the metastatic lesion. Judging from an image included in the article [84], the volume of the metastatic lesion can roughly be estimated as 1 cm^3, i. e., approximately 10^9 cells. Then, the associated doubling time of the metastatic growth is 4.1 days, which is again very fast, yet theoretically possible. Note also that assuming the same scenario for the first clinical case would lead to a prohibitively low doubling time.

The most frequent source of wounding associated with cancer treatment is surgery and radiation therapy for a primary tumor. The effects of these treatments and concomitant injury on metastasis will be discussed at length in Sections 5.2–5.4.

4 The dogmas of oncology

In this chapter, I examine some uncritically adopted, ossified notions related to the natural history of cancer and its diagnosis that hold sway in theoretical and practical oncology. Those associated with cancer treatment will be discussed in the next chapter. This chapter develops and expands upon some of the ideas initially formulated in my work [85].

4.1 Linear progression theory: the central dogma of oncology

Empirical observations of human cancer over more than 2500 years have led to a paradigm of its linear progression. It posits that once a solid cancer becomes symptomatic, its progression in time is irreversible and follows its anatomic spread from the primary tumor site to local lymph nodes to regional lymph nodes and finally through metastatic dissemination to distant organs and tissues.

Because primary breast tumor is a common malignancy that is generally easier to diagnose and observe than other solid tumors, breast cancer has become by far the most studied type of cancer and somewhat of a model emblematic of other solid cancers. The first scientific, by modern standards, theory of breast cancer origination and progression was put forward by Rudolf Virchow (1821–1902), a tireless and transformative German medical doctor and pathologist. Based on his post-mortem examination of scores of breast cancer patients and pioneering extensive use of microscopy, he came to a conclusion that breast cancer is caused by systematic irritation or inflammation of breast tissue and starts from a single focus [86]. He found that subsequently the tumor expands and spreads through the flow of lymph to lymph nodes in accordance with their anatomic sequence.

Following this theory, treatment of breast cancer since the late 19th century has focused on resection of the primary tumor and as much of the surrounding tissue and as many affected lymph nodes as possible and practicable. This has led to a sequence of increasingly more radical breast cancer surgeries with radical mastectomy on the one end and its various extensions involving excision of proximal and regional lymph nodes and chest muscles on the other end. The primary driving force behind this development was the US surgeon William Halsted (1852–1922), who designed and perfected these surgical procedures and advocated them to his numerous disciples and followers. Due to Halsted's charisma, his revolutionizing influence on surgery, patient care and medical education in the US, and his perch as one of the founding members of Johns Hopkins School of Medicine, the linear progression theory exerted an outsized influence on medical thinking and surgical practice in the treatment of breast cancer and far beyond. In many overt and subtle ways, the linear progression paradigm continues to live on to this day, permeating the theory and shaping the practice of oncology.

https://doi.org/10.1515/9783111334035-005

The principal challenges to the linear progression theory and methods of cancer treatment informed by it came from two insights into the natural history of breast cancer and other solid tumors.

The first of them was born of extensive experimental studies of breast cancer on animal models by a notable US cancer biologist and oncologist Bernard Fisher (1918–2019) and his coworkers in the 1950s–1970s, reviewed in [87]. Based on the results of this work, Fisher concluded that, contrary to the linear progression postulate, seeding of metastases via hematogenous and lymphatic routes can render breast cancer systemic long before the primary tumor becomes detectable or symptomatic and spreads to local lymph nodes. I will call this remarkable phenomenon the *Fisher effect*. A noteworthy clinical implication of Fisher's systemic theory of breast cancer is that the extent of surgery would have only minor impact on disease-free and overall survival of patients with invasive breast cancer. To validate this striking hypothesis, Fisher initiated and directed in the 1970s–1990s numerous clinical trials conducted by the Pittsburgh-based National Surgical Adjuvant Breast and Bowel Project (NSABP), which he founded and chaired. The results of these trials confirmed the tested hypothesis unequivocally [88].

This landmark finding places the long-term outcome of primary breast tumor resection squarely into the hands of the state of metastasis immediately after surgery. If no metastases are present then most likely the patient will be cured. If, on the other hand, tumor cells with metastatic potential were released into the bloodstream during surgery or if at the time of primary tumor resection solitary metastatic cancer cells or avascular micrometastases were already lodged at secondary sites in the state of dormancy or slow growth, then the patient's survival would depend on whether these metastases will ever progress to the stage of vascular, actively growing secondary tumors over the patient's lifetime. Finally, if at the time of surgery some of the metastases had already progressed to the vascular stage then the patient would most likely develop metastatic relapse.

The Fisher's systemic theory of breast cancer progression implies that clinical variables pertaining to the stage of the disease, such as the number of affected lymph nodes, that have long been thought to bear high long-term prognostic significance, are mostly associated with loco-regional short-term treatment outcomes.

Definitive results of the NSABP trials clearly suggested that the extent of surgery for primary breast cancer could be scaled back and limited to lumpectomy augmented with adjuvant or neoadjuvant systemic treatments, mostly chemo-, hormonal and immunotherapy, without a detriment to the patient's long-term survival. In reality, however, due to fierce resistance of the surgery establishment, the transition from the Halstedian paradigm of primary breast cancer treatment to the Fisherian one took almost 50 years, which unnecessarily subjected an untold number of women to disfiguring surgery. In his review paper published in 1999 [88], Fisher went even further and prophesied about the future of breast cancer treatment: "*... it is likely that surgery for the disease will continue to diminish in importance ...*" Thus, vis-a-vis breast cancer, surgery for primary tumor remains one of the last redoubts of the Halstedian linear progression theory, which continues to dominate the landscape of breast cancer oncology. As will be argued in the next chapter, along with benefits, excision of a metastasizing primary tumor carries significant risks.

No revolutionary figure comparable to Bernard Fisher in stature, passion and influence has emerged among researchers and practitioners studying and treating solid malignancies other than breast cancer. As a result, these areas of oncology still remain under a strong influence of the linear progression theory.

The second challenge to the linear progression theory originated from the groundbreaking work of Judah Folkman on tumor angiogenesis that spanned almost the four decades of 1970–2008 [16]. It resulted in a discovery that upon reaching a microscopic diameter of about 1–2 mm, a primary or secondary tumor hits a hard barrier to its continued growth due to limitations on the supply of nutrients, oxygen and growth factors through diffusion alone (the *Folkman effect*), see Section 3.3. To ensure further growth, the tumor has to induce angiogenesis resulting in the creation of a network of capillaries providing an adequate supply of vital chemicals [42]. If tumor cells do not exhibit angiogenic phenotype or if their microenvironment is dominated by angiogenesis inhibitors, the tumor would maintain the state of dormancy due to a dynamic equilibrium between cell proliferation, quiescence and apoptosis [69].

Folkman's theory of angiogenesis-driven tumor growth contravenes the linear progression theory on two fronts:

(1) It suggests that a vascular primary tumor can start shedding blood-borne metastases before it reaches a detectable size and/or becomes symptomatic through lymph node involvement and other clinical signs. Also, recall from Subsection 3.5.2 that hematogenous and lymphatic dissemination routes are not mutually exclusive because the lymph eventually drains into systemic circulation. In summary, breast cancer and other malignancies may disseminate long before their primary source is discovered, which provides a biological underpinning to Fisher's systemic theory of breast cancer. The time window for metastasis seeding while the disease is still subclinical can be quite long. For example, suppose a spherical tumor with the Folkman's diameter of 1.5 mm at angiogenesis completion was detected when its volume reached 1 cm^3, a typical lower end value for primary breast tumor volume at diagnosis. Assume also that the tumor was growing exponentially with the doubling time of 100 days (a representative value for moderately fast growing primary breast tumors [43]). Then, a simple computation based on the formulas from Section 7.2 would show that the start of the tumor's vascular growth and its detection are about 2.5 years apart. That's the amount of time the tumor was surreptitiously seeding metastases without being detected!

(2) The Folkman's theory uncovered an angiogenesis-dependent mechanism by which small primary tumors and micrometastases can remain dormant. Recall from Section 3.6 that the dormant state of cancer has two main forms: (a) quiescent solitary cancer cells or their small clumps and (b) small avascular primary or secondary tumors in a state of dynamic equilibrium maintained due to the dominance of angio-

genesis inhibitors over angiogenesis promoters [69], competition with other cells for limited resources, refractory microenvironment, noninvasive (*in situ*) phenotype or other reasons.

Importantly, as was argued in Section 3.6, dormancy is a natural stable state for many types of cancer. Thus, in a stark departure from the linear progression theory, an unstoppable march from the locoregional to systemic phase is not a necessary feature of cancer development. In fact, cancer can remain dormant or even spontaneously regress.

The linear progression theory was challenged along other lines as well (see, e. g., a seminal early paper [89]). However, due to its simplicity, intuitive appeal and an entrenched network of exponents continuously renewed through medical education and mentorship, it largely remains to this day a central dogma of practical oncology and continues to inform cancer treatment.

4.2 Three spin-offs of the linear progression theory

The linear progression theory has spawned many influential ideas and practices that acquired an independent life of their own and are rarely traced back to their conceptual antecedent. Three of them are discussed next.

4.2.1 Local vs. systemic disease

The linear progression theory draws a fairly rigid demarkation line between local and systemic disease. According to this theory, the onset of a systemic disease is a relatively late event in the natural history of cancer occurring when the onslaught of cancer cells from the invading primary tumor overwhelms local and later regional lymph nodes by exceeding their capacity to filter out and inactivate cancer cells. This graphic image, inspired by Virchow's views on breast cancer progression described in Section 4.1, has captivated several generations of cancer researchers and oncologists. Empirical evidence, however, suggests that this picture is misleading. First, this image of cancer cell assault on lymph node bastions predicts that patients diagnosed at the earliest stages of the disease with no signs of lymph node involvement and who had their primary tumor resected would be guaranteed a cure, barring the possibility of cancer cell release into the circulation during surgery. In reality, a considerable fraction of such patients develop distant metastases even when surgeons take pains to reduce perioperative escape of cancer cells into the bloodstream. Second, circulating tumor cells (CTC) (see Subsection 3.5.2) can be shed into the bloodstream as soon as the tumor of origin becomes vascular. They are routinely discovered in blood specimens of early-stage cancer patients, which clearly demonstrates that cancer is not confined to primary tumor and its microenvironment anymore and therefore contravenes the notion of universal late onset of systemic cancer.

Nowhere in the world of oncology is the mantra of local disease and local control ringing louder than in the realm of cancer radiotherapy. Hundreds of thousands of articles and numerous books have been published on the subject of local control, i. e., eliminating as many clonogenic cancer cells of the primary tumor as possible, within the limits imposed on radiation damage to normal cells and vital organs. To be sure, achieving this goal could lead, with some luck, to local cure and would reduce the number of metastases seeded by the primary tumor. However, this would typically do nothing to thwart progression of metastases disseminated prior to the start, or in the course, of radiation treatment.

Even worse, there exists a much graver risk associated with radiotherapy that is almost entirely ignored by radiation oncologists—acceleration of metastasis caused by ablation of the primary tumor by radiation. This exceedingly important phenomenon and a similar effect associated with surgical excision of the primary tumor will be discussed at length in Sections 5.2–5.4.

The idea of viewing cancer as local disease until it spreads to distant sites is anachronistic because it contradicts the vast body of knowledge about cancer that has been accumulated over several recent decades. Even when anatomically localized, the primary tumor is engaged in a host of systemic interactions:

(1) Immunogenic tumors attract cells of the immune system, including T lymphocytes, macrophages, natural killer cells, neutrophils and dendritic cells [78], often to such an extent that these cells constitute a considerable fraction of tumor mass and become abundant in the tumor microenvironment.
(2) Likewise, many tumors are capable of recruiting progenitor cells from the bone marrow, which helps create pro-angiogenic and pro-inflammatory microenvironment beneficial to tumor growth, invasion and metastasis [90, 91].
(3) As was explained in Section 3.7, systemic inflammation tends to create a propitious environment for cancer progression.
(4) Frequently occurring subtypes of several common cancers, such as cancer of the breast, ovary, uterus and prostate, depend on systemically produced sex hormones for their growth and development.
(5) As medical procedures, surgery and radiation treatment of primary tumor or, importantly, directed against *any other target in the body* elicit pro-inflammatory, pro-angiogenic, immunosuppressive and metastasis-boosting systemic responses (see Sections 5.2–5.4).
(6) As soon as primary tumor becomes vascular, it can start generating circulating tumor cells (CTCs) that may seed metastases throughout the body and even reseed the primary tumor and already existing vascular metastases [92].
(7) Actively growing malignant tumors consume a lot of nutrients, especially glucose, which alters the patient's metabolism and can lead to severe loss of muscle mass and fat, a systemic metabolic condition termed *cachexia*.

In summary, upon reaching a certain microscopic size (and potentially prior to becoming detectable or manifesting symptomatically), a primary tumor becomes an active player in the complex game of systemic interactions and effects.

4.2.2 Cancer staging

An important summary measure received by cancer patients at diagnosis is the stage of their disease. The most widely used staging system applicable to most solid cancers is the so-called TNM classification, where T followed by a number and often augmented by a letter characterizes the size of the primary tumor and the extent of its invasion into the stroma and surrounding tissues, N followed by a number stands for the number of lymph nodes involved in the cancer process, and M followed by 0 or 1 is the indicator of metastatic dissemination with M0 being "no metastases discovered." Alternatively, the cancer stage can be truncated to a single number 0–4, where stages 0–3 represent M0 combined with a certain aggregation of TN (with stage 0, primary tumor *in situ*, being the most favorable and stage 3 the most unfavorable), while stage 4 is M1. For several types of cancer, more detailed classifications involving histological and molecular characteristics of the disease have been developed. Clearly, the notion of linear progression underlies all these staging systems.

The accuracy of cancer staging depends critically on the sensitivity and specificity of imaging technology as well as on the experience and expertise of both image readers and pathologists who examine biopsy samples; chance factors associated with needle biopsy also play a role. As a cancer patient's disease progresses, the stage may change. However, the initial stage is conventionally viewed as a sort of patient's permanent cancer ID. The main purpose of cancer staging is to guide treatment, as a result of which the initial treatment plan is heavily influenced by cancer stage assigned at diagnosis.

For millennia, medicine prided itself on being an empirical science that shuns theorizing about the unobservable. Accordingly, cancer stage is descriptive of the *apparent*, or observable, state of the disease. Recall from Section 3.5 that in 50–75 % of cancer patients their primary tumor had metastasized before it became detectable, a finding dubbed the Fisher effect in Section 4.1. For such patients, the initial stage of their cancer, even the earliest one, such as T1N0M0, would in reality be T1N0M1. This would also make a world of difference in treatment: While the apparent stage suggests local treatment, typically surgery and/or radiotherapy, perhaps combined with systemic adjuvant therapies, the actual stage would rather point to a systemic treatment as the first-line therapy. Furthermore, treating metastatic cancer on the false premise of localized disease could bring about the most dreaded scenario, discussed in Sections 5.2 and 5.4, where local treatment accelerates metastasis. Finally, for metastasized tumors classified (or rather misclassified) as M0, the stage formula is silent about the most clinically significant characteristic of metastatic cancer, specifically, whether metastases are dormant or actively growing. In the former case, a reasonable course of action would likely be either low-dose, e. g., metronomic (see Section 5.1) systemic treatment aimed at keeping primary tumor growth in check or just watchful waiting. In contrast, the latter case would warrant a more aggressive systemic treatment against both primary tumor and metastases.

Thus, built into the conventional staging system is an overly optimistic assessment of the extent of cancer spread in a sizable subset of cancer patients, which systematically misleads the patients and their doctors alike regarding the required treatment and prognosis.

4.2.3 Early cancer detection and the mass cancer screening debacle

The linear progression theory has another influential, and on the face of it self-evident, consequence that reigns supreme in oncology—that cancer should be detected and treated as soon as possible (compare with Section 1.1). The idea is that early cancer discovery followed by early treatment would increase the probability of cure and reduce mortality. This has brought about a massive and costly public health effort aimed at early detection of breast, prostate and colorectal cancers. As elsewhere in oncology, breast cancer with its mass mammography screening program initiated in the mid-1980s was at the forefront.

The reality of mammographic screening, however, diverged from these expectations. Numerous large-scale clinical trials conducted in the 1960s–1990s consistently showed little or no survival benefit of mammography relative to the control (no-mammography) arm [93]. This posed an imminent threat to the pro-mammography medical establishment, medical industry's vested interests and influential patient advocacy groups that ardently promoted mammography. Their fierce resistance has brought about a quarter century of "mammography wars," described in colorful detail in [93, 94]. While they were raging, the mass mammography continued unabated.

One of the main reasons for the dubious value of mammography is that a large fraction of women with invasive breast cancer, which were supposed to benefit from mammography the most, fall into the Fisher effect category. For such women, mammography-based early detection of their primary tumor comes way too late because their cancer has already metastasized.

In an even more troubling development, mammography trials have led to an ostensibly counterintuitive observation that mass screening for breast cancer is associated with *increased mortality* in certain categories of women, a phenomenon that came to be known as the *mammography paradox*. As one striking example, a thorough meta-analysis of seven large randomized mammography trials found that women aged 40–49 years at study entry had higher cumulative mortality than in the control group for 10 years of follow-up in a row [95] (for mortality data in individual trials, see [96] and references therein).

A key to explaining the mammography paradox is the fact that early breast cancer detection triggers early treatment, and in most cases the first line of treatment is surgery for the primary tumor, typically followed by radiotherapy. As was mentioned, and will be explicated in Sections 5.2–5.4, this causes accelerated progression of subclinical metastases already present at the time of primary tumor detection in a considerable fraction of breast cancer patients, which results in excess mortality reported by cancer epidemiologists. An additional contributing factor is earlier release of cancer cells from the primary tumor into the bloodstream during surgery, compared to matching no-mammography patients diagnosed and treated later.

Increased mortality would alone be sufficient for putting the brakes on mass mammography screening. However, what actually derailed it was another striking phenomenon—massive *overdiagnosis* of breast cancer [97], that is, discovery on a large scale of clinically insignificant breast lesions. These include tumors that are (1) borderline between benign and malignant, (2) regressing on their own, (3) representing noninvasive types precursory to breast cancer such as ductal and lobular carcinoma *in situ* (DCIS and LCIS) or (4) invasive breast cancers of a dormant, indolent or slowly growing variety that, if left untreated, would be unlikely to surface during the patient's lifetime or otherwise be the cause of death. Due to the lack of diagnostic tools for distinguishing clinically significant from insignificant early-stage breast tumors with any reasonable accuracy, early breast cancer patients with a given histological/molecular subtype of the disease are handled more or less uniformly. And this is how overdiagnosis translates into *overtreatment*. As a result, hundreds of thousands women globally were subjected unnecessarily to disfiguring, toxic and debilitating treatment by surgery, radiation and chemotherapy, which in many cases has likely shortened their lives.

After the dust of the mammography wars had settled, mass mammographic screening for breast cancer was dramatically scaled back. What was left of a once forceful, ambitious and expensive mass mammography program varies by the country and whom you ask. However, a typical residual recommendation is that women aged 40–74 with a family history of breast cancer or those carrying certain mutations in BRCA1 or BRCA2 tumor suppressor genes should periodically receive mammography.

A similar fate, and for the same reasons of overdiagnosis and overtreatment, befell mass prostate cancer screening based on monitoring the serum concentration of prostate-specific antigen (PSA) [76]. In the words of Richard Ablin [98], who discovered PSA in 1970,

> I never dreamed that my discovery four decades ago would lead to such a profit-driven public health disaster. The medical community must confront reality and stop the inappropriate use of P.S.A. screening. Doing so would save billions of dollars and rescue millions of men from unnecessary, debilitating treatments.

Finally, the jury is still out on the net balance of risks and benefits of mass colonoscopy screening for colorectal cancer [8, Chapter IX]. Negative effects of colonoscopy could be due, among many other reasons, to risks associated with bowel cleansing required as a preparation for colonoscopy. This may lead to serious metabolic conditions such as hyponatraemia and hypokalaemia caused by the loss of electrolytes. Additionally, the attendant massive dehydration causes blood hyperviscosity, which can result in life-threatening cardiovascular events. For example, I personally know of two cases of severe stroke occurring shortly after pre-colonoscopy bowel purge.

4.3 The independence principle

The *independence principle* states that different concurrent primary and secondary tumors in the same host evolve independently. This notion complements the linear progression theory, which considers each tumor local until a relatively late point in its natural history when it will have disseminated to distant sites. The independence principle also dovetails with the conventional view of cancer as an autonomously growing entity driven by its evolving genotype and constrained by the supply of nutrients, oxygen and growth factors. It is a curious historical fact that, although substantial empirical evidence against the independence principle had first come to light in the early 20th century and has kept accumulating ever since, it still remains an influential idea in oncology.

The first definitive proof of inter-tumor interaction is due to the work of Paul Ehrlich (1854–1915), one of the founders of modern medicine and immunology and the laureate of a Nobel Prize in Physiology or Medicine of 1908. His seminal study of interaction between tumors was conducted at the Royal Institute for Experimental Therapy in Frankfurt am Main and published in 1906 [99]. The two main experimental findings, among many others, reported in that article can be summarized as follows:

(1) In mice and rats that were inoculated with cancer cells and developed a viable tumor, subsequently implanted second tumors of the same or different kind are rejected by the host.
(2) In the presence of a primary tumor (sarcoma or carcinoma) implanted in mice, lung metastases it has produced don't grow beyond a certain microscopic size.

The Ehrlich's pioneering work initiated a series of similar studies under varying experimental conditions including a selection of different host species, types of induced primary tumor, kinds of cancer cells grafted to tumor-bearing animals and the number of cancer cells in the graft. They confirmed the paper's first finding unequivocally. The first among these studies appeared as early as in 1907 [100]. The general conclusion of these and numerous subsequent experimental and clinical investigations was that *large tumors suppress the growth of smaller ones*, as summarized in a comprehensive review [101].

The second finding of the Ehrlich's paper was apparently the earliest experimental demonstration of the metastasis-suppressing effect of the primary tumor. For future reference, I will call this fundamental principle the *Ehrlich effect*. Its experimental basis was extensively discussed and summarized in [101]. Clinical confirmation and implications of the Ehrlich effect will be addressed in Section 5.2. Unexpectedly, as will be shown in Section 9.2, this principle can be proven mathematically under minimal, biologically plausible assumptions. This demonstrates that the homeostatic effect of primary tumor on metastases is rooted in very basic structural and kinetic properties of the processes of metastasis formation, dissemination and growth.

Rejection of tumors resulting from inoculation of tumor-bearing animals with cancer cells has the appearance of immunization of the host against cancer cells by the existing tumor. This is the reason why the phenomenon was dubbed “concomitant tumor immunity” or “concomitant tumor resistance” (see e. g. [101, 102]). Although the immune system can indeed get activated in response to antigens expressed by tumor cells making the host refractory to the second tumor challenge, the same effect, although often to a lesser extent, is also manifested by non-immunogenic tumors [101]. That is why this immunological terminology is not widely used anymore.

What is, then, the immunity-independent mechanism driving inter-tumor interaction? Such a mechanism was hypothesized by Richmond Prehn [103] (see also [104]). The key idea is that the dynamics of primary and secondary tumors depends on the balance between generation and disintegration of growth and angiogenic factors as well as of inhibitors of growth and angiogenesis. Importantly, the half-life of these factors is typically shorter than that of the corresponding inhibitors [46]. The more easily degradable growth and angiogenic factors are produced by tumors and their microenvironment and exert their influence on the tumors and vasculature mostly locally and spread primarily by diffusion. By contrast, the more stable growth and angiogenesis inhibitors are produced both locally and systemically and, when released into the bloodstream, may reach remote primary and secondary tumors and suppress their growth and vascularization.

Note also that the aforementioned mechanism of inter-tumor interaction makes it plausible to hypothesize that, if present, growth- and angiogenesis-suppressing effects of larger primary or secondary tumors on smaller ones within the same localized organ is not a factor of major importance.

The phenomenon of inter-tumor interaction is yet another facet of the systemic nature of cancer discussed in Subsection 4.2.1. Likewise, there is no such thing as “local treatment” of a metastasizing primary tumor. In fact, any intervention against a primary tumor not only reduces or prevents the seeding of new metastases but can also stimulate progression of the previously disseminated ones. In particular, primary tumor resection leads to abrupt cessation of its suppressing effect on metastases enabling their escape from dormancy, vascularization and active growth. The same effect, albeit perhaps a more protracted one, can result from radiation therapy. The all-important subject of such metastatic saltation will be taken up in Sections 5.2–5.4.

5 Cancer treatments and their effects

When confronted with the elusiveness of the victory in the War on Cancer documented in Chapter 2, people frequently ask in bewilderment how has this become possible given all the amazing feats of science and engineering like landing astronauts on the moon and creating such technological marvels as personal computers, the internet, cell phones, GPS and AI. Such questions belie a major misunderstanding of the nature of cancer. The aforementioned technological breakthroughs solved *fixed* problems in the sense that no matter how complex these problems don't change when attempts are made to solve them. By contrast, attempts to treat cancer change, and frequently worsen, the course of the disease. The general reasons are three-fold, at a minimum:

(1) Clinically significant cancer is a systemic disease, see Subsection 4.2.1 and Section 4.3. While local treatment can bring about temporary relief, the effects of such treatment on metastasis, discussed in detail in Sections 5.2–5.4, often exacerbate the disease and reduce overall survival of cancer patients.
(2) Genetic diversity and instability of the genomes of cancer cells give rise to fast-paced selection processes within the treated cancer cell population. As cancer cells sensitive to the treating agent are eliminated, the residual tumor is being gradually taken over by the lineages of resistant survivors. The resistant cell population is heterogeneous. It may contain cancer stem cells and/or quiescent cells that are constitutively refractory to radiation and systemic treatments (see Section 3.4). Additionally, some dividing differentiated cancer cells can be resistant due to their genetic or phenotypic attributes. Finally, hypoxic cells are also refractory to radiation and various systemic treatments, but their resistance may be transient—as their oxygenation level improves following elimination of their sensitive competitors, they can become susceptible to the administered treatment. Cancer resistance to systemic treatments will be further discussed in Section 5.5.
(3) Another universal phenomenon rooted in evolution and selection is accelerated repopulation of the residual tumor post-treatment with increasingly faster proliferating cancer cells. This mechanism of resistance to treatment will be elucidated in Chapter 11 (see also [105]).

Treating cancer can be likened to playing multidimensional chess against a grandmaster trained over hundreds of millions of years of evolution. Thus, understanding cancer as an evolutionary process has momentous importance for cancer treatment [106, 107]. In particular, any fixed, predetermined treatment strategy, such as the MTD approach introduced in Section 1.1, is likely doomed to fail.

The goal of cancer treatment is either (1) curative or (2) to thwart or inhibit cancer progression or (3) palliative, i. e., to achieve symptomatic relief and ensure better quality of a patient's life. Strictly speaking, cure means elimination of all cancer cells. In the vast majority of cases of invasive solid cancer, attaining such a cure is unrealistic.

https://doi.org/10.1515/9783111334035-006

Perhaps even more significantly, the event of strict cure is unobservable. Therefore, in most contexts in this book, cure means the absence of *detectable* cancer deposits in the body and their clinical manifestations over a patient's lifetime post-treatment.

5.1 Modes of cancer treatment: a brief overview

Cancer treatments fall into two broad categories—local and systemic. Local treatments are directed against primary tumor or large isolated metastases and chiefly comprise surgery and various modalities of radiation therapy. Contrary to a common belief among some oncologists and cancer patients, local treatments have far-reaching systemic implications consequential for patients' overall survival. This subject was already touched upon in Section 4.3 and will be discussed more thoroughly in Sections 5.2–5.4.

The intent of *surgery* can be life-saving (i. e., removal of a tumor that threatens a vital organ or function), curative, diagnostic, preventative (for example, excision of a precancerous lesion), debulking (e. g., partial resection of a large tumor) or palliative.

The two principal modes of *radiation therapy* are *external beam radiation* and *brachytherapy*. The former uses one or multiple external sources of radiation to deliver photons, electrons, protons, heavier ions or neutrons to the tumor. External beam radiation is delivered in a few fractions, often on business days with weekend breaks. A significant progress has been achieved over recent decades in the design of physical methods of radiation delivery. As a result, a large single dose of radiation (up to 10 Gy or even greater) can be delivered to a specific tumor-containing region within the body, while incurring controllable, limited damage to normal tissues and organs. Brachytherapy consists of placing a source of ionizing radiation within, or in the vicinity of, a tumor either permanently or for a relatively long period of time. The dose rate of radiation emitted by the inserted radioactive seeds decreases exponentially with time.

The most widely used systemic cancer treatments are cytotoxic chemotherapy, hormonal therapy, antiangiogenic therapy, immunotherapy and targeted therapy. These treatments are called systemic because they are aimed at all cells or molecules in the body sharing certain features.

Cytotoxic chemotherapy often targets the processes of DNA replication and repair, RNA synthesis or the cell's molecular machinery operating during mitosis. These processes occur in *all* actively dividing cells, which is why cytotoxic chemotherapy frequently causes severe side effects to normal organs and tissues containing such cells. Examples are skin, lining of the intestines, bone marrow, hair follicles, epithelial cells in the mouth and cells in the outer layer of the adrenal cortex.

Hormonal therapy drugs are administered to patients whose cancer cells depend for their growth and division on sex hormones, which bind to special receptors on the membrane of cancer cells. These drugs block or inhibit sex hormones, or prevent them from binding to the receptors.

Antiangiogenic therapies interfere with various aspects of angiogenesis. Some of them act as angiogenesis inhibitors, while others inactivate various signaling molecules such as vascular endothelial growth factor (VEGF) that trigger angiogenesis or their receptors. Recall that binding of VEGF molecules to their receptors on the membrane of endothelial cells causes the latter to proliferate and create new capillaries.

Immunotherapy against solid tumors is a large group of diverse anticancer interventions that employ or mimic the action of cells, molecular agents or processes of the immune system to kill cancer cells. This is achieved through a variety of mechanisms such as helping the immune system to recognize cancer cells, enhancing the immune system's overall operation, blocking its natural inhibitors that prevent autoimmune reactions, and counteracting the many ways by which cancer cells evade immune surveillance. Many immunotherapies act by augmenting the existent assets and capabilities of the immune system rather than by employing foreign agents; for this reason, they are called *biological treatments*. One kind of cancer immunotherapy consists of immunizing a patient to a specific tumor-derived antigen that trains T-cells to recognize it as foreign. A more traditional approach is to immunize a patient against cancer-causing viruses such as human papillomavirus (HPV) that can engender cervical cancer (and a few other cancers) and hepatitis B virus (HBV) that can cause liver cancer. The reader can glean more information about cancer immunotherapy from the literature (see e. g. [108, 109]).

Finally, *targeted therapy* is an umbrella category comprising treatments that target all cancer cells (or co-opted normal cells in the tumor microenvironment) with a specific identifiable molecular feature, i. e., carrying a certain mutation or expressing a particular protein on the cell membrane. Many hormonal and antiangiogenic treatments as well as some immunotherapies belong to the class of targeted therapies. The purpose of the latter is to kill cancer cells, to restrict or block their growth, division or proliferation, or to inhibit their metabolism. Targeted therapies, especially those aimed at cancer cells carrying specific mutations, are more selective compared to cytotoxic chemotherapy and therefore can be viewed as a refinement of chemotherapy along the lines of *precision (or personalized) medicine*. In particular, targeted therapies have a reduced cross-reactivity with normal cells, which potentially leads to fewer and less severe side effects. The article [110] is a good source of additional information on targeted therapies.

Treatments are administered to cancer patients either as a stand-alone therapy or in combination—concurrently or sequentially. The most frequent first-line therapy for solid cancers is surgery. To eliminate residual and disseminated cancer cells, other therapies are often deployed post-surgery, in which case they are called *adjuvant treatments*. Sometimes it is therapeutically advantageous to administer them before surgery, e. g., to reduce the size of the tumor and thereby the extent of surgery. Such therapies are termed *neoadjuvant*.

5.2 The elephant in the room: surgery-induced acceleration of metastasis

As every oncologist and veterinarian would attest, cancer patients and tumor-bearing animals seldom present with clinically manifest metastases. This observation is corroborated by clinical studies. For example, it was found that among 1,042 stage I, II and III breast cancer patients only 0 %, 3 % and 7 %, respectively, had bone metastases at presentation [111] (to provide context to this data, it should be noted that more than a half of patients with clinically confirmed metastatic breast cancer have bone metastases). Overall, less than 5 % of breast cancer patients display metastases at diagnosis [68].

The rationale for these and other similar clinical observations is the all-important Ehrlich effect, discussed in Section 4.3, i. e., that the primary tumor often suppresses progression of metastases. As was mentioned there, the effect can be explained by the disparity between shorter half-life of growth and angiogenic factors produced by the tumor and its microenvironment and the longer half-life of their locally and systemically generated inhibitors , which results in the dominance of the inhibitors at distant metastatic sites [103, 104]. Hence, a note to cancer patients: *your primary tumor is likely your limited warranty against metastases!*

The Ehrlich effect makes it natural to expect that extirpation of a primary tumor would accelerate metastatic progression. In fact, surgery for primary tumor removes a major source of growth and angiogenesis inhibitors, which could potentially throw angiogenic switch at the sites of dormant metastases and cause their escape from dormancy, vascularization and aggressive growth. Additionally, surgery-induced inflammation leads to local vasodilation, which facilitates intravasation of residual cancer cells or those disseminated in the course of surgery and feeds them into the metastatic pipeline.

The first direct experimental observation of the surgery-induced acceleration of metastasis in mice was reported in 1910 [112]. This study revealed that the frequency of development of large visceral metastases was much higher in mice with resected primary tumor of the mammary gland than in those mice whose primary tumor was left intact. The striking phenomenon of rapid outgrowth of metastases following primary tumor excision was later confirmed by a wealth of other empirical studies conducted on several animal models and involving many different types of primary tumor and a variety of metastatic sites; this body of work was reviewed in [101, 113, 114, 104].

Another mechanism by which excision of the primary tumor can accelerate metastatic progression applies specifically to immunogenic cancers. In this case, removal of the primary tumor eliminates a massive source of antigens presented by cancer cells, which may weaken the immune response and thus allow metastases to evade or overcome immune surveillance. This mechanism acts synergistically with the abrogation of the Ehrlich effect.

In the clinical setting, explosive outgrowth of metastases following resection of a primary tumor (or large secondary tumors) was reported in a multitude of case studies. Here are a few representative well-documented published clinical cases:

(1) Excision of the primary adenocarcinoma of the pancreas (Whipple procedure) in a 55-year-old female patient caused surfacing of numerous previously undetected liver metastases within 34 days after the surgery [115].
(2) Two male patients aged 63 and 88 presented with extremely large melanomas on their upper arm but without evidence of distant metastases. However, in less than 2 months and in 6 months, respectively, after resection of their primary tumor, the patients developed multiple distant metastases [116].
(3) A 58-year-old woman was diagnosed with primary squamous cell carcinoma, a rare type of breast cancer, with no evidence of local, regional or distant dissemination. The patient was treated with modified radical mastectomy. However, about 5 months post-surgery, CT of the head and chest X-ray showed metastatic lesions in her brain and lungs [117].

These and countless other clinical cases demonstrate that in a large fraction of patients metastases surface within a few weeks, months or years after excision of the primary tumor. Also, the same phenomenon seems to be a matter of common knowledge among veterinarians. This leads to the following question: *Is this just a coincidence or is there a cause-and-effect relationship between (a) the presence of a primary tumor and metastatic dormancy; and (b) primary tumor resection and rapid outgrowth of metastases?*

Although experimental and clinical data accumulated over the last 120 years provide profuse biomedical evidence supporting the suppressive effect of primary tumor and stimulating effect of its ablation on metastases, more definitive general conclusions applicable to human cancers have been so far elusive, for at least four reasons:
(1) While in experimental animal models both effects were established beyond reasonable doubt, using similar investigative methods in human subjects would be unethical.
(2) Dormant micrometastases and critical microevents that trigger origination of metastases, their escape from dormancy, vascularization and progression to detectable secondary tumors in humans are largely unobservable.
(3) Due to the length of time over which metastasis runs its natural course (which, as was argued in Section 3.5, may include extended periods of dormancy), such randomly occurring formative microevents are often separated by months, years or even decades from their clinical manifestations, which greatly complicates establishing cause-and-effect relationships.
(4) Owing to enormous inter-patient variation in the course of cancer progression and response to treatment, the existing clinical evidence does not, and cannot, universally support the aforementioned hypothetical causal relationship. In fact, some cancer patients develop overt clinical metastases while a primary tumor is in place (see, e. g., Chapter 10), while in many others metastases remain subclinical and undetectable over long periods of time after removal of the primary tumor or even never manifest at all over the patients' lifetime.

This leads to the next question: *Can one establish a definitive relationship between primary tumor and its ablation and the growth of metastases?* Unexpectedly, the answer to this question is affirmative! I will approach it along two complementary routes—biological and mathematical. From the biological perspective, the question is if there are known mechanisms by which surgery could affect metastasis beyond abrogation of the Ehrlich effect. Such mechanisms will be described in the next section. Some of them are triggered specifically by surgical removal of the primary tumor, while others result from *any* surgery and other injurious interventions.

The fruit born by the mathematical route is remarkable; see Chapter 9 for details. Firstly, this approach enables formulation of the relationship of interest in *precise mathematical form*. Secondly, I will show that under minimal biological and mathematical assumptions the dual suppression/acceleration phenomenon is a necessary mathematical consequence of very general structural features of metastasis as a biological process (see also [118]). In particular, although additional impetus to metastasis produced by surgery as a medical procedure enhances the acceleration phenomenon, the latter is bound to manifest even without this extra boost.

5.3 Effects of surgical procedure on metastases

Effects of the presence of primary tumor and its excision on metastases manifest, respectively, as inhibition and stimulation of angiogenesis and cell proliferation. However, as subsequently described, these seemingly simple effects are a combination of several disparate phenomena with their own distinct mechanisms.

Surgery for a primary or secondary tumor is an invasive procedure that invariably entails a certain amount of mechanical manipulation of the tumor. It also involves excision and inflicting other damage on proximal blood vessels. Thus, resection of a primary tumor often leads to a massive release of tumor cells, potentially including those capable of spawning metastases, into the tumor environment, lymphatics and the bloodstream (see [119, 104, 65] and references therein). Empirical evidence for the significance of this effect in the case of prostate cancer was presented in [120]. That squeezing and palpation of primary tumor produces metastases has been known for more than a century [121].

Apart from triggering a surge in CTCs associated with surgical insult to a primary tumor, there are a number of metastasis-promoting mechanisms associated with *any* open or laparoscopic surgery, not necessarily related to primary tumor and rooted in the nature of this medical procedure:

(1) A major effect of surgery is *wounding*, which, as was explained in detail in Section 3.8, causes a spike in local and systemic production of growth and angiogenic factors required for wound healing. Some of these substances can reach distant metastatic sites and stimulate the growth and vascularization of metastases. The

highest concentration of these agents occurs at the site of injury, which causes accelerated progression of subclinical micrometastases present there as well as formation of new metastatic foci facilitated by enhanced entrapment and extravasation of CTCs. The systemic pro-metastatic environment created by surgical trauma may persist for a few days after surgery.

(2) A universal physiologic reaction to wounding is local *inflammation*, which forges conditions for tissue regeneration and wound healing. One of the most important among them is vasodilation, which enables trafficking of assorted cells of the immune system to the inflammation site. As was argued in Section 3.6, such inflammation tends to locally promote cancer including metastasis.

(3) Surgery is accompanied by anesthesia, analgesia and often blood transfusion and hyperthermia. These systemic interventions and the resulting stress elicit powerful metabolic, neurovascular and endocrine responses bringing about *immunosuppression* [122], which can last for a few weeks post-surgery [104]. Under certain conditions, such weakening of the immune system can produce a signal strong enough to trigger escape of metastases from their state of dormancy. An elaborate study [123] identified some of these conditions and quantified the metastasis-promoting effect in mice.

The magnitude of the surgery-driven boost to metastasis can be expected to be proportional to the extent of surgery; for supporting experimental evidence, see Section 3.8. Thus, from this perspective, laparoscopic surgery when feasible is preferable to the open one. However, it should be kept in mind that even a minor surgical procedure such as an open or fine-needle biopsy [81] or implantation of needles containing seeds of a radioactive material into a tumor for the purpose of brachytherapy can have a measurable metastasis-stimulating effect.

It cannot be emphasized strongly enough that the three aforementioned specific effects of surgery apply to *all* surgeries including those unrelated to cancer. That these interventions can give a boost to metastasis is a consideration that cancer patients and their families are urged to heed. Convincing evidence showing that wounds, including incidental surgeries, can worsen survival of cancer patients was presented in a cohort study involving 418 patients with advanced cancer [124]. As another example, a significantly elevated risk of metastatic recurrence of breast cancer was reported for a group of 125 women who underwent delayed large flap breast reconstruction after mastectomy, as compared to a group of 182 individually matched patients who received mastectomy alone [125].

What was said previously about metastasis-promoting effects of surgery applies in equal measure to primary tumor recurrence. Surgical removal of the primary tumor can have a strong proliferative effect on residual tumor cells due to a surge in the production of growth and angiogenic factors, inflammation, immunosuppression and reduced competition among these cancer cells for space and vital chemicals.

Finally, the aforementioned effects of surgery as a medical procedure act synergistically with abrogation of the Ehrlich effect, which is primarily due to production of growth and angiogenesis inhibitors by the primary tumor and its microenvironment. Thus, primary tumor excision shifts the balance of influences at the sites of dormant metastases toward growth and vascularization.

5.4 What about radiation therapy?

The homeostatic effect of primary tumor on metastases and its annulment following primary tumor removal are clearly independent of exactly how the primary tumor was removed. In particular, the dual metastasis suppression/acceleration principle, established for surgical removal of the primary tumor in Sections 4.3, 5.2 and 5.3, must also hold true for its ablation by radiation. However, unlike surgery where the principle rests on a solid edifice of experimental and clinical observations, published empirical evidence in the case of radiation is surprisingly sketchy. It essentially consists of a few early reports on metastasis-accelerating effects of primary tumor irradiation in the mouse and rat models published since the early 1940s, reviewed in [126], and just a handful of more recent studies. One of them is a detailed experimental murine study by Judah Folkman and coworkers [69] addressing the effects of primary tumor irradiation on metastasis and angiogenesis at the metastatic site. A complex interplay between primary tumor eradication by radiation and subsequent explosive outgrowth of metastases versus their protracted dormancy as mediated by the competition between angiogenic factors and angiogenesis inhibitors in mice was investigated in a seminal paper [127]. Finally, putative molecular mechanisms underpinning the interaction between primary tumor irradiation and various aspects of metastasis in animal models were reviewed in [128]. A few additional references can be gleaned from [129]. Thus, relatively little scientific light has been shed on the problem of radiation-induced acceleration of metastasis, which allowed the vast, well-oiled radiation-therapy enterprise to operate without a comprehensive critical evaluation of the long-term effects of radiation treatment.

Such a gap in the amount of empirical knowledge between the effects of surgery and radiotherapy on metastasis and the fact that metastasis-promoting effects of radiation have not been studied in earnest is bewildering, for at least two reasons. First, radiation therapy is one of the cornerstones of cancer treatment, with more than half of cancer patients receiving radiation at some point in the course of their treatment. Second, the literature on cancer radiotherapy includes many hundreds of thousands of articles addressing all conceivable other aspects of this treatment modality, such as physical methods and techniques of radiation delivery, treatment planning, radiation dosimetry, modeling of irradiated cell survival, comparison and optimization of the regimens of radiation treatment, and the assessment of radiotherapy's side effects including toxicity and damage to normal organs and tissues.

The principal therapeutic theme hammered out in this voluminous literature is *local control*, i. e., elimination of the maximum number of clonogenic cancer cells comprising the primary tumor. However, achieving local control provides a clear benefit to the patient only if no subclinical metastases are present during radiation therapy. Due to the Fisher effect (see Section 4.1), the latter condition is not met by a considerable fraction of cancer patients with invasive cancer. Furthermore, the condition is virtually impossible to test at the time when such testing could make a difference, i. e., before the start of radiation treatment. And finally and importantly, in those cases where seeding of viable metastases has occurred prior to the end of radiation therapy, pursuit of local control is likely to precipitate metastatic relapse and thus shorten the patient's residual lifetime.

The differences between surgery and radiation therapy as medical procedures are manifold. For one thing, surgery is effectively an instantaneous event while radiation treatment, including external beam fractionated radiotherapy and brachytherapy, can take up a few weeks or months. For another thing, surgery permanently eliminates cancer cells (unless a resected tumor recurs), while radiation only inactivates cancer cells clonogenically without killing them. However, vis-a-vis effects on metastasis, those caused by surgery and radiation are exceedingly similar, for both treatment modes negate the Ehrlich effect, produce wounding and inflammation, diminish the immune response due to elimination of the antigen-bearing immunogenic primary tumor and also are procedurally immunosuppressive with radiation typically having a stronger and longer lasting impact. In particular, *any* significant local or whole-body radiation exposure due to medical, diagnostic, environmental, professional or any other reason is likely to have metastasis-promoting effects. For a review of such effects in animal models, see [129] and references therein.

5.5 Drug resistance

In 1907 Paul Ehrlich introduced the concept of "magic bullet" (Zauberkugel in German). By this he meant an agent that can cure an infectious disease without incurring significant harm to the patient. In 1909 he developed the first such magic bullet—Salvarsan—for treating syphilis. He thought the same is achievable for cancer treatment with chemotherapy, the term he coined. This proved impossible, and the principal reason is *drug resistance.*

The reality of cancer therapy is that every systemic treatment, such as cytotoxic chemo-, antiangiogenic, hormonal, immuno- and targeted therapy, sooner or later loses its efficacy. This happens due to the selection, survival and persistence of pre-existing or emerging cancer cells that are refractory to the given therapeutic agent. As sensitive cells are progressively eliminated by the therapeutic agent, the clones spawned by the surviving resistant cells take over the residual tumor and start to aggressively proliferate, which leads to treatment failure. This phenomenon is commonly called drug resistance.

Drug resistance comprises several nonmutually exclusive mechanisms:

(1) As a protective measure against harmful substances, cells in most organisms have the ability to transport toxic agents across the cell membrane. Due to specific mutations in relevant genes, cancer cells can enhance this basic efflux capability to the degree that makes them resistant to many, and often virtually all, anti-cancer agents.
(2) Mutations and metabolic changes in cancer cells can endow them with the ability to inhibit or degrade cancer drugs, or alter their targets [130].
(3) The aim of many chemotherapy and targeted therapy drugs is to disrupt DNA integrity, replication and repair, which if successful would bring about cell death through one of the two common mechanisms—apoptosis (programmed cell death) or autophagy (internal lysis and recycling of cellular components). Some cancer cells develop the ability to enhance DNA repair and inhibit both cell-death pathways, which would confer on them resistance to this class of anticancer agents.

Finally, extensive experimental evidence gained from animal studies and reviewed in [129] suggests that under certain conditions all systemic treatments without exception can induce and enhance metastasis.

5.6 Front loading principle: the central dogma of cancer treatment

Taken collectively, the notions of early cancer diagnosis and that cancer should be hit as hard and as soon as possible constitute a unified paradigm that can be called the *front loading principle*. The principle seems self-evident because it ostensibly has the greatest chance to prevent the cancer's further growth and spread over any alternative strategy. For anticancer interventions, which, unlike surgery and some immuno- and targeted therapies, have a well-defined dose, i. e., for radiation and various chemical agents, this translates into the *Maximum Tolerated Dose* (MTD) principle, which prescribes administration of the agent's maximum dose a patient can tolerate (compare with Section 1.1).

The front loading principle dominates the thinking of oncologists and cancer patients alike. What is seldom realized is that it is deeply rooted in the linear progression theory, and where the latter theory fails (see Section 4.1), so may the former principle as well.

Is the front loading principle universally true for solid cancers? To answer this question, it is instructive to analyze its hidden foundations. In doing so, I will follow Henri Poincaré (1854–1912), a genius French mathematician, theoretical physicist and philosopher who was the first to keenly understand the fundamental importance of hypotheses and assumptions for the validity of scientific research [2], a subject to be further discussed in Section 6.1.

The validity of the front loading principle rests on a number of implicit assumptions, specifically that (1) cancer does not regress spontaneously; (2) it will manifest clinically during a patient's lifetime; (3) cancer detected early can be reliably diagnosed, characterized and staged, which is a prerequisite for successful treatment; (4) in particular, cancer did not produce subclinical metastases prior to primary tumor detection; and (5) cancer treatment does not exacerbate the disease.

It has been known long ago that, as universal statements, all these assumptions are false:

(1) Although spontaneous regression of cancer is hard to observe systematically, such clinical cases have been reported and brought into the medical mainstream as early as in the 1960s [131–133]. Some of the cancers that are prone to regress on their own without treatment include renal cell carcinoma, melanoma, testicular cancer, neuroblastoma (a childhood cancer originating in the adrenal glands) and non-Hodgkin's lymphoma. The rate of spontaneous breast cancer regression was estimated in an important study [134], which compared the rates of invasive breast cancer detection in two closely matched groups of Norwegian women, altogether comprising more than 229,000 women followed from 1992–2001. Women in the first group were given biannual mammography, while those in the control group received mammography only at the end of the 6-year observation period. The comparison revealed that the mammography group produced 22 % excess cancer cases over the control group. A careful analysis conducted in [134] showed that this effect can only plausibly be attributed to breast cancer regression in the control group. Although sporadic cancer regression still remains a *terra incognita*, it is safe to hypothesize that it is enabled, among other mechanisms, by the activity of the immune system and the regulatory role of tumor microenvironment. A large body of experimental evidence reviewed and analyzed in [32–35] suggests that healthy microenvironment can inhibit cancer progression and even reprogram cells with malignant phenotype back into normal cells through epigenetic mechanisms (see also Sections 3.1 and 3.2).

(2) Extensive theoretical and empirical evidence reviewed in Section 3.6 suggests that primary and secondary tumors can indefinitely remain in a dormant or indolent subclinical state. The ubiquity of tumor dormancy is confirmed by a wealth of autopsy studies exemplified in Section 3.6. Furthermore, solitary cancer cells can indefinitely remain quiescent.

(3) Due to its sampling nature, needle biopsy is unreliable. Furthermore, as every pathologist knows, distinguishing between various benign lesions, cancer *in situ* and invasive malignancies as well as scoring histological grade in early stages of the disease may prove difficult and liable to false positive and false negative diagnoses. Most importantly, no methods for reliably telling an aggressive, life-threatening early stage cancer with high metastatic potential from the one that can be safely ignored are currently available for most types of cancer.

(4) Recall from Section 4.1 that the work of Bernard Fisher and his colleagues proved beyond a reasonable doubt that, in a large fraction of patients with invasive breast cancer, by the time primary breast tumor becomes clinically detectable, it has already metastasized. This conclusion was corroborated through mathematical modeling based on various parametric versions of the general model of metastatic cancer progression explicated in Sections 8.1 and 8.2 (see also Section 9.1), with parameters estimated from site-specific volumes of metastases collected from breast, prostate and lung cancer patients [135–139].
(5) Finally, that cancer treatment including surgery and radiation therapy can give boost to metastasis was extensively discussed in Sections 5.2–5.4.

The same assumptions 1–5 make or break mammography and PSA screening. Had they been carefully formulated and closely scrutinized, the disastrous rush to mass screening could have been averted. Instead, early cancer detection effort should be focused on the search for those categories of patients for whom the benefits of screening outweigh the risks.

It is also worth mentioning that as far as pursuit of local control is concerned, the front loading principle for fractionated cancer radiotherapy can be rigorously proven under very general, well-defined biological and mathematical conditions [140–142]. Moreover, under the assumption that radiation-induced normal tissue toxicity can adequately be accounted for by imposing fixed upper limits on the total dose and dose per fraction, this implies optimality of the uniform fractionation schedules consisting of equal doses separated by equal time intervals [142].

What are the alternatives to MTD cancer therapy? One of them is *metronomic treatment*, i. e., protracted administration of low-dose chemotherapy, which is clearly an exact opposite of the MTD approach. The metronomic treatment was pioneered by my colleague and friend Dr. Michael Retsky who successfully tested it in the mid-1990s on his own colon cancer. Here are a few details of this remarkable story, published in [143–145].

Michael Retsky is a physicist and an innovative, visionary cancer researcher. In 1994 he was diagnosed with stage IIIc colon cancer that had penetrated the bowel wall and spread to four lymph nodes. After surgical removal of the primary tumor, he decided to use long-term low-dose chemotherapy to prevent primary tumor recurrence and metastasis. His computer simulations of tumor growth suggested that this treatment would be superior to standard high-dose chemotherapy. The schedule of administration of 5-fluoruracil, a common colon cancer chemotherapy drug, was designed by the oncologist William Hrushesky MD and modified by Michael Retsky. The course of the treatment was also discussed with the renowned oncologist Judah Folkman, introduced earlier in this book in Chapters 1, 3 and 4. Michael Retsky administered the drug himself every night for about 6 hours using a portable pump. The overall duration of the treatment was 2.5 years. The side effects were minimal, and he was able to work and exercise daily. And most importantly, he never relapsed.

Part II: **Mathematical modeling in biomedical sciences**

6 Mathematical modeling: basic principles and a new methodology

6.1 The role of assumptions in scientific research

That logic, including careful formulation of assumptions, is critical for the correctness of all sorts of arguments in mathematics, science and far beyond has been recognized since the times of Pythagoras and Aristotle. However, it was Henri Poincaré who, as was noted in Section 5.6, was the first to realize the paramount importance of assumptions and hypotheses for the rigorous development of science [2]. He was the last universalist who knew both contemporary mathematics and physics in their entirety. Among many other things, Poincaré discovered special relativity and published his account of it in 1904, a year before Einstein. However, unlike Einstein, Poincaré didn't believe in objective, immutable laws of nature—he rather believed in hypotheses and their empirically verifiable consequences. That's probably the reason, along with the fact that he published his paper in an obscure Italian journal, that it is Einstein who is credited with the creation of the special relativity theory.

From the formal logic perspective, every proposition, except for statements of fact such as $2 + 3 = 5$, has the form $P \Rightarrow Q$, where P is the assumptions (or premises), Q is the conclusions and $\Rightarrow$ represents implication. In a broader setting of theoretical and empirical sciences, the symbol $\Rightarrow$ signifies the method by which conclusions are derived from the assumptions, including logic, mathematical proofs, theoretical arguments, computations, experiments and statistical analysis of experimental data. In logic, the implication $P \Rightarrow Q$ is true if and only if either P is false or both P and Q are true. Thus, without rigorously stating the assumptions and examining their correctness, the truth value of a scientific study cannot be determined.

Furthermore, for a study to be logically and scientifically correct, its assumptions must be valid, complete and noncontradictory. As was mentioned in Section 1.4, assumptions behind experimental and theoretical biomedical studies are rarely spelled out either formally or informally. As a result, the validity and the scope of generality of the results and conclusions of such studies are often uncertain.

Poincaré's ideas about assumptions and hypotheses were laid down in his landmark book [2], whose first edition was published in 1902. Apparently, these ideas had appeared so much ahead of their time that even nowadays they have not been fully recognized and taken to heart by the scientific community.

6.2 Mathematical models as axiomatic systems

For an experimental scientist, all theoretical constructs—concepts, principles, rules, methods, hypotheses and interpretations—are liable to change as new experimental findings emerge that do not fit the old theories. Such changes of theoretical framework

https://doi.org/10.1515/9783111334035-008

constitute the evolution of (and sometimes revolutions in) science. This only makes it more tempting to allow the same flexibility in mathematical modeling by adding, removing or altering model assumptions in the process of model building, deriving model-based formulas, conducting data analysis or formulating results. It is precisely such manipulations that could compromise scientific research, an outcome I witnessed on numerous occasions in the publications I have read. Once the assumptions of a mathematical model are stated and agreed upon, they become an axiomatic system from which implications are derived with the same mathematical rigor one would expect in pure mathematics. Of course, model assumptions may change as new data, theories and hypotheses come to light. This change, in turn, would engender new models and new axiomatic systems.

Unlike experimental sciences, mathematics, when done correctly, makes a transition from the assumptions of theorems (P) to their conclusions (Q) with impeccable accuracy, which gives mathematical models the quality of a solid rock in the fluid sea of empirical sciences. A fundamental epistemological difference between them is that in empirical sciences, at least in principle, every conclusion, theoretical result or conjecture is open to experimental verification, while mathematics has no such external, empirical criterion of truth. The only means available to a mathematician is rigorous noncontradictory arguments based on axioms, definitions, formal logic, previously established theorems and, of course, a good measure of intuition and inspiration to know what the correct P and Q should be, and a creative impulse to find a valid path from P to Q.

No one understood the role of axioms in mathematics, science and other realms of human activity better than John von Neumann (1903–1957), one of the greatest mathematicians and scientists to have ever set foot on Earth [146]. He was gifted with an almost supernatural ability to create and rigorously analyze elaborate axiomatic systems that captured the essence of the fields of science and practice as diverse as logic, functional analysis, quantum mechanics, nuclear physics, game theory, economics, design of computers, military strategy, logistics, cellular automata and the design of self-replicating machines.

6.3 Mechanistic vs. phenomenological models

A general principle driving empirical sciences (and minds) is, “the more details the better.” Mathematical models of biological processes aiming to embody this principle are called *mechanistic* because they seek to describe mathematically microscopic, typically molecular, mechanisms of these processes in organisms ranging from cells to humans. Although motivated by a noble goal of achieving a more complete knowledge of biological processes, the principle of mechanistic modeling has a number of shortcomings:

(1) The postulated mechanisms may be known only partially and hypothetically, in which case the proposed mechanistic models are only provisional.

(2) Microscopic processes described by mechanistic models are often unobservable. To account for this, the models and algorithms implementing them typically depend on a multitude of unknown parameters that have to be computed or estimated from data. In many situations, including the single-patient setting discussed in this book, the available data is collected on a more macroscopic level and may have considerable separation in time and space from the causative microscopic events and processes the model seeks to describe. Quite frequently, due to technological or ethical reasons as well as prohibitive costs, such data is insufficient for estimation of model parameters.
(3) Microscopic biological processes are highly interrelated, which may cause the same model parameters to appear in various combinations in several components of the model and in relevant equations. As a result, it may, and often does, happen that different sets of model parameters produce exactly the same model output, i. e., an observable quantity whose sample values form a dataset collected for estimation of model parameters. In this case, model parameters are inestimable from the data. This ubiquitous yet underappreciated devastating phenomenon is called *model non-identifiability*. It is elucidated below in Section 6.5 and exemplified in Chapters 9 and 10.

The phenomenological approach of this book, described in Section 1.2, provides an attractive alternative to mechanistic modeling of cancer—*phenomenological models*. They deal with relatively simple and clinically relevant quantitative characteristics of cancer, such as timing and rates of cancer-related processes, the sizes of various cancer cell populations and the probabilities of critical events driving cancer progression. The output of a phenomenological model usually represents an observable, macroscopic, quantitative manifestation of the underlying microscopic processes. Importantly, phenomenological models can be formulated independently of the detailed mechanisms of these processes, be it known, partially known or unknown. A very general phenomenological model descriptive of metastatic cancer progression and the effects of treatment is presented in Chapter 8, while its more specific parametric versions are instantiated in Chapters 9 and 10.

It should be kept in mind that the distinction between mechanistic and phenomenological models is relative. As a rule of thumb valid for this book, mathematical models describing subcellular processes, and especially when doing so on the molecular level, are viewed as mechanistic, while those dealing with cells and their populations, organs and tissues, and whole-body effects are considered phenomenological. Some phenomenological models employed in this book are non-identifiable; however, their non-identifiability is more tractable than that of more complex multi-parametric mechanistic models in that non-identifiable models discussed in the book can be re-parameterized through a smaller set of biologically meaningful parameters expressed as simple combinations of the original parameters.

The following example, whose concept is borrowed from [19], illustrates the power of phenomenological models. Consider the response of a homogeneous clonogenic cancer cell population in vitro or in vivo to uniform fractionated radiation, i. e., to a number of short pulses of ionizing radiation carrying equal doses and separated by equal time intervals. Let's assume that the duration of the inter-dose intervals is at least a few hours, as is the case for a typical external beam radiation cancer therapy. Suppose the goal is to compute the probability that all cells in the population are inactivated by radiation. This probability is conventionally called the *tumor control probability* (TCP). Recall that a therapeutic dose of radiation doesn't physically kill cancer cells but rather clonogenically inactivates them, that is, makes them incapable of spawning a tumor.

The processes leading to cell inactivation are extremely complex and consist of several stages [147]:

(1) Formation of primary DNA lesions as a result of energy deposition by the particles of ionizing radiation or their secondary particles passing in the vicinity of a cell's DNA. Typical primary lesions consist of either damage to one or several bases on one strand of the DNA or simultaneous damage to two complementary bases on the opposite strands of the DNA, which produces a *double-strand break* (DSB).
(2) Repair, and occasionally misrepair, of some of the primary lesions through complex enzymatic processes. Isolated single-strand breaks are usually successfully repaired due to the complementarity of the two strands of the DNA; however, DSBs are less likely to be repaired. In the mitosis phase of the cell cycle, an unrepaired DSB can be seen under a microscope as a broken-off piece of an arm on one of the cell's chromosomes.
(3) Misrejoining of a pair of DSBs on the same or different chromosomes, which often leads to the formation of a *lethal chromosomal aberration*.

Inactivation of a cell by radiation is an end result of the presence of either lethal unrepaired or irreparable DSBs or, most frequently, of lethal chromosomal aberrations.

Of note, damage repair processes operate on the time scale from minutes to about an hour, so that by the time of the exposure to the next fraction of radiation the transient processes of inactivation and recovery of damaged cells caused by the previous dose will have been completed. As a result, no matter how complex the underlying biological processes may be, cell inactivation can be characterized with reasonable accuracy by a single phenomenological parameter—inactivation probability, p, for a single cell as a function of radiation dose, d, per fraction. In practice, p can be estimated experimentally by the fraction of inactivated cells in a large homogeneous population in vitro exposed to dose d divided by the *plating efficiency*, i. e., the surviving fraction of similarly cultured control (unirradiated) cells of the same kind.

Denote by N the number of cells in the population subjected to fractionated radiation and by n the number of fractions of radiation, and let P be the desired TCP. Assuming that cells in the population are inactivated by radiation independently of each other and with the same probability p per fraction, we find by applying basic rules of probability that $P = [1 - (1 - p)^n]^N$. By contrast, computing the probability P mechanistically by following the processes of formation of primary damage to DNA, its repair and binary misrejoining of DSBs would go well beyond the means of modern radiation biology.

Empirical scientists might dismiss these argument as a "mathematical trick." However, such "tricks," rooted in biological insight, lie at the heart of successful mathematical modeling.

The computation reveals that phenomenological models are *parsimonious* in that they are based on a small number of biologically realistic assumptions, are structurally minimalistic and involve a small number of unknown parameters, while still describing the outcomes of biological processes of interest with reasonable accuracy. This is yet another significant advantage of phenomenological models over mechanistic ones.

As was explained in Section 1.2, this book favors the phenomenological approach and is focused on a single patient rather than a population. Another crucial dichotomy faced by a modeler of biomedical processes is whether to use deterministic or stochastic models. This methodological choice is dissected in the next section.

6.4 The determinism vs. chance dilemma

During the Age of Enlightenment, inspired by its universalist ideas and the central role that mathematics played in physics and astronomy, other sciences including biology, medicine, demography and epidemiology became increasingly receptive to quantitative methods. However, there is an important distinction: While physics has precise universal laws typically expressed in the form of differential equations, no such laws have ever been discovered in biomedical or social sciences. That is why, to make quantitative inference from data, biomedical and social scientists resorted to statistics.

Over the last 100 years, the use of statistical methods has gradually become a mandatory component of biomedical research. Nowadays, no biomedical study involving experimental data can be published nor a grant proposal funded without an inclusion of statistical data analysis. Such a compliance pressure (or should we call it statistical diktat?) has caused biomedical scientists to adopt, mostly unwittingly, the assumption that every event occurring in a cell or a multicellular organism, including a human or animal subject, depends in essential ways on chance and likewise that every unknown quantity, measurable or otherwise, is a random variable.

That this assumption is not merely philosophical is clear: A nonrandom event either occurs or does not occur, and its detection is a matter of a single observation, while a genuinely random event only occurs with a certain probability whose estimation requires a large number of repeated observations. Formally, one could argue that a constant is a particular case of a random variable (i. e., the one with a degenerate distribution), which would seem to imply that determinism is a particular case of randomness. However, when applied to deterministic quantities, many concepts and results from probability become wrong, trivial or meaningless. For example, probability density functions of nonrandom variables don't exist. Also, such variables are automatically independent and are identically distributed if and only if they are identical. Likewise, for a degenerate distribution, the Law of Large Numbers (LLN) [148, Section 10.5] and the Central Limit Theorem (CLT) [148, Section 10.6], two foundational and extensively used results in probability and statistics, become trivial and utterly uninformative.

It is true that many classes of biological processes are decidedly random, such as:

(1) Purely random processes similar to flipping a coin or rolling a die. A classic example is passing on of gene variants forming an allele from heterozygous parents to their offspring in humans, animals or plants.
(2) Biological processes triggered by microevents governed by stochastic laws of quantum mechanics. For example, as was discussed in the previous section, this is the case for inactivation of a cell by radiation, where lethal damage, such as formation of an unrepaired DSB or a chromosomal aberration, is an end result of a complex sequence of ultramicroscopic random events.
(3) Low probability-high impact random microevents. Examples include genomic events leading to mutagenesis, formation of the first malignant clonogenic cell and shedding of a viable metastasis off a primary tumor.
(4) Randomly changing discrete quantities, e. g., the size of a small cell population. This is especially relevant to cancer, whose natural history is essentially driven by the dynamics and evolution of a small subpopulation of clonogenic cells (or cancer stem cells)—see Section 3.4. For example, the outcome of cancer treatment can be determined by survival of just a handful of clonogenic cells, potentially even a single one.

It is more intriguing that certain classes of biological processes display highly predictable, deterministic behavior. Here are some examples:

(1) Biological processes that are largely physical or chemical in nature and, if viewed macroscopically, are essentially deterministic. This includes diffusion, molecular transport, photo- and chemotaxis, the action of molecular motors, generation and transmission of neural signals, dynamics of action potentials, blood circulation, etc.
(2) Processes subject to physiologic homeostasis that cause many biochemical and biophysical measurements in an individual subject under normal conditions to be fairly stable. Examples are pH, concentrations of critical electrolytes such as Na, K and Ca in human blood, body temperature, cardiac output at rest and many others.
(3) Operation of biochemical systems forming a molecular basis of life. What we know about their functioning suggests that they essentially act as deterministic machines governed by differential equations of biochemical kinetics. If initial concentrations of all molecular agents, kinetic constants and external conditions for any such system are known, then the future states of the system can be predicted with great accuracy. Such a predictable operation within a wide range of external conditions is the reason why the genetic apparatus of a cell, which is nothing more than an extremely complex, self-regulating biochemical and biophysical system, displays such

a great fidelity in preservation and replication of the genome as well as in transcription, translation and adaptive regulation of gene expression. Additional features of biochemical systems, including the presence of activation thresholds, inhibitors and negative feedback loops, ensure stable and predictable execution of biological functions even in randomly changing environments, which contributes to physiologic homeostasis.

(4) Normal embryonic development with its remarkable precision, stability and predictability despite considerable fluctuations in the variables descriptive of the mother's biochemical and physiological condition and changes in the external environment.

Thus, the deterministic side of the modeling dilemma enjoys a strong backing from basic science.

Deterministic behavior of biochemical and biophysical systems is a collective result of an extremely large number of random quantum mechanical ultramicroscopic events. Therefore, before making an assumption about randomness of the observed macroscopic effects and embarking on statistical analysis of relevant data, one has to identify specific reasons that would explain why stochasticity reemerges in the particular setting and think about the practicality of taking it into account. Or is such stochasticity merely an illusion masking essentially deterministic causation?

Deterministic models of closed biological systems have the following uniqueness property: The state of the system described by such a model at any moment of time is completely determined by its initial state. However, dependence of the final state of such a system on the initial conditions can be very sensitive to minute perturbations of the latter, which would make the system dynamics *chaotic*. Complex, self-organizing, open biological systems including cancer generally don't have the uniqueness property. Therefore, deterministic models are too rigid to account for the full extent of complexity and variability associated with cancer progression and response to treatment.

In summary, the choice between deterministic and stochastic approaches to mathematical modeling of biological systems should follow the preponderance of scientific evidence regarding the nature of the phenomenon of interest. If such evidence is inconclusive then both approaches could be pursued competitively and the results of their application compared. Alternatively, one can devise models that combine deterministic and stochastic components. Examples of such hybrid models are presented in Chapters 8–10.

6.5 The devil in the corner: model non-identifiability

In November 1995, Dr. Andrei Yakovlev, my friend and collaborator introduced in Section 1.4, called my office in Detroit to discuss the two-stage model of carcinogenesis. This elegant model, developed by Moolgavkar, Venzon and Knudson [149, 150] and for this reason also called the MVK model, posits the following two-stage process of spontaneous or induced carcinogenesis in humans or animals. First, susceptible stem cells (see Section 3.4) acquire one premalignant mutation according to a Poisson process (described in the appendix) with rate ν, thus forming a population of *initiated cells*, which undergoes proliferation with rates of cell division α and death (or differentiation) β. Second, initiated cells acquire with rate μ a second mutation through asymmetric division, whereby an initiated cell divides into two cells—one initiated and another one carrying the additional second mutation. Acquisition of the latter converts an initiated cell into a fully malignant cell that grows into a detectable tumor over some deterministic or random time. Since this time is typically small relative to the time required for the emergence of the first malignant cell, the latter time can be viewed as the observed time to malignant tumor. The distribution of this time was computed in closed form as a function of parameters ν, α, β, μ [151, 152].

This computation opened up a tantalizing prospect of estimating these four unobservable, biologically important parameters from time-to-tumor data. No attempts, however, have succeeded in doing so, and Andrei Yakovlev wondered why. His intuition was that the problem was not in the set-up of the experiments or statistical analysis of time-to-tumor data, but in the structure of the model itself. On the same day, I called him back with the results: Even if the distribution of the time to the first malignant cell is fully known, the four model parameters are not jointly identifiable from this distribution; in fact, only three combinations of these four parameters turned out to be identifiable. These results were published in [153] (and, in a more heuristic way, independently discovered in [154]). That was my first encounter, also described in [19], with the phenomenon of model non-identifiability; many more have followed.

Consider a deterministic or stochastic model of a physical, biological or other process that has a certain output, which can be a number, a function or a probability distribution. Suppose the model depends on n unknown parameters represented as an n-dimensional vector $\theta = (\theta_1, \theta_2, \dots, \theta_n)$. If any two distinct parameter vectors produce distinct outputs, the model is called (structurally) *identifiable*. In other words, the model is *non-identifiable* if and only if there exist two distinct vectors of model parameters that generate exactly the same output (typically, in this case there are infinitely many parameter vectors with the same property). Thus, identifiability is an intrinsic, structural property of the model.

Let me illustrate the notion of model non-identifiability with a simple but realistic example from physics (this example is borrowed from [155]). Imagine a mass m suspended on an ideal spring with spring constant k. Pulling the mass down or pushing it up and perhaps additionally giving it a jolt sets the system into an oscillatory motion around the point of static equilibrium. The oscillation of the mass is described by the second Newton's law, which in the absence of air resistance has the form

$$mX''(t) - kX(t) = 0, \tag{6.1}$$

where $X(t)$ is the position of the mass at time t on the vertical axis relative to the point of static equilibrium. Differential equation (6.1) has the unique solution

$$X(t) = x_0 \cos(\omega t) + \frac{v_0}{\omega} \sin(\omega t) \quad \text{with } \omega = \sqrt{\frac{k}{m}},$$

where $x_0 = X(0)$ is the initial position of the mass, $v_0 = X'(0)$ is its initial velocity and ω is the frequency of the oscillation.

Function $X(t)$, the model output, represents a simple harmonic oscillation and depends on the vector of four parameters, $\theta = (m, k, x_0, v_0)$. However, it is clear that observation of the oscillation process alone won't enable the determination of parameters m and k separately; what can only be determined is their combination $\omega^2 = k/m$ (in fact, equation (6.1) implies that $\omega^2 = X''(0)/X(0)$). Thus, model (6.1) is non-identifiable, and the simplest identifiable vector of its parameters that completely determines the output is $(k/m, x_0, v_0)$.

As shown in [155], every non-identifiable model can be rendered identifiable by reparameterization, i. e., expressing the model through a new set of $r < n$ identifiable parameters represented as functions of the original n parameters. Notice that in this example of harmonic oscillation, one has $n = 4$ and $r = 3$, and the new identifiable parameters x_0 and v_0 are the same as the original ones, while the remaining new parameter, k/m, is the ratio of two original parameters. In many situations, however, the functions expressing new identifiable parameters through the original ones are more complex.

Therefore, every non-identifiable model is over-parameterized. The identifiability requirement sets up a natural upper limit to the complexity of a model used to describe a particular output. In other words, if the number of model parameters exceeds the upper limit, the description of the output by the model is redundant. This serves as a good illustration of the *principle of parsimony* referred to in Section 6.3. One way to make a non-identifiable model identifiable without changing its parameter vector is to augment the model with new independent observable outputs depending on the same model parameters. The principal difficulty faced by this approach lies in finding such new outputs.

One of the principal sources of new knowledge obtainable through mathematical modeling is estimates of unknown and unobservable biologically or clinically important model parameters. With these parameters at hand, researchers can run the model under various scenarios and predict the outcomes far beyond what can be, or has been, observed. However, there is a major precondition to realizing this benefit of mathematical modeling—the model should be identifiable. In fact, the most troublesome aspect of non-identifiable models is that their parameters cannot even in principle be estimated from the data, regardless of the method of parameter estimation. If attempted, estimates of model parameters would vary erratically depending on such irrelevant factors as the selection of optimization software and its settings and initialization of the vector of model parameters. Quite often, model parameters are estimated through a single, unsupervised run of a standard statistical software, which normally won't produce any red flags, thus causing unsuspecting scientists to believe that what they have obtained are true model parameters.

Thus, prior to parameter estimation, one has to make sure the model is identifiable, and if not, to re-parameterize the model through identifiable parameters. In practice, this approach is fraught with two difficulties: (1) detecting model non-identifiability and computing identifiable parameters is often a daunting analytical task; and (2) identifiable parameters, even if found, may not be as informative and readily interpretable as the original ones.

It should also be pointed out that even if a model is theoretically (or structurally) identifiable, estimation of its parameters using statistical methods may produce poor results due to large variance of the estimators, numerical instability of the estimation procedure, or poor data quality. This phenomenon is often called *practical non-identifiability*.

My experience suggests that a large fraction of models employed in biomedical sciences are non-identifiable, which contributes to generation of false knowledge and irreplicable scientific findings (see Sections 12.2–12.5). A suspicion that a model is non-identifiable arises when estimation of model parameters proves problematic, as was the case with the MVK model. Deciding whether this is due to structural or practical non-identifiability requires extensive analytical, statistical and numerical work including the use of many methods and algorithms of parameter estimation, running them on numerous datasets, and trying multiple initializations of model parameters.

Finally, non-identifiability of a model does not preclude assessing its adequacy by computing various measures of goodness-of-fit to the data. If a researcher's focus is on the quality of fit to the data and if it is found that a model with a particular parameter vector fits the data well, existence of other parameter vectors producing the same fit would not disqualify the model.

6.6 A new methodology

By the grace of nature, the universal laws of physics have precise mathematical form [156]. In molecular biology, many microscopic processes that are essentially physical or chemical in nature, such as the action of molecular motors, kinetics of biochemical reactions and propagation of action potentials, can also be described fairly accurately by mathematical models. By contrast, in the biology of cells, organs, tissues and whole organisms as well as in medicine, no universal quantitative laws have been discovered so far. In their stead, biomedical sciences make qualitative or quantitative statements about biological objects or processes that are based on measurements, observations, theoretical arguments, experience, intuition or rejection of alternatives and are believed to be true for organisms or patients of a certain kind. I will here call such statements, perhaps for lack of better term, *natural laws*.

To illustrate difficulties with the formulation and justification of natural laws, consider a statement, often made by cancer researchers and practitioners, that systematic consumption of certain foods, e. g., red meat products, increases the risk of a specific cancer. Four interrelated impediments make verification of this statement challenging. First, biological mechanisms behind this putative cause-and-effect relationship remain largely unknown. Second, effects of a diet on the risk of cancer are subject-specific, so that the statement may be true for some individuals and false or uncertain for others. Such an heterogeneity is a great hindrance to rigorous statistical analysis aimed at confirming the association of interest (see Sections 12.6–12.9). Third, establishing this association is typically based on the *relative risk*, i. e., the ratio of the proportions of individuals in a population who have developed cancer among those with and without a particular diet habit. Such comparisons are methodologically problematic because cancer risk depends on many other, and often more important, factors potentially correlated with the diet such as genetic makeup, family history of cancer, age, BMI, amount of exercise, exposure to environmental, lifestyle or occupational hazards and many others. Fourth, the gap between statistical association and causation is a formidable one to fill [157].

The question I take up in this section is as follows: *Could natural laws in the biomedical sciences be formulated in precise mathematical terms and discovered or confirmed unequivocally, under certain realistic assumptions, through mathematical modeling and statistical analysis?* Surprising as it is, the answer to this question is affirmative, and the key to it is a new methodology that I now set out to describe. This methodology makes it possible for mathematical modeling to provide, in certain cases, definitive answers to systemic biomedical questions that elude empirical resolution. One striking example is the discovery in Chapter 9 of a natural law concerning the effects of primary tumor and its removal on the rate of growth of metastases seeded by the primary tumor.

Mathematical modeling of biological systems of any kind faces two principal challenges. The first is the enormous complexity of biological objects and processes including their evolution and interaction with each other and the environment. As biology and medicine uncover new levels of complexity in molecular mechanisms of life and disease, mechanistic mathematical models attempting to catch up with these developments are destined to become insurmountably complex and to gradually lose their mathematical tractability and eventually also computational feasibility. As a result, in the grand scheme of things, mathematical models have only played so far an auxiliary role in biomedical sciences. The second challenge is great variability and heterogeneity of biological systems. Accounting for this requires mathematical models to have stochastic components and involve a multitude of adjustable parameters. The two challenges greatly limit the utility of detailed mechanistic models in biomedical sciences.

These challenges are especially prominent in cancer research and treatment, which pose even greater difficulties in the formulation of natural laws. Over the last century, scientific understanding of cancer has been revolutionized by many discoveries, such as

(1) the role of mutations in cancer origination and progression; (2) aberrant regulation of growth, cell cycle, proliferation and apoptosis in cancer cells; (3) their metabolic plasticity; (4) the role of angiogenesis in malignant tumor growth; (5) principal features of the metastatic cascade; (6) significance of primary and secondary tumor dormancy; (7) complex interactions between cancer cells and the immune system; (8) critical role of tumor microenvironment as well as of local and systemic interactions among different types of cancer and normal cells; (9) important role of inflammation and injury in cancer origination and progression; (10) dependence of several types and subtypes of cancer on hormones for tumor growth; and (11) identification of cancer stem cells. These and many other discoveries have considerably changed the landscape of oncology. In spite of this, they failed to bring about a commensurate revolution in cancer treatment. Why? A likely answer is that many important aspects of cancer have not been discovered yet! This is one of the reasons why answering systemic questions about cancer cannot fully rely on mathematical models based on specific biological mechanisms. This, combined with the insurmountable complexity of mathematical models accounting even for well-established mechanisms, calls for a different approach.

Here, I propose an alternative methodology for mathematical modeling of biomedical processes. It is based on two ideas. The first is rooted in the phenomenological spirit of this book and consists of building mathematical models that, on the one hand, are firmly grounded in well-established basic biomedical knowledge but, on the other hand, eschew mechanistic details and are general enough to account for many mechanisms, both known and unknown. The simplicity and generality of such models, representing two of the mathematics' most notable hallmarks and strengths, offer a greater chance to enable closed form solutions and rigorous theoretical analysis than complex and highly specific mechanistic models. Such analytic solutions enable detailed exploration of the behavior of the model and its output over the entire parameter space, a job for which more complex models with parameters estimated from the data are decidedly ill-suited. The idea of building such general models was first conceptualized and advocated in my book chapter [158].

Mathematical models depend on numerical and functional parameters, and the former can be estimated from observations. One of the most appealing ways to do so is to select parameter values that maximize the model-based probability of observations or, in the case of absolutely continuous observables, their joint probability density function (pdf). This time-tested method of parameter estimation, known as the *principle of maximum likelihood*, goes back to Gauss, Lagrange, Euler, Daniel Bernoulli and Laplace [159]. Specifically, if $x_1, x_2, \dots, x_n$ are observations and θ is an unknown vector of model parameters, then the method of maximum likelihood aims to maximize the *likelihood function*

$$\mathcal{L}(\theta) = p(\theta; x_1, x_2, \dots, x_n),$$

where $p(\theta; x_1, x_2, \ldots, x_n)$ is the joint probability of the observations if the latter are discrete or the value of their joint pdf if they are absolutely continuous, computed for a model with parameter θ. In many experimental settings, observations are sample values of independent random variables resulting from independent replications of the same observation or measurement procedure. In this case, if $p(\theta; x)$ is the probability of a discrete observation x or the value of the pdf of an absolutely continuous observable at x, then the likelihood function takes on a simpler form

$$\mathcal{L}(\theta) = \Pi_{j=1}^{n} p(\theta; x_j). \tag{6.2}$$

As a rule, the likelihood-maximizing values of parameters depend on observations. However, occasionally it may happen that some of them are universal, that is, the same for all admissible observations. Every such universal parameter value is, therefore, a property of the model rather than a function of observations. Thus, if the model is general enough and depends only on a minimal set of realistic assumptions, then one can hope that a universal parameter value thus discovered represents a general pattern pertaining to the class of biomedical systems described by the model, i. e., a natural law. Note that this likelihood-maximizing state of the system or pathway of the process does not exclude other possibilities; however, they are less likely to occur.

Identifying such universal parameter values, if they exist, is the second idea underlying the new approach to mathematical modeling of biomedical phenomena. To the best of my knowledge, article [118] represents the first implementation of this idea. The principal limitation of the new method is a possible nonexistence of model parameters with universal maximum likelihood estimates (MLEs).

Finally, a statistical remark is in order. Imagine a synthetic dataset generated by a model with a fixed set of parameters. Then one would expect the MLEs of numerical parameters based on such data to converge, as the sample size increases indefinitely, to the parameter values used to generate the data, which would prevent the existence of universal MLEs. However, this convergence property, called *consistency of the MLEs*, is only true if the model satisfies certain regularity conditions (see e. g. [160, p. 202]). Therefore, to make possible data-independent MLEs, the model must not meet the regularity conditions. Such irregularity can be suspected for the models whose distributional output (e. g., the joint pdf of observations) has discontinuities or depends in a discontinuous fashion on model parameters.

In Chapters 8 and 9, the new methodology will be applied to cancer metastasis and produce under minimal, and fairly realistic, mathematical and biomedical assumptions a definitive answer to the two questions of great importance posed in Section 5.2. In spite of a wealth of experimental and clinical data amassed over the last 120 years, these questions have stubbornly evaded conceptual resolution.

7 The laws of tumor growth

Progression of a solid cancer consists of three principal stages: (1) growth of the primary tumor; (2) seeding of metastases by the primary tumor at various distant sites; and (3) growth of metastases in some of these secondary sites. In this chapter, I describe general mathematical forms of primary or secondary tumor growth, two of the most widely used specific growth laws, and biological assumptions underpinning the general and specific models of tumor growth. There are other growth laws that are significant either because they fit a wide range of experimental and clinical data well or are derived from compelling first principles (see e. g. [161, 162]). However, as elsewhere in this book, I will only discuss those specific growth laws that are actually used in subsequent chapters for discovery or illustration of important principles.

Recall that malignant tumors in humans and animals usually originate from one initiator cancer cell or a few such cells. Just like normal cells, cancer cells divide at the end of the cell cycle producing two daughter cells. However, unlike normal cells whose proliferation is tightly controlled by internal and external signals, cancer cells have the ability to evade or inhibit these signals and proliferate in a more independent fashion. In spite of this, growing malignant tumors encounter a hard barrier to their growth; overcoming it requires angiogenesis (see a detailed discussion in Section 3.3). If, due to internal and/or external conditions, angiogenesis is thwarted, the tumor may remain dormant as a result of dynamic equilibrium between tumor cell proliferation, quiescence and death or even regress (see Section 3.6).

Following the completion of angiogenesis, the law of growth of a vascularized tumor may change significantly, compared to the growth of the same previously avascular tumor. Thus, growth of a primary or secondary tumor may consist of several phases governed by different growth laws or may even include periods of dormancy. This lends support to the hypothesis of intermittent tumor growth, which was first proposed by my colleague Michael Retsky and his coworkers [163, 164].

No rule in biology is without exceptions. In particular, if a tumor resides in a blood-vessel rich environment such as the lungs or on the surface of a blood vessel, the neoangiogenesis requirement for sustained tumor growth can be expected to be less stringent. In this case, the tumor growth law can be assumed to be the same from the moment of tumor origination onward. Tumor growth under such special circumstances is studied in Chapter 10. Another exception is chondrosarcomas (tumors of the cartilage tissue of the bones), whose growth is to a large extent angiogenesis-independent.

As was explained in Section 3.4, cancer cells within a malignant tumor are heterogeneous in many respects: (1) some of them are clonogenic, others are not; (2) some cancer cells are actively dividing, while others are quiescent due to overcrowding, hypoxia, undernourishment or being cancer stem cells; and (3) cancer cells differ in their spatial position within the tumor, which may affect their viability, proliferative behavior and motility. Additionally, cancerous tumors are infiltrated to a variable degree by

https://doi.org/10.1515/9783111334035-009

nonmalignant stromal and vascular endothelial cells as well as by various types of cells of the immune system (see Section 3.7). Thus, when a volumetric tumor measurement is taken, the observed gross tumor volume may exceed the total volume of cancer cells, even more so for the total volume of the subpopulation of clonogenic cells. This fact has important implications for mathematical modeling of tumor growth and metastasis (see Chapters 8–11).

7.1 General mathematical formulation of tumor growth laws

Growth of a cell population is described quantitatively by the formula

$$N(t) = f(t; N_0), \tag{7.1}$$

where $N(t)$ is tumor size (i. e., the number of cells comprising the tumor) at time t, N_0 is the initial size of the tumor at time t_0, and f is an increasing function of variable t. If N_0 is fixed, I will often write $N(t) = f(t)$. It will be assumed without loss of generality that $t_0 = 0$, unless stated otherwise. Strictly speaking, the population size $N(t)$ in (7.1) only takes integer values. However, for a large cell population, the unit jumps of population size occurring at the times of cell division or death are negligible. Accordingly, function f will be assumed continuous (see also a discussion in the beginning of the next section).

Descendants of any among N_0 cells present at time t_0 form a *clone* generated by a given initiator cell. If the proliferative characteristics of the initiator cells are identical and if their clones grow under similar conditions and independently of each other, then

$$N(t) = N_0 g(t), \tag{7.2}$$

where $g(t) = f(t; 1)$ is the growth law for a single clone. Formula (7.2) will be referred to as the *clonal growth model*, while formula (7.1) is said to represent the *general growth model*.

In Chapters 8–11, equations (7.1) and (7.2) and their special cases will be applied to the growth of cancer cell populations. From a practical standpoint, it is more convenient to deal with tumor volume rather than size because volume is readily measurable. Note that tumor volume is proportional to tumor size, where the coefficient of proportionality is the volume of a single cell, assumed for simplicity the same for all cells in the population of interest and constant in time. Therefore, the dynamics of tumor volume is described by equations very similar to (7.1) or (7.2). In what follows, I will be switching back and forth freely between tumor size and volume, but the choice will be clear from the context.

7.2 Exponential growth

If cells in a certain population divide after a fixed amount of time, say, 1 day, then in a clone generated by one initiator cell, there will be 2 cells after one day, 4 cells after two days and in general, 2^n cells after n days. In reality, the duration of the cell cycle varies somewhat between both initiator cells and their offspring, so that after a few generations, the cells in the population will start to cycle asynchronously. Therefore, in a large population the growth law can be assumed a continuous function of time rather than a discrete one with jumps occurring at certain specific time points.

Consider a large population of cells that are identical, or close to such, in all respects relevant to cell proliferation and death. Suppose also that cells within the population divide and die independently of each other. Biologically, cell division occurs at the end of the cell cycle, and the same is typically true for cell death. However, if cells are cycling asynchronously, which is the case in the vast majority of experimental and natural settings (with the exception of cell populations irradiated under certain experimental protocols where cells can get temporarily arrested in the same most radiosensitive phases of the cell cycle, see e. g. [165]), one can ignore cell cycling and assume as an approximation that each cell can divide or die at any given time. Note, however, that because every cell must grow from half the normal size at birth to the normal size and go through all the phases of the cell cycle before it can divide at the end of the cell cycle in the phase called *mitosis*, the duration of the cell cycle cannot be shorter than a certain minimum amount of time (e. g., in human cells this lower limit is about 20 hrs).

Let b be the rate of cell division, also termed the *birth rate*. Mathematically, this means that the probability $P(t, \Delta t)$ of the event that a cell present at time t will divide into two daughter cells between t and $t+\Delta t$, where Δt is a positive sufficiently small time increment, is given by

$$P(t, \Delta t) = b\,\Delta t + o(\Delta t). \tag{7.3}$$

Here, $o(\Delta t)$ is any function of Δt such that $o(\Delta t)/\Delta t \to 0$ as $\Delta t \to 0$. According to (7.3), the probability that a cell will divide during a short time interval $[t, t+\Delta t]$ is approximately proportional to Δt. Similarly, by definition of the *death rate*, d, the probability, $Q(t, \Delta t)$, that a cell will die during a small time interval $[t, t + \Delta t]$ satisfies the equation

$$Q(t, \Delta t) = d\,\Delta t + o(\Delta t). \tag{7.4}$$

If the processes of cell division and death are stationary (in other words, homogeneous in time), the probabilities $P(t, \Delta t)$ and $Q(t, \Delta t)$ depend on Δt alone. They will be denoted by $P(\Delta t)$ and $Q(\Delta t)$, respectively. In this case, the rates b and d are constant rather than functions of time.

Consider the behavior of a cell present at time t over a short observation period $[t, t+\Delta t]$. Since cell cycle duration is bounded below, no more than one event of cell division or death can happen to the cell of interest. Thus, there are only three possibilities for the outcome of our observation: (1) the cell remained intact; (2) the cell divided into two daughter cells; (3) the cell died.

Under the stated assumptions, observing the fate of any of $N(t)$ cells present at time t over the interval $[t, t+\Delta t]$ can be viewed as $N(t)$ independent replications of the same random experiment with the three outcomes. The event of cell division leads to a net increase of the population size by one cell, while the event of cell death decreases the population size by one cell. Therefore, the increment, $N(t+\Delta t) - N(t)$, of the size of the cell population over the interval $[t, t+\Delta t]$ can be represented in the form

$$N(t+\Delta t) - N(t) = N_+(t, t+\Delta t) - N_-(t, t+\Delta t),$$

where $N_+(t, t+\Delta t)$ and $N_-(t, t+\Delta t)$ are the respective numbers of cells in the population that divided or died between t and $t+\Delta t$. According to the empirical definition of probability, which in the setting at hand is a particular case of the Law of Large Numbers [148, Section 10.5], the empirical frequencies of cell division and death in a large cell population are close to their theoretical probabilities:

$$\frac{N_+(t, t+\Delta t)}{N(t)} \simeq P(\Delta t) \quad \text{and} \quad \frac{N_-(t, t+\Delta t)}{N(t)} \simeq Q(\Delta t).$$

Therefore,

$$N(t+\Delta t) - N(t) \simeq N(t)[P(\Delta t) - Q(\Delta t)].$$

Dividing both sides of this equation by Δt, taking the limit as $\Delta t \to 0$ and using (7.3) and (7.4) yields

$$N'(t) = (b-d)N(t). \tag{7.5}$$

Thus, the dynamics of the cell population is governed by the differential equation

$$N'(t) = \lambda N(t), \tag{7.6}$$

where $\lambda = b - d$ is the *net proliferation rate* per cell.

The solution, $N(t)$, of equation (7.6) is easy to find. In fact, setting $M(t) = e^{-\lambda t}N(t)$, we have in view of (7.6)

$$M'(t) = -\lambda e^{-\lambda t}N(t) + e^{-\lambda t}N'(t) = e^{-\lambda t}[N'(t) - \lambda N(t)] = 0.$$

Therefore, function $M(t)$ is constant: $M(t) = C$ for all $t \geq 0$. This implies that $N(t) = Ce^{-\lambda t}$, $t \geq 0$. Finally, setting here $t = 0$, we find that $C = N(0) = N_0$. Therefore,

$$N(t) = N_0 e^{\lambda t}. \tag{7.7}$$

This equation represents *exponential growth* of a cell population if $\lambda > 0$ and *exponential decay* if $\lambda < 0$.

I now make a few comments about the meaning, applicability and remarkable properties of the exponential law:

(1) In the case $\lambda < 0$, formula (7.7) can only be used when N_0 is sufficiently large and only as long as the population remains large enough. The kinetics of small populations of cells and other organisms is better described by stochastic processes rather than ordinary differential equations (ODEs).

(2) The assumptions underlying the derivation of the exponential growth law (7.7) imply that this law of population kinetics must be clonal, that is, have a general from (7.2). Expectedly, this is the case for formula (7.7), where the function $g(t) = e^{\lambda t}$ with $\lambda > 0$ represents the size at time t of a clone generated by a single initiator cell present at $t_0 = 0$.

(3) Equation (7.6) states that the rate of change of the population size is proportional to the current size of the population or, in other words, that the net per cell proliferation rate is constant: $N'/N = \lambda$. This represents one of the simplest and most basic patterns in nature and society. That is the reason why formula (7.7) provides an adequate description of the kinetics of many cell populations in vitro and in vivo, various animal and even human populations, many other processes in biology and far beyond. Importantly for this book, it was found that the exponential law provides a good approximation to the dynamics of various treated and untreated tumors both in experimental [166] and clinical [167] settings, especially at the initial stages of tumor growth, where interaction between cancer cells including competition for space and vital material resources can often be deemed negligible.

(4) An equivalent way to represent the exponential law (7.7) is to express it through the *doubling time*, that is, time $T > 0$ such that $N(t + T) = 2N(t)$. Solving the equation

$$N_0 e^{\lambda(t+T)} = 2N_0 e^{\lambda t}$$

for T yields

$$T = \frac{\log 2}{\lambda}.$$

Remarkably, T depends neither on t nor on N_0! Thus, the size of any exponentially growing population doubles over every time interval of duration T. Expressing the growth rate through the doubling time, $\lambda = (\log 2)/T$, converts the exponential law (7.7) into the following equivalent form

$$N(t) = N_0\, 2^{t/T}.$$

(5) A remarkable property of the exponential kinetics described by formula (7.7) is that it is *self-similar*, i. e., has the same mathematical form when initialized at any time $t_0 > 0$:

$$N(t) = N(t_0)e^{\lambda(t-t_0)}, \quad t \geq t_0.$$

In fact, in view of (7.7),

$$N(t) = N_0 e^{\lambda[t_0+(t-t_0)]} = N_0 e^{\lambda t_0} e^{\lambda(t-t_0)} = N(t_0)e^{\lambda(t-t_0)}.$$

The self-similarity property can also be expressed as

$$N(t) = \frac{N(t_0)}{N_0} \cdot N(t-t_0), \quad t \geq t_0. \tag{7.8}$$

Furthermore, (7.7) is the only continuous function that has the self-similarity property (7.8) for all $t_0 \geq 0$. To see this, represent (7.8) in an equivalent form

$$\frac{N(t)}{N_0} = \frac{N(t_0)}{N_0} \cdot \frac{N(t-t_0)}{N_0}, \quad t \geq t_0.$$

Then, for the function $h(t) = \log[N(t)/N_0]$, we have by setting $u = t_0$ and $v = t - t_0$

$$h(u+v) = h(u) + h(v) \quad \text{for all } u, v \geq 0. \tag{7.9}$$

This formula expresses the *additivity property* of function h and is called the *Cauchy equation*, named after the great French mathematician Augustin-Louis Cauchy (1789–1857). He showed in his treatise [168] that every continuous solution of equation (7.9) is a linear function: $h(u) = \lambda u$ for some real number λ. Equivalently, $N(t) = N_0 e^{\lambda t}$, as claimed.

What can be said about the range of values for the growth rate λ for an exponentially growing cell population, e. g., a malignant tumor? The fastest growth occurs in the absence of cell death and quiescence, i. e., when cells go through the cell cycle continuously without any delay or inhibition. If τ is the length of the cell cycle, then under the stated conditions the size of the population doubles after τ units of time so that the maximum value of λ is $(\log 2)/\tau$ (see the previous discussion of the doubling time). Note, however, that due to cell death and quiescence, population growth can be arbitrarily slow. For human cells, a typical cell cycle duration is about $\tau = 24$ hrs. In the absence of cell death and quiescence, this would translate into the birth rate $b = (\log 2)/\tau \simeq 0.693\,\text{day}^{-1}$. In reality, human tumors grow at a much slower pace. For example, a tumor with the doubling time $\tau = 20$ days is considered very fast growing. For such a tumor, we find from the equation $b - d = (\log 2)/\tau$ with the above-specified value of b that the death rate d constitutes 95 % of the birth rate b.

7.3 Gompertzian growth

As a saying popular among mathematical modelers has it, “everything that grows, slows.” In particular, due to limited space and material resources, the growth of a cell population cannot proceed indefinitely and at some point must saturate. How can one describe this mathematically?

The idea is to convert the differential equation (7.5) (or equivalently, (7.6)) into a more realistic one by incorporating into its right-hand side (RHS) an additional term accounting for the interaction between cells. The latter includes, in particular, contact inhibition, cell-to-cell signaling and competition for space, nutrients, oxygen and growth factors. Assuming that each cell interacts with a fixed number of other cells leads to an extra term that is proportional to $N = N(t)$ so that the new RHS in (7.5) becomes $bN-dN-cN = (b-d-c)N$, which brings us back to the original equation (7.6). The other extreme, where each cell is allowed to interact with all, or a fixed fraction of, other cells, gives rise to the *logistic growth* governed by an equation of the form $y' = \alpha y - \beta y^2$ with α, $\beta > 0$. A more realistic assumption is that a cell can interact with a potentially unlimited number of other cells but still much less than their total number. One especially useful and widely employed population growth equation arises when the interaction term is proportional to $N \log N$. In this case, equation (7.6) becomes

$$N'(t) = \lambda N(t) - \beta N(t) \log N(t), \tag{7.10}$$

where it is assumed that the *intrinsic net per cell growth rate* λ and the *growth inhibition coefficient* β are positive constants.

To solve equation (7.10), we divide it by $N(t)$ and set $y(t) = \log N(t)$ to obtain

$$y'(t) = \lambda - \beta y(t). \tag{7.11}$$

This linear differential equation has a general solution

$$y(t) = \frac{\lambda}{\beta} + Ce^{-\beta t} \tag{7.12}$$

with an arbitrary constant C. The latter can be found from the initial condition $y(0) = \log N_0$, which in view of (7.12) yields $C = \log N_0 - \lambda/\beta$. This implies, after some algebra, that

$$N(t) = N_0^{\exp\{-\beta t\}} \exp\left\{\frac{\lambda}{\beta}(1 - \exp\{-\beta t\})\right\}. \tag{7.13}$$

This function is referred to as the *Gompertz function*. It is named after the British actuary Benjamin Gompertz (1779–1865), who discovered it in an effort to describe human mortality as a function of age [169].

I now turn to discussing a few remarkable properties of the *Gompertz growth law* (7.13).

(1) Setting in (7.13) $N_0 = 1$ leads to the Gompertz growth law for a clone originating from a single cell:

$$g(t) = \exp\left\{\frac{\lambda}{\beta}(1 - \exp\{-\beta t\})\right\}. \tag{7.14}$$

Observe that the Gompertz law (7.13) is of the general form (7.1) and, unlike the exponential law, does not belong to the class of clonal growth laws described by equation (7.2). Interestingly, however, the size at any given time $t > 0$ of a population whose growth is governed by the Gompertz law (7.13) is identical to the size at the time t of a population of $N_0^{\exp\{-\beta t\}}$ noninteracting clones whose growth follows the clonal model (7.2) with function g specified in (7.14).

(2) Application of the Taylor formula $e^{-x} = 1 - x + o(x)$ with $x = \exp\{-\beta t\}$ to formula (7.13) leads to two conclusions: (a) on the initial interval of time where βt is sufficiently small, the Gompertz law (7.13) is very close to the exponential law (7.7); and (b) the Gompertz law (7.13) degenerates into the exponential law (7.7) as $\beta \to 0$ (the same can also be expected on the basis of equation (7.10)).

(3) It follows from (7.13) that the limiting size of the population as $t \to \infty$ is

$$K = \exp\left\{\frac{\lambda}{\beta}\right\}, \tag{7.15}$$

a finite quantity independent of N_0. Thus, the Gompertz law represents saturated growth. The upper limit, K, of the size of a growing population depends on the ratio, λ/β, of its kinetic parameters and thereby both on the intrinsic characteristics of the organisms forming the population and on the environment, which provides resources for the growing population. However, K is called, somewhat inaccurately, the *carrying capacity of the environment*. The Gompertz law (7.13) can alternatively be represented through parameters K and β as

$$N(t) = K\left(\frac{N_0}{K}\right)^{\exp\{-\beta t\}}. \tag{7.16}$$

In all practically interesting cases of tumor growth, the carrying capacity is very large, which means that the intrinsic net growth rate λ is considerably larger than the growth inhibition coefficient β.

(4) It follows from equation (7.11) that for $N_0 < K$ one has $N' > 0$, i. e., as expected, the size of the cell population increases (the same can be also inferred directly from (7.16)). Notice, however, that the same equation (7.11) implies that the *per cell growth rate* N'/N decreases from $\lambda - \beta \log N_0 = \beta \log(K/N_0)$ at $t = 0$ to 0 as $t \to \infty$.

(5) Differentiation of equation (7.10) yields

$$N'' = N'(\lambda - \beta - \beta \log N),$$

which shows that $N'' = 0$ if and only if $\log N = \lambda/\beta - 1$ or equivalently $N = K/e$. Thus, the inflection point, where the rate, N', of population growth switches from an increasing pattern to a decreasing one and therefore attainsing its maximum value, occurs when the population size reaches about 37 % of the carrying capacity. It follows from (7.10) and (7.15), with a little bit of algebra, that this maximum value is $K\beta/e$. The Gompertz growth curve is convex as long as $N < K/e$ ($N'' > 0$) and concave when $N > K/e$ ($N'' < 0$) with the transition occurring at the inflexion point.

Finally, recall that equation (7.10) is based on very general considerations of population growth and its inhibition through interaction of the members of the population between themselves, including competition for space and vital chemicals, and with their environment. This explains why the pattern of Gompertz growth is descriptive of the dynamics of many cell and animal populations as well as many other processes both within and beyond the realm of biomedicine. The adequacy of the Gompertz law as a descriptor of tumor growth has been confirmed empirically for many experimental [170, 171] and clinical [172] tumors.

8 A general mathematical model of metastatic cancer

In this chapter, I present, in the spirit of phenomenological approach adopted in this book, a very general mathematical model focused on well-established clinically significant processes associated with metastasis, while avoiding explicit description of their specific mechanisms. For a review of the biology of metastasis, see Section 3.5.

The first model of this kind was proposed in [173] and further developed in [174, 136, 118]. Various parametric versions of the model were applied to individual-patient data on the volumes of metastases detected in a given secondary site for the purpose of inference on the natural history of cancer and the effects of treatment (see [135–137, 139, 175]). The model explicated in this chapter is obtained from the very general model described in [118] by dispensing with any specific functional form of the dependence on the law of primary tumor growth of the rate of metastasis shedding off the primary tumor.

The model embodies a hybrid approach in that it combines deterministic laws of growth of metastases in a given site before and after primary-tumor resection with a stochastic description of metastasis-related processes that clearly depend on chance [176], such as seeding of metastases, their survival and dormancy in the site of interest. Two features of the model make it very general: (1) The rate of metastasis shedding is an arbitrary function of time; and (2) the duration of metastatic latency has an essentially arbitrary absolutely continuous probability distribution. Thus, the model largely avoids the step of initial parameterization that would make it rigid at the outset.

Once the angiogenic switch is activated and angiogenic factors, secreted by a tumor and its microenvironment and produced by various cells circulating in the blood, induce endothelial cell proliferation resulting in sprouting of proximal capillaries and their migration toward the tumor, neoangiogenesis is completed within a few days [177, 42]. This period is very short relative to the duration of other processes associated with tumor progression and metastasis. Therefore, to streamline mathematical modeling, tumor vascularization will be viewed as effectively instantaneous and the time of its occurrence will be termed *tumor inception*. The notion of inception applies in equal measure to both primary and secondary tumors. Vis-a-vis primary tumors, the significance of inception is two-fold: Firstly, it is the earliest time a tumor may start shedding hematogenous metastases and, secondly, following tumor inception, a vascularized primary tumor typically grows faster, and therefore according to a different law, compared to the avascular phase (recall also that prior to inception, a tumor can remain dormant over some period of time).

8.1 Model formulation

The model described below will be instrumental in Chapter 9, where it will lead to the discovery of a natural law concerning the relationship between the presence and re-

https://doi.org/10.1515/9783111334035-010

section of a primary tumor or its ablation by radiation on the one hand and the rate of growth of metastases on the other hand. This natural law serves as a guiding principle illuminating the large body of experimental and clinical knowledge described in Sections 4.3 and 5.2–5.4. The model will be applied in Chapter 9 to a generic individual patient with metastatic cancer whose primary tumor had been removed by local treatment and whose metastases were detected and measured at a later time.

Surgery and radiation therapy for a primary tumor are rarely given to cancer patients with overt metastatic disease, unless the primary tumor itself is life-threatening due to its large size, anatomic location or debilitating effects on the patients' health. A mathematical model addressing full or partial primary tumor resection in the confirmed presence of metastases will be described in Chapter 10 and applied to four cases of renal cancer with lung metastases, which will lead to interesting conclusions about some unobservable aspects of the natural history of the patients' disease.

In the model outline that follows, each component and relevant assumptions are described separately. The model utilizes Poisson processes and some of their properties. Definitions and relevant results on Poisson processes are provided, along with detailed proofs, in the appendix.

Primary tumor inception and observables

Let T be the unobservable individual patient's age at primary tumor inception. Denote by V the known patient's age at primary tumor resection or completion of its treatment by radiation and by W a later age at which metastases were detected and measured in a given distant secondary site. Thus, $0 < T < V < W$ (see Figure 8.1). Let m be the smallest measurable tumor size in the site in question. In general, m is site- and patient-specific and depends on the imaging technology used to survey metastases. Denote by $x_1, x_2, \dots, x_n$, where $m \le x_1 < x_2 < \dots < x_n$, the observed sizes of the detected metastases. Such data can be obtained through laborious reading of CT/PET images, as exemplified in [173, 135–137, 139, 175].

Generation of metastases

It is assumed that metastasis shedding off the primary tumor is governed by a Poisson process with rate $r(t)$, where time t is counted from the age T of primary tumor inception. This means (see Section A.2 in the appendix and [178, pp. 270–273]) that (1) the numbers of metastases shed over nonoverlapping time intervals are stochastically independent and (2) the number of metastases shed over any interval $[s, t]$ is a Poisson distributed random variable with the expected value $\int_s^t r(u)du$.

I assume that function r is continuous and positive on the interval $[0, V - T]$. In particular, function r may have a peak at around the time $V - T$ to account for a possible release of cancer cells from the primary tumor into its environment and the bloodstream during surgery. It is also assumed that $r(t) = 0$ for $t > V - T$. This reflects the simple fact

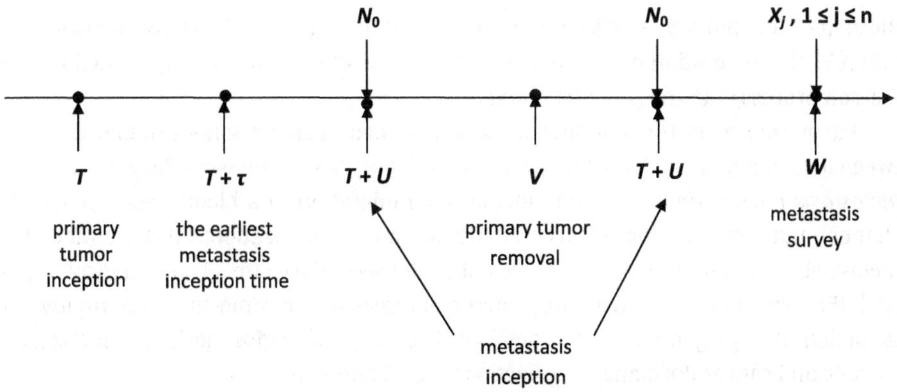

Figure 8.1: Timeline of the natural history of metastatic cancer and its treatment in an individual patient. All times are represented as ages counted from the birth of the patient. $T + U$ is the age at inception of a particular metastasis. Note that the inception may occur either before or after primary tumor ablation by surgery or radiation. Numbers with arrows above the timeline represent the sizes of metastases at the indicated time points. For more details, see Section 8.1.
The figure was reproduced with permission from Hanin L, Rose J. Suppression of metastasis by primary tumor and acceleration of metastasis following primary tumor resection: A natural law? Bull Math Biol 2018, 80(3), 519–539.

that primary tumor ablation removes the source of new metastases. Implicit in the latter assumption is the understanding that the removed primary tumor is nonrecurrent.

Secondary metastasizing

It is assumed that formation of "metastasis of metastasis" to a given site, both from other sites and from within, is negligible. Although conclusive experimental evidence for or against secondary metastasizing has not been found so far [179], arguments based on analyzing both experimental and clinical data suggest that metastases rarely metastasize (see also an earlier study [81]). As one specific example, the authors of [180] investigated the metastatic potential of spontaneously occurring lung metastases from breast cancer in mice by reimplanting them into the mammary gland of *syngeneic* (genetically identical) hosts. While all these metastatic cells produced primary breast tumors, only about 30 % of the latter metastasized. On the clinical side, an overall conclusion from a detailed analysis of the natural history of the disease in thousands of breast cancer patients is that secondary metastasis is uncommon [181]. Finally, from both mathematical modeling and practical standpoints, neglecting secondary metastasis seems a necessary choice because in clinical settings the generational number of a metastasis is unobservable, thus making primary and secondary metastases indistinguishable.

Inception of metastases

It is assumed that metastases shed off by the primary tumor survive and give rise to clinically detectable secondary tumors in a given site independently of each other with the same probability $q > 0$; such metastases will be called *viable*. Therefore (see Section A.3), the generation of viable metastases in the site of interest is governed by the Poisson process with the rate $\mu(t) = qr(t)$.

Furthermore, each viable metastasis is assumed to spend some random time between detachment from the primary tumor and inception in the secondary site, termed *metastasis latency time*. This time includes: (1) migration to a blood vessel or lymph channel and intravasation; (2) free circulation and extravasation; (3) dormancy of a metastasis as a solitary cancer cell lodged in the secondary site; (4) initial growth period; (5) dormancy as an avascular micrometastasis in the same site; and, finally, (6) induction of angiogenesis. (For a detailed discussion of angiogenesis, the metastatic cascade and cancer dormancy, see Sections 3.3, 3.5 and 3.6.)

Latency times of viable metastases bound for a given site are thought of as independent and identically distributed (iid) random variables with some continuous probability density function (pdf) f and the corresponding cumulative distribution function (cdf) F. As shown in Section A.5, the resulting delayed Poisson process is again a Poisson process with the rate

$$\lambda(t) = \int_0^t \mu(s)f(t-s)ds = q \int_0^{\min\{t,\, V-T\}} r(s)f(t-s)ds. \tag{8.1}$$

It is also assumed for simplicity that the growth of all vascular metastases in the site in question starts from the *same*, yet not necessarily known, initial size, N_0, at inception. This implies that the duration of metastatic latency is bounded below by a certain minimal time $\tau > 0$ during which a metastasis can reach the size N_0 if it grows from a single cell at a maximum possible rate immediately after seeding in the secondary site. Then $f(t) = 0$ for $0 \le t \le \tau$ and $f(t) > 0$ for $t > \tau$.

Although the exact value of τ is of no particular importance, τ is thought to be sufficiently small, so that $T+\tau < V$ (see Figure 8.1). To justify this assumption, observe that in the absence of cell death and quiescence, the maximum tumor growth rate corresponds to the doubling time of about 1 day, a typical cell-cycle duration for human cells. To estimate N_0, let's use the largest Folkman diameter $d = 2$ mm, whose volumetric equivalent for a spherical tumor is $\pi d^3/6 \simeq 4.19\,\text{mm}^3$. A standard size-to-volume conversion for tumor cells proceeds from 10^6 cells per mm^3, which leads to the estimate $N_0 = 4.19 \times 10^6$ cells at metastasis inception. Then formula (7.7) yields $\tau \simeq 22$ days, which is indeed very small compared to the time, $V-T$, between the primary tumor inception and its ablation by surgery or radiation, which typically spans many months or even years.

Finally, a standard tumor volume measurability threshold m corresponds to metastatic diameter of about 4–5 mm, while the diameter of a metastasis at inception is close to the Folkman's avascular limit of about 1–2 mm. Therefore, it is assumed that $m > N_0$.

Growth of metastases

Denote by U the random inception time of a particular metastasis relative to the age T of the primary tumor inception, so that $T + U$ is the patient's age at metastasis inception (see Figure 8.1). Let $\Psi_U(t)$ be the size of the metastasis at time t counted from the inception age $T + U$. Note that $\Psi_U(t)$ accounts for the *total* number of cells comprising the metastasis, including but not necessarily limited to clonogenic cells or even cancer cells for that matter. The reason is that volumetric measurements for the detected metastases represent their *total volumes* at the patient's age W. Recall also that $\Psi_U(0) = N_0$.

As highlighted in Sections 5.2–5.4, extirpation of a primary tumor by surgery or radiation can have a dramatic effect on the rate of growth of metastases. To assess this effect quantitatively, one component of the model—the laws of growth of metastases before and after primary tumor removal—needs to be parameterized. Quite often nowadays, clinical metastases are detected early when they are likely to be still in the exponential phase of their growth or close to such. For this reason, it is assumed that after inception, all viable vascular metastases in the given site grow exponentially with the same two net growth rates, γ_0 and γ_1, not necessarily distinct, before and after primary tumor ablation, respectively. As a reminder from Section 7.2, the exponential growth function $N(t) = N_0 \exp\{\gamma t\}$ has the following self-similarity property: for every $t_0 \geq 0$, one has $N(t) = N(t_0)\exp\{\gamma(t-t_0)\}$ for all $t \geq t_0$ (and moreover, this is the only continuous growth law with this property). This enables a natural combination of two exponential growth laws. Specifically, consideration of the cases, where metastasis inception occurs before or after extirpation of the primary tumor and whether the current patient's age, $t+T+U$, where t is the time elapsed since metastasis inception, is smaller or greater than V leads to the following formula for $\Psi_U(t)$:

$$\Psi_U(t) = \begin{cases} N_0 \exp\{\gamma_0 t\} \\ \quad \text{if } T + U < V \text{ and } 0 \leq t \leq V - T - U \\ N_0 \exp\{\gamma_0(V - T - U)\} \exp\{\gamma_1[t - (V - T - U)]\} \\ \quad \text{if } T + U < V < t + T + U \\ N_0 \exp\{\gamma_1 t\} \\ \quad \text{if } T + U \geq V \text{ and } t \geq 0. \end{cases} \tag{8.2}$$

In a simpler setting where $\gamma_1 = \gamma_0$ studied in [173], $\Psi_U(t)$ is a function of t alone, independent of the inception time U. However, if the rate of metastatic growth is affected by eradication of the primary tumor ($\gamma_1 \neq \gamma_0$), this is not true anymore.

Effects of treatment

Primary tumor ablation is assumed to affect metastases only through the rates of their growth (and not through changes in the distribution of their latency times). This assumption is plausible because dormant tumors are known to be refractory to all kinds of biochemical and immunological signals, including those resulting from surgery as well as other cancer treatments such as radiation and cytotoxic chemotherapy, which are primarily effective against actively proliferating cancer cells [179, 182].

8.2 Distribution of the sizes of metastases

Let random variable X represent the size of a particular metastasis with inception time U detected in a given site and measured at age W. Then the total progression time from inception to detection for this metastasis is $W - T - U$. According to (8.2),

$$X = \Psi_U(W - T - U) = \begin{cases} N_0 \exp\{\gamma_0(V - T - U)\} \exp\{\gamma_1(W - V)\} & \text{if } T + U < V \\ N_0 \exp\{\gamma_1(W - T - U)\} & \text{if } T + U \geq V. \end{cases}$$

Importantly, this formula implies that the function Ψ_U, which relates the size X of a metastasis at patient's age W to its progression time, is actually independent of random variable U:

$$X = \Psi(W - T - U), \tag{8.3}$$

where

$$\Psi(y) = \begin{cases} N_0 \exp\{\gamma_1 y\} & \text{if } 0 \leq y \leq W - V \\ N_0 \exp\{\gamma_0[y - (W - V)]\} \exp\{\gamma_1(W - V)\} & \text{if } W - V < y \leq W - T - \tau \end{cases} \tag{8.4}$$

(recall that the shortest metastasis inception time allowed by the model is τ (see Section 8.1), so that the longest possible progression time y is $W - T - \tau$, as indicated in (8.4)).

Notice that function Ψ is increasing, continuous, piecewise differentiable and satisfies the condition $\Psi(0) = N_0$. The inverse function, $\delta = \Psi^{-1}$, is given by

$$\delta(x) = \begin{cases} \gamma_1^{-1} \log \frac{x}{N_0} & \text{if } N_0 \leq x \leq A \\ \gamma_0^{-1} \log \frac{x}{N_0} + (W - V)(1 - \gamma_1/\gamma_0) & \text{if } A < x \leq M, \end{cases} \tag{8.5}$$

where $A = N_0 \exp\{\gamma_1(W - V)\}$ is the size at age W of a hypothetical metastasis whose inception occurred at age V, and

$$M = N_0 \exp\{\gamma_0(V - T - \tau)\} \exp\{\gamma_1(W - V)\} \tag{8.6}$$

is the size at age W of a notional metastasis whose inception with size N_0 occurred over the shortest latency period possible, i. e., at age $T + \tau$ (see Figure 8.1). Observe that M represents the theoretical upper limit for the size of a metastasis at age W allowed by the model. Clearly, $N_0 < A < M$.

Formula (8.3) enables computation of the unobservable patient's age at inception of a particular metastasis from its observed or hypothetical size, x, at age W. In fact, setting $X = x$ in formula (8.3), we obtain

$$T + U = W - \delta(x).$$

According to (8.3), the sizes of metastases at age W are a fixed nonrandom transformation Ψ of their inception times U, which, under our model, follow a Poisson process with the rate given by (8.1). Therefore, the joint distribution of site-specific sizes of metastases at age W can be expressed through the joint distribution of metastasis inception times.

The following well-known theorem furnishes a remarkable formula for the conditional joint distribution of the event occurrence times in an arbitrary Poisson process conditional on their number. For a proof of this theorem, see Section A.4.

Theorem 8.1. *Let $t > 0$ and λ be a nonnegative continuous function on $[0, \infty)$ such that $\int_0^t \lambda(s)ds > 0$. Suppose random variables $T_1, T_2, \ldots, T_n$, where $0 \le T_1 < T_2 < \cdots < T_n \le t$, be the times of successive events in a Poisson process $X(s)$ with rate λ that have occurred by time t. Then the joint distribution of $T_1, T_2, \ldots, T_n$ conditional on their number n is absolutely continuous, and its joint pdf is given by the formula*

$$p_{T_1,T_2,\ldots,T_n|X(t)=n}(t_1, t_2, \ldots, t_n) = \frac{n!}{[\int_0^t \lambda(s)ds]^n} \Pi_{j=1}^n \lambda(t_j) \quad \text{for } 0 \le t_1 < t_2 < \cdots < t_n \le t \tag{8.7}$$

and 0 otherwise.

Remark 8.1. In various settings utilizing Poisson processes, event occurrence times $U_1, U_2, \ldots, U_n$ don't necessarily have an a priori natural ordering as in Theorem 8.1. In this case, $(T_1, T_2, \ldots, T_n)$ represents the vector of *order statistics* for the random vector $(U_1, U_2, \ldots, U_n)$. Then, according to a well-known result about the joint distribution of order statistics, see, e. g., [148, Section 10.3], Theorem 8.1 can be also stated as follows:

Under the assumptions of Theorem 8.1, random vector $(T_1, T_2, \ldots, T_n)$ is equidistributed, conditional on n, with the vector of order statistics for a random sample of size n drawn from the distribution with pdf

$$\frac{\lambda(u)}{\int_0^t \lambda(s)ds}, \quad 0 \le u \le t,$$

and 0, otherwise.

Everything is now put in place to formulate and prove the main result of this chapter.

Theorem 8.2. *Let $X_1, X_2, \ldots, X_n$, where $m \le X_1 < X_2 < \cdots < X_n$, be site-specific sizes of metastases detected at age W. Then, under the model described in Section 8.1, random* *vector* $(X_1, X_2, \ldots, X_n)$ *is equidistributed, conditional on n, with the vector of order statistics for a random sample of size n drawn from an absolutely continuous distribution with pdf*

$$p(x) = \delta'(x)\frac{\int_0^{\min\{W-T-\delta(x),\,V-T\}} r(s)f[W-T-\delta(x)-s]ds}{\int_0^{\min\{W-T-\delta(m),\,V-T\}} r(s)F[W-T-\delta(m)-s]ds}, \quad m \le x \le M, \tag{8.8}$$

and $p(x) = 0$ *for* $x \notin [m, M]$, *where* $\delta(x)$ *is given by* (8.5).

Proof. In this proof, all probabilities are taken conditional on n, which is therefore assumed fixed. Observe that, in view of (8.3) inception times $t_1, t_2, \ldots, t_n$ of detected metastases with respective observed sizes, $m \le x_1 < x_2 < \cdots < x_n$ are decreasing and satisfy the inequalities $0 \le t_n < t_{n-1} < \cdots < t_1 \le W - T - \delta(m)$. In accordance with the model, inception of viable metastases is governed by the Poisson process with rate λ given by formula (8.1). Applying Remark 8.1 to Theorem 8.1 with $t = W - T - \delta(m)$, we find that random vector $(T_n, T_{n-1}, \ldots, T_1)$ of inception times for metastases with respective sizes $X_1, X_2, \ldots, X_n$ is equidistributed with the vector of order statistics for a random sample of size n drawn from the distribution with pdf

$$\frac{\lambda(u)}{\int_0^t \lambda(v)dv} = \frac{\lambda(u)}{\int_0^t [\int_0^{\min\{v,V-T\}} r(s)f(v-s)ds]dv}, \quad 0 \le u \le t.$$

Changing the order of integration in the repeated integral in the denominator of this formula, considering two cases, $0 \le t \le V - T$ and $t > V - T$, and combining them in a single formula yields

$$\begin{aligned}\int_0^t \left[\int_0^{\min\{v,V-T\}} r(s)f(v-s)ds\right]dv &= \int_0^{\min\{t,V-T\}} r(s)\left[\int_s^t f(v-s)dv\right]ds \\ &= \int_0^{\min\{t,V-T\}} r(s)F(t-s)ds.\end{aligned} \tag{8.9}$$

Thus, the pdf underlying the distribution of inception times of detected metastases has the form

$$\frac{\lambda(u)}{\int_0^{\min\{W-T-\delta(m),\,V-T\}} r(s)F(t-s)ds}, \quad 0 \le u \le W - T - \delta(m). \tag{8.10}$$

Observe that formula (8.3) can equivalently be represented as $U = W - T - \delta(X)$. Then, by the standard pdf transformation formula [148, p. 153], the relationship between pdfs of random variables X and U is

$$p_X(x) = \delta'(x)p_U[W - T - \delta(x)].$$

In combination with (8.1) and (8.10), this leads directly to formula (8.8). □

Formula (8.8) can be represented in a more specific form. In view of (8.5), $W - T - \delta(x) \leq V - T$ if and only if

$$x \geq \Psi(W - V) = N_0 \exp\{\gamma_1(W - V)\} = A.$$

Therefore, in the case $A \leq m$ formula (8.8) becomes

$$p(x) = (\gamma_0 x)^{-1} \frac{\int_0^{W-T-\delta(x)} r(s) f[W - T - \delta(x) - s] ds}{\int_0^{W-T-\delta(m)} r(s) F[W - T - \delta(m) - s] ds}, \quad m \leq x \leq M, \tag{8.11}$$

while if $A > m$ then

$$p(x) = \begin{cases} (\gamma_1 x)^{-1} \frac{\int_0^{V-T} r(s) f[W-T-\delta(x)-s] ds}{\int_0^{V-T} r(s) F[W-T-\delta(m)-s] ds}, & m \leq x < A, \\ (\gamma_0 x)^{-1} \frac{\int_0^{W-T-\delta(x)} r(s) f[W-T-\delta(x)-s] ds}{\int_0^{V-T} r(s) F[W-T-\delta(m)-s] ds}, & A \leq x \leq M. \end{cases} \tag{8.12}$$

Formulas (8.11) and (8.12) represent the desired more specific version of the general formula (8.8). Notice that the first and second formulas in (8.12) account for metastases whose inception occurred after and before primary tumor removal, respectively.

8.3 Useful consequences of Theorem 8.2

In this section, I discuss Theorem 8.2 from various angles and draw a few corollaries.

Inventory of model parameters

Pdf (8.8) depends on functional parameters r and f, adjustable numerical parameters γ_0 and γ_1 and biological quantities T, N_0, τ, m. The latter quantities are assumed fixed; however, the first three of them are unknown and unobservable. Notice, however, that pdf (8.8) is free of the metastasis survival probability q and the number of detected metastases (sample size) n.

Continuity properties of the pdf

From (8.5), we find that $\delta(M) = W - T - \tau$. This implies, in view of our assumption about the support of pdf f (see Section 8.1), that $p(M-) = 0$. Thus, pdf p is continuous at point M. By contrast, pdf p has a jump discontinuity at point m as well as at point $A > m$, unless $\gamma_0 = \gamma_1$. This is the reason why model (8.8) generally does not meet the regularity conditions for the consistency of maximum likelihood estimators (MLEs). This observation is critical for the application in Chapter 9 of the new methodology developed in Section 6.6 to the model introduced in Section 8.1.

The expected number of viable metastases

To compute the expected value of the number, Y, of detectable metastases in the site of interest at age W, note that because the model-based sizes of such metastases range between m and M, their progression times $W - T - U$ fall somewhere between $\delta(m)$ and $\delta(M) = W - T - \tau$. Therefore, their inception times U satisfy the inequalities $\tau \le U \le W - T - \delta(m)$. According to the model, the inception times follow a Poisson process with the rate λ given by formula (8.1). Then, a computation similar to (8.9) produces the following result:

$$\mathbb{E}Y = \int_{\tau}^{W-T-\delta(m)} \lambda(t)dt = q \int_{\tau}^{W-T-\delta(m)} \left[\int_{0}^{\min\{t,V-T\}} r(s)f(t-s)ds \right] dt$$

$$= q \int_{0}^{\min\{W-T-\delta(m),V-T\}} r(s)F[W-T-\delta(m)-s]ds.$$

Likewise, by replacing in this argument m with N_0, one finds the expected value for the number, Z, of *all* post-inception metastases, both occult and detectable, to be

$$\mathbb{E}Z = q \int_{0}^{V-T} r(s)F(W-T-s)ds.$$

Both expected values involve the factor q that is absent from the distribution (8.8). Thus, they cannot be estimated from the volumes of detected metastases.

The probability of metastasis inception before primary tumor removal

To do this computation correctly, one has to specify the relevant concept of "probability" (playing fast and loose with this term is a source of much confusion and error in many a biomedical study dealing with biological events and processes involving chance). The probability in this case is conditional on n and governed by the pdf specified in (8.8). It is instructive to think about this probability in terms of the following random experiment: n sizes of metastases are sampled randomly and independently from the interval $[m, M]$ in accordance with the distribution (8.8). For each generated size x, formula (8.3) uniquely determines the inception time U of a metastasis that has reached the size x at the patient's age W. We are interested in the frequency, over a large number of replications of the sampling experiment, of the event that $T + U < V$, that is, in computing the quantity $\eta := \Pr(T + U < V)$, where V, as above, is the patient's age at primary tumor ablation by surgical excision or radiation. Recall that A is the size of a hypothetical metastasis whose inception occurred at the age V. Therefore $T + U < V$ if and only if $x > A$. If $A < m$ then clearly $\eta = 1$. In the case $A \ge m$ a straightforward integration of the pdf p given by the first formula in (8.12) over the interval $[m, A]$ with the help of (8.5) and a change of variable $s = \delta(x)$ yields

$$\begin{aligned}
\eta &= \int_A^M p(x)dx = 1 - \int_m^A p(x)dx \\
&= 1 - \frac{\int_0^{V-T} r(s)[F(W-T-\delta(m)-s) - F(V-T-s)]ds}{\int_0^{V-T} r(s)F[W-T-\delta(m)-s]ds} \\
&= \frac{\int_0^{V-T} r(s)F(V-T-s)ds}{\int_0^{V-T} r(s)F[W-T-\delta(m)-s]ds}. \qquad (8.13)
\end{aligned}$$

In view of formula (8.5), $\delta(m)$ is independent of γ_0, the rate of growth of metastases prior to primary tumor ablation. Then (8.13) implies that the same is true for the probability η. This observation will be instrumental in Section 9.2.

8.4 Implications for parameter estimation

The rate r of the Poisson process of metastasis shedding off the primary tumor generally depends on the current primary tumor size and is therefore a function of time (such Poisson processes are called *nonstationary*). As a result, detection of metastases in the site of interest cannot be viewed as a sequence of independent replications of the same random experiment. The upshot is that site-specific sizes of metastases at age W do not form a random sample from any probability distribution (see also Example 12.1 in Section 12.6). However, it follows from Theorem 8.2 that, remarkably, the distribution of any symmetric (i. e., rearrangement-invariant) statistic based on observations $x_1, x_2, \ldots, x_n$ is identical to the distribution of the same statistic based on a random sample of size n drawn from the pdf p given by formula (8.8). One such symmetric statistic is the joint likelihood of observations

$$\mathcal{L}(x_1, x_2, \ldots, x_n) = \Pi_{j=1}^n p(x_j), \qquad (8.14)$$

(compare this with formula (6.1)). Thus, pdf p serves, for the purpose of maximum likelihood computation and estimation, as a surrogate of the nonexistent distribution of the "size of a detectable metastasis at age W." It is also worth mentioning that in the case where $A > m$, if one of the observations x_j coincides with A then, in order to maximize the likelihood, the larger of the two one-sided limits of pdf p at $x = A$ should be employed. Maximum likelihood estimation will produce noteworthy results in Chapters 9 and 10.

Part III: **Mathematical solutions**

9 Effects of primary tumor and its ablation on the growth of metastases: a natural law

As promised earlier in Chapters 1, 4, 5 and 8, in this chapter I uncover a surprisingly clear-cut principle, or a natural law, that underlies the seemingly intractable relationship between primary tumor and its eradication on the one hand and the growth of its secondary tumors on the other hand.

9.1 A discovery against all odds: a scientific journey with a personal touch

Around 2011, Jason Rose, my doctoral student at Idaho State University, was reviewing a mathematical model of metastatic cancer progression, which I had previously developed in [174], and applying it to clinical data analyzed in my joint work with Dr. Olga Korosteleva [135]. The model represents a fully parameterized special case of the general model described in Section 8.1. The additional simplifying and/or specializing assumptions of the model are as follows: (1) A primary tumor grows exponentially at a constant rate β from a single malignant initiator cell that emerged at an unknown and unobservable patient's age T up until excision of the primary tumor at age V; (2) the Poisson rate, $r(t)$, of metastases shedding off the primary tumor is proportional to some power of the current primary tumor size $N(t)$,

$$r(t) = \alpha N^{\theta}(t), \quad 0 \le t \le V - T, \tag{9.1}$$

with some constants $\alpha > 0$ and $\theta \ge 0$; (3) latency times of metastases bound for a given secondary site are iid random variables exponentially distributed with an expected value $\rho > 0$, i. e., with the pdf $f(t) = \rho^{-1}e^{-t/\rho}$, $t \ge 0$; and (4) following the latency period, metastases lodged in a given site grow exponentially from a single initiator cell at a rate γ_0 before primary tumor resection and γ_1 thereafter. The idea to describe metastatic dissemination using Poisson processes whose rate depends on the primary tumor size was first proposed in [183].

Assumption (9.1) deserves a closer look. Clearly, the rate $r(t)$ is proportional to the unobservable current size, $M(t)$, of the population of metastases-generating cells within the primary tumor. As explained in Section 3.5, such cells share a very special set of properties (in particular, they have to be clonogenic) and therefore are expected to form a relatively small subpopulation of the primary tumor. Assumption (9.1), then, posits that $M(t)$ is proportional to $N^{\theta}(t)$. In the case $\theta > 1$, the fraction, $M(t)/N(t) = \alpha N^{\theta-1}(t)$, of metastases-producing cells increases with primary tumor size, which points to an especially aggressive metastasizing.

Parameter θ characterizes the size (and, indirectly, spatial position within the primary tumor) of the subpopulation of metastases-producing cancer cells. Two values of

https://doi.org/10.1515/9783111334035-012

θ seem to possess some a priori plausibility. If a fixed, typically small, fraction of cells within a growing tumor have metastatic potential, then one would expect that $\theta = 1$. Another pertinent consideration is that blood-borne metastases are formed when tumor cells migrate to, and intravasate into, the capillaries that perfuse the surface of the tumor. Therefore, for spherical tumors, θ can be expected to be close to 2/3. This number may further be modified by the *fractal dimension* of the capillary network that characterizes how densely the capillaries permeate the tumor surface. As will transpire in the next section and Chapter 10, the value of θ estimated from real-world clinical data may diverge considerably from these theoretical guesses.

The just-described parametric model was applied in [135] to a case of metastatic breast cancer that can be summarized as follows:

> At age 74 a patient was diagnosed at the Memorial Sloan Kettering Cancer Center (MSKCC) in New York City with stage III estrogen receptor positive primary breast cancer, and the volume of the primary tumor was found to be $S = 10.3\,\text{cm}^3$. The patient was treated and followed up at MSKCC. Shortly after the diagnosis, she underwent radical surgery and was put on an adjuvant hormonal therapy with tamoxifen. At age 82, $n = 31$ bone metastases were discovered and their volumes measured through laborious reading of CT/PET images. These volumes, expressed in cm^3 and rounded to two decimal places, were
> 1.69, 1.98, 2.01, 2.04, 2.14, 2.20, 2.46, 3.05, 3.18, 3.31, 3.37, 3.48, 3.52, 3.57, 4.22, 4.34, 4.73, 5.04, 5.08, 5.25, 5.45, 5.64, 6.36, 6.55, 7.39, 9.01, 9.21, 11.15, 12.71, 13.81, 22.96.
> Additionally, six metastases were discovered in other sites.

The same clinical case was analyzed in an earlier study [173] published in 2006, which I coauthored with Jason and Dr. Marco Zaider, my friend and collaborator who worked at the time at MSKCC and performed the cited volumetric measurements. In that study, *the same* rate of growth of metastases was assumed before and after primary tumor excision ($\gamma_1 = \gamma_0$). Around 2008, I became aware of the publications [126, 113] propounding two closely related hypotheses that the growth of metastases is (1) suppressed by a primary tumor and (2) accelerated by primary tumor resection (for a thorough discussion of these striking phenomena, see Sections 4.3, 5.2, 5.3 and references cited therein). To test these hypotheses, I decided to reanalyze the same data but this time around assuming two metastases growth rates, γ_0 and γ_1, the first before and the second after primary tumor resection.

Using the approach developed in [173], I expressed in closed form the pdf underlying site-specific volumes of metastases for the more general model with the two metastases growth rates [174]. The model depends on five biological parameters, $(\beta, \theta, \rho, \gamma_0, \gamma_1)$, whose identifiability was ascertained in [174] (for a detailed discussion of identifiability and its critical role for parameter estimation, see Section 6.5). The maximum likelihood estimates (MLEs) of these parameters computed from the volumes of $n = 31$ bone metastases in [135] were biologically plausible without any adjustment or calibration, and the model with optimal parameters provided an exceptionally good fit to the empirical distribution of the volumes of bone metastases (see Figure 3 in article [135]). Furthermore, log-likelihood profiles, where all parameters except the one of interest were fixed at their optimal values, while the remaining parameter ranged over its entire domain, displayed a clear-cut global maximum, signaling that the global maximum of the likelihood as a function of all five parameters was attained. This conclusion was validated in multiple ways including examination of intermediate log-likelihood profiles, running different optimization algorithms, and employing a variety of initial approximations to model parameters.

The following MLEs of model parameters were obtained in [135]:

$$\beta = 0.717\,\text{year}^{-1}, \quad \theta = 0.025, \quad \rho = 79.52\,\text{years}, \quad \gamma_0 = 0.083\,\text{year}^{-1}, \quad \gamma_1 = 2.676\,\text{year}^{-1}.$$

This leads to a number of clinically significant conclusions about unobservable aspects of the natural history of cancer for the patient in question:

(1) Pre-surgery growth of metastases was extremely slow with doubling times of 8.4 years. In fact, such growth is so slow that the metastases could be called dormant for all practical purposes. Therefore, the model supports the notion of metastatic dormancy (see Section 3.6) and confirms the Ehrlich effect, discussed in Section 4.3. After surgery, this indolent growth gave way to a much faster one, yet in absolute terms still moderate, with a doubling time of 94.5 days. Note that $\gamma_1/\gamma_0 \simeq 32.2$. In summary, the model suggests that the primary tumor suppressed the growth of bone metastases, while its resection dramatically accelerated this process, even in spite of metastatic growth-inhibiting effects of tamoxifen administered to the patient after surgery.

(2) The primary tumor was growing very slowly with a doubling time of 353 days. Availability of the volume, S, of the primary tumor at or about the time of surgery enables estimation of the patient's age, T_1, at primary tumor inception with an initial volume N_0. In fact, the equation $N_0 \exp\{\beta(V - T_1)\} = S$ implies that

$$V - T_1 = \frac{1}{\beta} \log \frac{S}{N_0}.$$

Let N_0 be the volume of a spherical tumor with the Folkman's diameter of 2 mm, i. e., $N_0 = 4.19 \times 10^{-3}\,\text{cm}^3$ (see Section 8.1). Then $V - T_1 \simeq 10.9$ years, so that $T_1 \simeq 63$ years. Thus, according to the model, inception of the primary tumor occurred about 11 years prior to diagnosis. It is worth noting that, although the model technically allows extrapolation of the primary tumor growth further back in time (and, in particular, computing the age, T, of tumor origination), doing so would be misleading due to the possibility of a change in the growth rate of the primary tumor around the inception time, potential tumor dormancy prior to inception, and the fact that the dynamics of small cell populations cannot adequately be described by exponential or any other deterministic growth law. In any case, origination of the primary tumor had likely occurred several decades prior to its detection.

(3) The very long mean latency time ρ for bone-bound metastases suggests that by the time of their detection and volumetric survey, the vast majority of these metastases were still dormant and undetectable.
(4) In accordance with the general model (see Section 8.2), the metastasis with the earliest seeding time was the one that reached the largest volume, $x_n = 22.96\,\mathrm{cm}^3$, at age W. Let T_2 be the patient's age at inception of this metastasis with the same volume N_0 as noted. The equation $N_0 \exp\{\gamma_1(W - T_2)\} = x_n$ then yields

$$W - T_2 = \frac{1}{\gamma_1} \log \frac{x_n}{N_0}.$$

From this formula, inception of the largest metastasis occurred about 3.2 years prior to metastasis survey and hence about 4.8 years after the excision of the primary tumor. Inception of other detected bone metastases, therefore, occurred at later times. Thus, at the time of surgery, all detected bone metastases were avascular, while at the time of their detection eight years later, they had reached considerable sizes unattainable for an avascular tumor. Therefore, a notable effect of primary tumor excision was likely turning on the angiogenic switch.
(5) The fact that the estimated value of θ is close to 0 suggests that the rate of the Poisson process of metastasis shedding is essentially constant regardless of the size of the primary tumor. Therefore, the population of metastases-producing cancer cells has an almost constant size $M(t) = aN^{\theta}(t)$ with some constant $a > 0$, notwithstanding the ongoing cell loss. In fact, for the estimated value of $\theta = 0.025$, it is easy to find that, over the period of about 11 years between primary tumor inception with the volume $N_0 = 4.19 \times 10^{-3}\,\mathrm{cm}^3$ and detection with the volume $S = 10.3\,\mathrm{cm}^3$, the size $M(t)$ has grown by less than 22 %, to be compared with the 2,458-fold increase of the primary tumor volume over the same period. This suggests that the population of metastases-producing cells has self-renewal capacity, e. g., through asymmetric division characteristic of cancer stem cells (see Section 3.4). Recall that breast cancer stem cells have been discovered experimentally [184, 49].

Conclusions 1–5 showcase the power of mathematical modeling and likelihood-based parameter estimation. They will serve as a template for uncovering clinically important unobservable features of the natural history of the disease in four cases of renal cancer in Chapter 10. However, as the ensuing course of events demonstrates, the validity of biomedical conclusions hinges not only on model adequacy and soundness of parameter estimation methodology, but also on subtle details of its numerical implementation.

In 2012 Jason brought to my attention that his numerical simulations for the five-parametric model applied to the same dataset were occasionally producing values of the likelihood function exceeding the global maximum. I initially attributed this to computational artifacts. However, in a few weeks, he came up with a mathematical proof that, for a certain data-dependent value of parameter γ_1, the likelihood as a function of γ_0, with the other three model parameters being fixed, tends to infinity as $\gamma_0 \to 0$. I examined the proof and found it to be correct.

After a fairly protracted period of shock and disbelief, I set out to find the reasons behind the phenomenon that Jason had discovered. The outcome proved even more shocking than the occurrence of infinite likelihood. It turned out that the same is true for a much more general model and for any admissible data set $x_1, x_2, \ldots, x_n$! This finding was published in our joint article [118]. Thus, the MLE $\gamma_0 = 0$ is universal (i. e., data-independent), which is a critical condition for applicability of the new methodology developed in Section 6.6.

The general model presented in [118] still involves an assumption that the Poisson rate of metastasis shedding is a continuous function of the current size of primary tumor, with formula (9.1) being one specific example of such relationship. As it turns out, even this assumption can be dispensed with, thus extending the universality phenomenon to the most general model described in Section 8.1. Mathematical formulation and immediate implications of this finding are provided in the next section.

9.2 The main result and its consequences

Because cell cycle duration has a lower limit, the growth rate of any cell population has a cap. Therefore, the net metastasis growth rates γ_0 and γ_1 are bounded above by some constant C. However, due to cell death and quiescence, they may approach zero. Let $G = (0, C) \times (0, C)$ be the set of all admissible pairs (γ_0, γ_1). Denote

$$B = \frac{\log(x_n/N_0)}{W - V}. \tag{9.2}$$

This quantity represents the rate of growth of a hypothetical metastasis whose inception occurred at the patient's age V of primary tumor resection or completion of radiation treatment and which reached the size x_n, the largest among the observed sizes of metastases, at age W. The following theorem summarizes extremal behavior of the likelihood as a function of the parameter vector (γ_0, γ_1).

Theorem 9.1. *Under the model of cancer progression described in Section* 8.1, *for any fixed functional parameters r, f, fixed numerical parameters T, N_0, τ, and for every data set $x_1, x_2, \ldots, x_n$ such that $m \le x_1 < x_2 < \cdots < x_n$, the supremum of the likelihood function $L(\gamma_0, \gamma_1)$ given by formula* (8.14) *over the set G is infinite. Furthermore, if $L(\gamma_0(k), \gamma_1(k)) \to \infty$ for some sequence $(\gamma_0(k), \gamma_1(k))$ in G, then $\gamma_0(k) \to 0$ and $\gamma_1(k) \to B$.*

The proof of Theorem 9.1 can be obtained by a minute modification of a detailed proof of a similar result given in [118].

Theorem 9.1 implies that the MLE of parameter vector (γ_0, γ_1) is $(0, B)$. Notice that for parameter γ_0, the MLE $\gamma_0 = 0$ is independent of the data! By contrast, in view of (9.2) the MLE $\gamma_1 = B$ for parameter γ_1 depends on the largest observation x_n.

Thus, in biomedical terms, Theorem 9.1 amounts to the following natural law:

The likelihood-maximizing scenario of metastatic cancer progression in an individual patient whose primary tumor was resected or ablated by radiation is invariably the same—suppression of metastatic growth while primary tumor is in place followed by an abrupt growth acceleration after primary tumor removal.

This finding provides a compelling explanation for the fact that the described scenario is very often observed in clinical and veterinary practice as well as in experimental animal studies. However, this most likely course of events does not prevent other scenarios—rapid outgrowth of metastases while primary tumor is still in place, delayed surfacing of metastases after primary tumor removal or indefinite metastatic dormancy–from frequent manifestation. These other scenarios, though, are expected to occur with smaller probability.

I now turn to a few immediate implications of Theorem 9.1. In the next section, I will review the assumptions behind Theorem 9.1, while its biomedical significance in a broader biological context will be a matter of concern in Section 9.4.

1. *The limiting model as $\gamma_0 \to 0$.* What is the distribution of the sizes of metastases in the limiting case $\gamma_0 = 0$? Suppose first that $A \geq m$, i. e., that a notional metastasis whose inception occurred at age V of primary tumor removal is detectable at age W (then, so are the metastases with earlier inception time). Notice that if $\gamma_0 = 0$, then in view of (8.5) and (8.6) $M = A = N_0 \exp\{\gamma_1(W - V)\}$ and $\delta(x) = \gamma_1^{-1} \log(x/N_0)$. As was discovered in Section 8.3, in the case $A \geq m$, the probability η, given by formula (8.13), of the event that inception of a viable metastasis in the site of interest occurred before age V is independent of γ_0, which means that formula (8.13) is inherited by the limiting model. Under the latter, following inception, all such metastases remain dormant until age V and grow at the rate γ_1 thereafter. Therefore, the limiting model-based probability distribution underlying the sizes of detectable metastases at age W is a mixture of a discrete and an absolutely continuous distributions. Specifically, with probability η, the size equals $A = N_0 \exp\{\gamma_1(W-V)\}$ and with probability $1-\eta$, it has, due to the first formula in (8.12) and (8.13), a properly normalized pdf

$$p(x) = (\gamma_1 x)^{-1} \frac{\int_0^{V-T} r(s) f[W - T - \gamma_1^{-1} \log(x/N_0) - s] ds}{\int_0^{V-T} r(s)[F(W - T - \gamma_1^{-1} \log(m/N_0) - s) - F(V - T - s)] ds}$$

for $m \leq x \leq A$ and 0 otherwise. Observe also that, in the case $A < m$, no metastases will ever become detectable at age W.

2. *The most likely pattern of metastatic volumes.* The just-described distribution of the sizes of metastases in the limiting case $\gamma_0 = 0$ with $\gamma_1 = B$ (which in view of Theorem 9.1 is the likelihood-maximizing value of parameter γ_1) suggests the following pattern of sizes of $n \geq 1$ metastases detected at age W:

   All those (say, k) metastases, $1 \leq k \leq n$, whose inception occurred before ablation of the primary tumor remained essentially dormant until age V and were growing at a rate γ_1 close to B thereafter, so that by age W they reached volumes close to the maximum observed volume x_n. The remaining $n - k$ metastases whose inception occurred after age V were growing at about the same rate $\gamma_1 = B$ and at age W attained more widely spread smaller volumes $x_1, x_2, \ldots, x_{n-k}$.

   Interestingly, this somewhat unexpected qualitative pattern describes fairly well what was actually observed in all the patients I have analyzed. This includes:
   (a) the breast cancer patient with bone metastases whose volumes were displayed in Section 9.1 ($n = 31, k = 1$);
   (b) two additional breast cancer patients analyzed in [135] ($n = 15, 20, k = 1$);
   (c) a prostate cancer patient analyzed in [136, 137] with bone metastases having the following volumes in cm^3 ($n = 36, k = 3$):
   1.40, 1.85, 2.05, 2.30, 2.48, 2.85, 3.20, 3.35, 3.43, 3.52, 4.24, 4.34, 5.14, 5.27, 6.26, 6.29, 6.61, 6.65, 6.66, 8.26, 8.68, 9.32, 10.40, 10.94, 11.31, 11.32, 13.49, 13.67, 14.33, 15.17, 15.39, 15.79, 16.85, 21.82, 25.91, 27.95;
   (d) four renal cancer patients with pulmonary metastases ($n = 13, k = 1$; $n = 15, k = 1$; $n = 53, k = 3$; $n = 60, k = 2$), see [175] and Section 10.1 in this book.
3. *A computational lesson.* Theorem 9.1 carries an important lesson in numerical analysis. Although optimization algorithms employed to obtain the results of [135] correctly found the global maximum of the likelihood in the *interior* of the parameter space, they missed a narrow infinite peak on the boundary and thus the true MLEs of model parameters. Therefore, when estimates of model parameters are computed through optimization of a certain criterion such as the likelihood or the sum of squared deviations of model-based predictions from the data (commonly referred to as the *least squares* criterion), along with the original model, one has to also optimize all its submodels arising on the boundary of the parameter space and other limiting cases. Chapter 10 furnishes another example emphasizing the importance of this principle.
4. *Comparison between the general and parametric models.* The general model from Section 8.1 and the resulting natural law are applicable, in particular, to the case of breast cancer patient examined in Section 9.1, which leads to a conclusion that, in all likelihood, the growth of her metastases was suppressed by the primary tumor and accelerated following its resection. Alternatively, the effect of the primary tumor and its excision on the growth of metastases in the same patient can be assessed through the more specific five-parametric model described in Section 9.1

with likelihood-maximizing parameters reported in the same section. Vis-a-vis parameter estimation, the principal difference between the results was that for the general model the likelihood-maximizing parameters belong to the boundary of the parameter space, while for the parametric model they were found in its interior. The fact that the conclusions reached by the two models are qualitatively identical is reassuring. Furthermore, on the quantitative side, the general model's MLEs of the two rates of growth of bone metastases, $\gamma_0 = 0$ and $\gamma_1 = 1.076\,\text{year}^{-1}$ (see formula (9.2)), and those for its parametric counterpart, $\gamma_0 = 0.083\,\text{year}^{-1}$ and $\gamma_1 = 2.676\,\text{year}^{-1}$, are in reasonable accord with each other.

9.3 A close look at the assumptions behind the natural law

The essence of Theorem 9.1 and the resulting natural law is that, under certain mathematical and biomedical assumptions, they hold true for every site-specific metastatic progression process involving: (1) Poisson dissemination of cancer cells interrupted by ablation of the primary tumor by surgery or radiation; (2) random independent survival of metastases; (3) their latency with random iid durations; and (4) exponential growth of metastases with two fixed rates, one before and one after removal of the primary tumor. Thus, the natural law is rooted in very basic temporal and kinetic aspects of metastasis and is applicable in equal measure to any other structurally similar process of biological or other nature. This may perhaps create an impression of a rabbit extracted from the hat. Therefore, it seems worthwhile to review the assumptions of the phenomenological model described in Section 8.1 and assess their generality and realism.

For starters, observe that the underlying model of cancer progression is grounded in three most significant clinical aspects of metastasis discovered in the second half of the 20th century. The first is a highly selective, multi-stage, stochastic nature of metastasis seeding (see Section 3.5). The second is a crucial observation, made in Section 4.1, that dissemination of blood-borne metastases may start long before primary tumor becomes detectable (the Fisher effect). The third feature is the ubiquity of metastatic dormancy in the form of solitary cancer cells or avascular micrometastases in a state of equilibrium between cell proliferation, quiescence and death (see Section 3.6).

The validity and generality of the natural law depends on how well the model assumptions agree with reality. Mathematical premises include, first, homogeneity and independence assumptions, i. e., that metastases bound for a given secondary site survive independently of each other with the same probability, that their latency times are iid random variables, that they undergo inception in the site with the same initial size N_0 and that they grow exponentially with the same constant pre- and post-surgery net rates γ_0 and γ_1, respectively. Second, we employed the assumption that metastases are shed off the primary tumor according to the Poisson process with rate $r(t)$. Due to arbitrariness of the rate function r, this essentially reduces to stochastic independence of the numbers of metastases shed over nonoverlapping time intervals and the condition that the probability of multiple metastases shed over an interval of small duration h is $o(h)$ (see [178, pp. 281–284]). Finally, I postulated in Section 8.1 certain qualitative properties (specifically, continuity and positivity) of functions r and f. All these mathematical assumptions are what the great Henri Poincaré, introduced in Sections 5.6 and 6.1, called *neutral hypotheses* [2]—they facilitate conceptualization and mathematical formalization of the phenomenon of interest without distorting its essence and unduly restricting its scope.

Biomedical assumptions of the model are minor and well-grounded in reality. One of them, that secondary metastasis is negligible, is corroborated by the existing evidence, reviewed in Section 8.1. Another assumption posits that resection of primary tumor or its ablation by radiation affects metastases through the rate of their growth rather than through a change in their latency times. This assumption is supported by the well-known fact that quiescent cancer cells and dormant microtumors are refractory to various microenvironmental and systemic signals as well as to most therapeutic interventions [182]. Interestingly, though, in the likelihood-maximizing limiting case of no metastatic growth prior to primary tumor removal at age V, this assumption amounts to de facto extension of metastatic latency until the age V.

Although the assumptions of the mathematical model of cancer progression described in Section 8.1 are quite modest and generic, they are still only an approximation to reality. As a result, the qualitative natural law formulated here is not expected to manifest literally for every type of cancer, every metastatic site and every patient, but rather as a prevalent trend.

9.4 Concluding remarks

The natural law formulated in Section 9.2 exposes the great cancer treatment gamble. On the one hand, removal of the primary tumor by surgery or radiation cuts off the supply of new metastatic cells (except those released during surgery) and thus reduces the number of metastases disseminated by the primary tumor. On the other hand, it is likely that ablation of the primary tumor will trigger vascularization of the already existing micrometastases and accelerate their growth. Therefore, devising genomic, molecular, histological or clinical biomarkers predictive of the response of occult metastases to extirpation of the primary tumor in an individual patient has a momentous clinical significance. However, because our current knowledge of the interaction between the primary tumor and metastases and of the responses of the latter to primary tumor resection or irradiation is so skimpy, designing such biomarkers seems at present to be a long shot.

Although the natural law was stated for an individual patient, it can be applied to, and validated in, the setting of patient cohorts and populations. As one example, the notion that surgery for primary breast tumor accelerates metastatic progression was confirmed through a fairly general mathematical model of the metastatic cascade accounting for inter-patient variation in the natural history of breast cancer [185]. Parameters of the model were estimated from a sample of metastatic relapse (or censoring) times for a cohort of 673 breast cancer patients treated with surgery.

The discovered natural law has potentially far-reaching consequences for cancer biology and clinical oncology. First, it underscores an urgent need to reevaluate the utility of surgery and radiotherapy for various types of cancer, stages of the disease and categories of cancer patients. Second, it calls for gaining definitive insight into biological mechanisms behind suppression of metastatic progression by primary tumor. Third, it calls for elucidating biophysical, biochemical and immunological mechanisms by which primary tumor ablation by surgery or radiation, or any unrelated surgery for that matter, causes metastases to escape from their state of dormancy, triggers angiogenesis and promotes metastatic growth.

Given that mechanisms by which primary tumor suppresses vascularization and growth of metastases identified so far are largely hypothetical, a general question arises as to how bearers of this trait were selected in the course of evolution. In most cases, a primary tumor is not lethal per se, while metastases are. Therefore, any spontaneously emerging heritable mechanism of metastases suppression by a primary tumor would confer on the bearers of this trait both survival and reproductive advantage over non-bearers, while also allowing the bearers to pass it on to their offspring. As a result, the forces of natural selection would have fixed such a mechanism making it dominant across the relevant population.

10 Reconstruction of the natural history of renal cell carcinoma from the volumes of lung metastases

In this chapter, I make good on two promises made earlier in the book. First, I demonstrate how a parametric version of the very general single-patient phenomenological model described in Section 8.1 can be employed to reconstruct clinically significant unobservable aspects of the natural history of metastatic cancer (unfortunately, only retrospectively, after metastases have been detected and measured). Second, taking a clue from the computational lesson on maximum likelihood estimation learned in Chapter 9, I describe and optimize all the submodels arising as particular or limiting cases of the parametric model. The results, described in Section 10.5 and presented in Tables 10.3–10.5, reinforce the lesson.

Unlike in Chapters 8 and 9, the current focus is on studying a relatively rare, yet by no means extraordinary, scenario where metastases are discovered concurrently with the primary tumor. Specifically, I analyze four cases of clear-cell subtype of renal cell carcinoma (RCC) where multiple lung metastases were detected and measured at or around the time of complete or partial resection of the primary tumor. The methodological approach and general line of exposition in this chapter follow the articles [139, 175].

RCC accounts for 2–3 % of all malignancies globally and has a 2:1 male to female occurrence ratio [21]. About 75–85 % of all RCCs belong to the clear cell histological subtype of epithelial origin (see e. g. [186–189]). Most commonly, RCC tumors metastasize to the lungs, which occurs in about 45 % of all RCC patients with distant metastases [190]. Renal cancer is one of the most insidious cancers in that it frequently progresses asymptomatically until late stages of the disease. In fact, historical data suggest that 25–35 % of RCC patients present with metastases at primary diagnosis [191, 188]. More recently, extensive use of diagnostic imaging including ultrasound, CT and MRI has increased the rate of accidental renal cancer discovery, thus reducing the fraction of patients with clinically manifest metastases at presentation [187, 188]. As one specific example, SEER data suggests that the rate of metastatic renal cancer incidence dropped from 32 % for the period 1973–1985 to 25 % for the next period 1986–1998 [191].

Any mathematical model of biomedical processes should be tailored to the data it seeks to analyze. Therefore, we start with describing the clinical cases of RCC patients and the observables.

10.1 Clinical cases and data

Analyzed in this chapter are clinical data for four clear-cell RCC patients with pulmonary metastases. Three of them were diagnosed and treated at the University Medical Center in Magdeburg, Germany, and one patient at the Martin Luther University Clinic in Halle, Germany. For each of these patients, the following data were collected:

https://doi.org/10.1515/9783111334035-013

- age U at which the volume of the primary tumor was measured;
- volume S of the primary tumor calculated from an MRI or CT scan;
- patient's age V at complete or partial primary tumor resection;
- patient's age W at metastases survey;
- number n of detected pulmonary metastases; and
- their volumes estimated from CT images.

The values of the clinical variables U, V, S, W, n are given in Table 10.1, while the volumes of pulmonary metastases rounded to the nearest mm^3 are displayed in Table 10.2. Observe from Table 10.1 that ages V and W are separated by no more than 33 days, while ages U and V are no more than 13 days apart. Therefore, in the model of the natural history of RCC described in the next section, it is assumed for simplicity that $U = V = W$.

Importantly, all four patients received no treatment between the diagnosis and resection of the primary tumor or metastatic survey, whichever occurred later.

Table 10.1: Data summary for four RCC patients.
The table is reproduced from Hanin L, Jandrig B, Pavlova L, Seidel K. The natural history of renal cell carcinoma with pulmonary metastases illuminated through mathematical modeling. Math Biosci 2019, 309, 118–130.

Patient #	Sex	*V*	*U*	*S* (mm^3)	*W*	*n*
1	M	55 y 300 d	55 y 295 d	931,890	55 y 294 d	13
2	M	49 y 14 d	49 y 14 d	199,662	49 y 12 d	15
3	M	45 y 145 d	45 y 132 d	2,082,880[a]	45 y 178 d	53
4	F	74 y 199 d	74 y 199 d	33,811	74 y 181 d	60

[a]This volumetric measurement was based on a CT image taken 7 days prior to partial resection of the primary tumor. According to the pathology report, the volume of the resected portion of the primary tumor was 623,083 mm^3.

All primary tumor volumes were obtained by first measuring three perpendicular tumor diameters (a, b, c) from MRI (or, in the case of patient 3, CT) images. The volume S of primary tumor was approximated by the volume of an ellipsoid with these diameters: $S \simeq \pi abc/6$. The volumes of pulmonary metastases were measured from CT images using the same method. However, determination of one of the diameters proved unreliable; therefore, its value was taken to be the arithmetic mean of the other two diameters.

It is assumed that the minimum diameter of a detectable spherical metastasis with measurable volume is $d_{\min} = 5$ mm [192]. Then the corresponding minimum volume, m, is given by $m = \pi d_{\min}^3/6 \simeq 65.45\,\text{mm}^3$. Only metastatic volumes exceeding m were reported for all patients. The volume of a single cell in the case of clear-cell RCC was measured to be $c = 4.8 \cdot 10^{-6}\,\text{mm}^3$. This value, assumed for both primary tumors and their lung metastases in all four patients, was used for converting tumor volume into tumor size.

Table 10.2: Volumes of lung metastases.
The table is reproduced from Hanin L, Jandrig B, Pavlova L, Seidel K. The natural history of renal cell carcinoma with pulmonary metastases illuminated through mathematical modeling. Math Biosci 2019, 309, 118–130.

The volumes of lung metastases below are rounded to the nearest mm^3. The total detected pulmonary metastatic burden, B, is based on the original (unrounded) volumes of metastases.
Patient 1 (n = 13)
68, 72, 90, 108, 133, 172, 179, 248, 490, 516, 650, 1877, 2949
$B = 7,552\ mm^3$
Patient 2 (n = 15)
69, 73, 74, 82, 91, 94, 104, 116, 118, 135, 172, 179, 203, 827, 12695
$B = 15,032\ mm^3$
Patient 3 (n = 53)
67, 70, 71, 75, 77, 85, 87, 110, 111, 129, 140, 150, 171, 173, 175, 195, 230, 266, 278, 312, 413, 484, 516, 568, 590, 593, 659, 681, 693, 797, 853, 876, 985, 1197, 1443, 1541, 1662, 1839, 1899, 2970, 3240, 4517, 4642, 5064, 5555, 10150, 11760, 13065, 13219, 14143, 26419, 35751, 66929
$B = 238,688\ mm^3$
Patient 4 (n = 60)
110, 127, 130, 140, 157, 206, 248, 252, 278, 281, 310, 316, 330, 360, 362, 363, 372, 511, 513, 564, 570, 595, 596, 596, 641, 663, 695, 700, 706, 864, 890, 923, 992, 1013, 1085, 1601, 1820, 1985, 2055, 2207, 2218, 2330, 2331, 2356, 2572, 2732, 2822, 3735, 4346, 4378, 4838, 4842, 6006, 6536, 8100, 9561, 9718, 14465, 26157, 47223
$B = 194,393\ mm^3$

The clinical data shown in Tables 10.1 and 10.2 reveals, somewhat counterintuitively, the lack of correlation between the primary tumor size at surgery and such natural measures of metastatic burden as the number of detected lung metastases, their total volume and the volume of the largest detected metastasis. In particular, the smallest primary tumor in patient 4 has generated the largest number of detectable metastases and the second largest total and maximum metastatic volumes, while patient 3's huge primary tumor has produced the second largest number of metastases, but still the largest total and maximum volumes. Additionally, these three indicators of metastatic burden for the two intermediate-volume primary tumors in patients 1 and 2 were much smaller than for patients 3 and 4.

10.2 A mathematical model of RCC

The extent to which metastatic progression follows the same angiogenesis-dependent pattern potentially involving a protracted period of dormancy as the process of primary tumor growth depends on many factors such as the type of cancer, cooperativity of the microenvironment of the metastatic site, the presence of the primary tumor, motility of metastatic cells and certainly the intrinsic aggressiveness of a particular metastatic phenotype. Therefore, a mathematical model seeking to describe the four clinical cases in question has to take into account the following biological circumstances:

(1) Metastases were seeded in the lungs that have extensive capillary networks rich in oxygen and nutrients. This may reduce the role of neoangiogenesis as a critical factor of metastatic cancer progression.
(2) The exterior of pulmonary blood vessels represents a natural conduit for metastatic cell migration and a propitious site for colony formation [69].
(3) By the time of primary tumor resection all four patients had developed a significant number of pulmonary metastatic lesions, while the largest among them had reached considerable size (see Table 10.2). Furthermore, this had likely occurred in spite of an inhibiting effect of the primary tumor on metastatic vascularization and growth (see Section 4.3). Therefore, metastasis in these patients represented a particularly aggressive phenotype.

These considerations lend support to the notion of concurrency of angiogenesis and metastatic growth. The model, described next, presumes that all pulmonary metastases grow starting from a single initiator cell and follow the same patient-specific growth law. However, the model allows for a latency period, albeit potentially a short one, between separation of an initiator metastatic cell from the primary kidney tumor and its inception in the lungs. As described in Section 3.5, this latency period includes migration from the primary tumor site to a blood vessel or lymph channel, intravasation, free circulation, extravasation into the lungs, migration within the lungs and potentially quiescence as a solitary cancer cell up until the moment of the start of its active proliferation.

The assumption $U = V = W$, made in Section 10.1, leads to a considerable simplification of the general model of metastatic cancer progression described in Section 8.1 because in this case the model does not have to account for post-surgery dynamics of metastases, which can be quite different, as we know from Sections 5.2, 5.3 and 9.2, from their pre-surgery dynamics. The general model of cancer natural history in the case $V = W$ has been thoroughly studied in [139].

Stated next are the mathematical assumptions of an individual-patient model of metastatic cancer progression tailored to the cited four clinical cases. It is obtained by appropriate simplification and specialization from the general model described in Section 8.1. Suitable parameterizations of the model will be described in Section 10.4.

Primary tumor growth

Denote by $\Phi(t)$ the size of the primary tumor at time t counted from the unobservable patient's age, T, of primary tumor inception. Let $\Phi(0) = N_0$, where N_0 is the Folkman's avascular limiting size of the primary tumor. It is assumed that up until the age, V, of primary tumor resection, Φ is an increasing continuous function. We further assume that clones generated by N_0 initiator cells do not interact with each other and expand according to the same growth law $g(t)$ with $g(0) = 1$. By contrast, tumor cells within each clone are allowed to interact due to their spatial proximity and the resulting signaling inhibition, competition for space and essential chemicals and other factors. Then

$$\Phi(t) = N_0 g(t), \quad 0 \le t \le V - T. \tag{10.1}$$

To utilize a term introduced in Section 7.1, formula (10.1) is a *clonal* growth model.

Metastasis formation

Metastases are shed off the primary tumor according to a Poisson process whose rate, $r(t)$, is proportional to some power, θ, of the current size of the primary tumor:

$$r(t) = a\Phi^{\theta}(t), \quad 0 \le t \le V - T,$$

where $a > 0$ and $\theta \ge 0$ (see formula (9.1) and the ensuing discussion).

Other assumptions regarding generation of metastases are identical to those in the general model. Specifically, metastases shed off by the primary tumor and bound for the lungs survive independently of each other with the same probability $q > 0$, while their latency times are iid random variables with a continuous pdf f and the corresponding cdf F. Then the rate of the resulting Poisson process of metastasis inception is

$$\nu(t) = qa \int_0^t \Phi^{\theta}(s) f(t-s)\,ds, \quad 0 \le t \le V - T$$

(compare with formula (8.1)). Finally, secondary metastasizing is presumed negligible.

Metastatic growth

All lung metastases are assumed to grow in accordance with the same law. In keeping with the notation from Chapter 8, we denote the growth function by $\Psi(t)$, where time t is counted from the patient's age at inception of a particular metastasis. We assume that Ψ is a differentiable function with $\Psi'(t) > 0$ for all $t \ge 0$ and that $\Psi(0) = 1$. We retain notation δ for the inverse function Ψ^{-1}.

10.3 Distribution of the sizes of metastases and its two special forms

We now specialize Theorem 8.2 for the particular case, where $W = V$, $\tau = 0$ and $M = \Psi(W - T)$. Observe that in this case M, the largest metastatic volume theoretically allowed by the model, represents the size of a hypothetical metastasis whose inception in the lungs occurred without delay at the earliest possible time, i. e., at time T of primary tumor inception. According to formula (8.8), the pdf underlying (in the sense of Theorem 8.2) the sizes of detectable metastases at age W has the following form:

$$p(x) = \delta'(x)\frac{\int_0^{W-T-\delta(x)} g^\theta(s)f[W-T-\delta(x)-s]ds}{\int_0^{W-T-\delta(m)} g^\theta(s)F[W-T-\delta(m)-s]ds}, \quad m \le x \le M, \tag{10.2}$$

and $p(x) = 0$ for $x \notin [m, M]$.

Distribution (10.2) is completely determined by numerical parameters T, θ and functional parameters g, f, Ψ. However, it is free of parameters a, q and is independent of the sample size n and the primary tumor size at inception N_0. Therefore, the values of a, q and N_0 cannot be inferred from the observed volumes of metastases. Just as for the general model, pdf p is continuous at point M with $p(M) = 0$ but has a jump discontinuity at point m.

As was pointed out in Section 8.4, Theorem 8.2 implies that the distribution of any *symmetric* statistic based on observed site-specific metastatic volumes $x_1, x_2, \ldots, x_n$, where $m \le x_1 < x_2 < \cdots < x_n$, is identical to the distribution of the same statistic based on a random sample of size n drawn from the pdf p given by formula (10.2). The upshot is that identifiable parameters of a suitably parameterized model of metastatic cancer progression discussed in this chapter can be estimated by maximizing the joint likelihood of observations

$$\mathcal{L}(x_1, x_2, \ldots, x_n) = \Pi_{k=1}^n p(x_k).$$

Another such statistic is the L^1 distance

$$K(x_1, x_2, \ldots, x_n) = \int_m^M |G(x) - G_e(x)| dx \tag{10.3}$$

between the theoretical cdf, G, corresponding to the pdf p and its empirical analog, G_e, based on observations $x_1, x_2, \ldots, x_n$. Functional K, which coincides with the *Kantorovich (or Wasserstein) distance* [193] between the two distributions, enables one to quantify the model's fit to the data.

I now turn to two special submodels of the more general model of the individual natural history of RCC outlined in Section 10.2 and the resulting specializations of the pdf (10.2). Other special and limiting cases of the model and distribution (10.2) require additional parameterization and will be a matter of our concern in Section 10.4.

Instantaneous seeding model

Because inception of pulmonary metastases was assumed to occur when they consist of just one cell, it is theoretically possible that metastatic latency time is very short compared to other processes associated with metastatic progression. The resulting limiting model is termed *instantaneous seeding (IS)* model. It follows from (10.2) that under the IS model

$$p(x) = \delta'(x)\frac{g^\theta[W-T-\delta(x)]}{\int_0^{W-T-\delta(m)} g^\theta(s)ds}, \quad m \le x \le M, \tag{10.4}$$

and $p(x) = 0$ elsewhere. A peculiar property of the IS model, as opposed to the more general model (10.2), is that

$$p(M) = \frac{\delta'(M)}{\int_0^{W-T-\delta(m)} g^\theta(s)ds} > 0,$$

which means that function p is discontinuous at point M.

Homogeneous model

A notable particular case of the model (10.2) occurs when $\theta = 0$. In this case, the pdf p is independent of the law of the primary tumor growth:

$$p(x) = \delta'(x)\frac{F[W - T - \delta(x)]}{\int_0^{W-T-\delta(m)} F(s)ds}, \quad m \le x \le M, \tag{10.5}$$

and $p(x) = 0$ otherwise. This formula will be referred to as the *homogeneous* model because, in the case $\theta = 0$, the Poisson process of metastasis shedding off the primary tumor is homogeneous. In particular, setting $\theta = 0$ in (10.4) yields the following *homogeneous IS* model:

$$p(x) = \frac{\delta'(x)}{W - T - \delta(m)}, \quad m \le x \le M. \tag{10.6}$$

10.4 Model parameterization

To fully parameterize model (10.2) and its submodels (10.4), (10.5) and (10.6), one has to assume a certain functional form for all, or some, of the following model components: (1) the law, g, of post-inception clonal growth of the primary tumor; (2) the pdf, f, of the metastases latency time; and (3) the growth law, Ψ, for lung metastases. All parameters built into the resulting models, described in the following, are patient-specific.

Because most of the lung metastases developed by the RCC patients analyzed in this chapter did not reach very large sizes at age W (see Table 10.2), it can be hypothesized that at that time they were still in the exponential phase of their growth. Therefore, compare with Sections 8.1 and 9.1, it is assumed that each lung metastasis grows exponentially with the same rate $\gamma > 0$. Then

$$\Psi(t) = e^{\gamma t}, \quad \delta(x) = \frac{\log x}{\gamma} \quad \text{and} \quad M = e^{\gamma(W-T)}.$$

As for the metastases latency time, it is assumed, similarly to Section 9.1, to be exponentially distributed with pdf $f(t) = \rho^{-1}\exp\{-t/\rho\}$, where time t for an individual metastasis is counted from its shedding off the primary tumor and $\rho > 0$ is the expected duration of latency, assumed the same for all viable lung metastases in a given patient. Our selection of the latency time distribution implies that longer latency times occur with smaller probability. Note that no biological considerations prevent ρ from being either very small or very large.

Finally, we consider the following two possibilities for the law of post-inception clonal expansion of the primary tumor:

(a) Exponential growth with rate $\beta > 0: \ g(t) = \exp\{\beta t\}$; and

(b) Gompertzian clonal growth (10.1) with

$$g(t) = \exp\left\{\frac{\beta}{\lambda}(1 - \exp\{-\lambda t\})\right\}, \tag{10.7}$$

where $\beta, \lambda > 0$. Recall from Section 7.3 that in this case, the limiting primary tumor size as $t \to \infty$ is $S(\infty) = N_0 \exp\{\beta/\lambda\}$ and that as $\lambda \to 0$ the Gompertz growth function (10.7) degenerates into the exponential law $g(t) = \exp\{\beta t\}$. The latter means that models (a) and (b) are *nested.*

As indicated in Section 7.3, the clonal growth law (10.7) is a solution of the ODE

$$y' = \beta y - \lambda y \log y, \quad y(0) = 1.$$

Therefore, β represents the intrinsic net rate of primary tumor cell proliferation, while λ can be interpreted as the growth inhibition coefficient. The inhibition is caused by intra-clone interaction between cancer cells including competition for space, nutrients, oxygen and growth factors; the action of local and systemic growth inhibitors and apoptosis promoters; interaction of cancer cells with the microenvironment and the immune system; and other factors.

10.4.1 Homogeneous model

With the stated parameterizations, the homogeneous model (10.5) takes on the form

$$p(x) = (Cx)^{-1}\left[1 - \left(\frac{x}{M}\right)^b\right], \quad m \le x \le M, \tag{10.8}$$

and 0 elsewhere, where $b = 1/(\gamma\rho)$ and

$$C = \log\frac{M}{m} - b^{-1}\left[1 - \left(\frac{m}{M}\right)^b\right]. \tag{10.9}$$

Here and in the following, letter C denotes various normalization constants. Model (10.8), (10.9) depends on parameters b and M alone. The corresponding cdf G, to be used for computing the Kantorovich distance (10.3), can be found from (10.8) by integration:

$$G(x) = C^{-1}\left\{\log\frac{x}{m} - b^{-1}\left[\left(\frac{x}{M}\right)^b - \left(\frac{m}{M}\right)^b\right]\right\}, \quad m \le x \le M.$$

Letting $\rho \to 0$ (or equivalently $b \to \infty$) in (10.8), (10.9) leads to the following 1-parametric version of the homogeneous IS model (10.6):

$$p(x) = \frac{1}{(\log \frac{M}{m})x}, \quad m \le x \le M, \tag{10.10}$$

whence by integration

$$G(x) = \frac{\log \frac{x}{m}}{\log \frac{M}{m}}, \quad m \le x \le M.$$

Another 1-parametric limiting form of the homogeneous model (10.8), (10.9) arises when $\rho \to \infty$ (or equivalently $b \to 0$). In fact, application of the l'Hôpital's rule to (10.8) and (10.9) yields

$$p(x) = \frac{2 \log \frac{M}{x}}{(\log^2 \frac{M}{m})x}, \quad m \le x \le M. \tag{10.11}$$

This model will be called the *homogeneous long-latency* model. From (10.11),

$$G(x) = 1 - \frac{\log^2 \frac{M}{x}}{\log^2 \frac{M}{m}}, \quad m \le x \le M.$$

10.4.2 Exponential growth of the primary tumor

For an exponentially growing primary tumor, a straightforward, although perhaps a little tedious, computation based on (10.2) produces the following formula (see also [139]):

$$p(x) = (Cx)^{-1}\left[\left(\frac{M}{x}\right)^a - \left(\frac{x}{M}\right)^b\right], \quad m \le x \le M, \tag{10.12}$$

and 0 otherwise, where model parameters M, a, b are given by

$$M = \exp\{\gamma(W - T)\}, \quad a = \frac{\beta\theta}{\gamma}, \quad b = \frac{1}{\rho\gamma} \tag{10.13}$$

and the normalization constant C is

$$C = a^{-1}\left[\left(\frac{M}{m}\right)^a - 1\right] - b^{-1}\left[1 - \left(\frac{m}{M}\right)^b\right]. \tag{10.14}$$

Then from (10.12) one obtains by integration

$$G(x) = C^{-1}\left\{a^{-1}\left[\left(\frac{M}{m}\right)^a - \left(\frac{M}{x}\right)^a\right] - b^{-1}\left[\left(\frac{x}{M}\right)^b - \left(\frac{m}{M}\right)^b\right]\right\}, \quad m \le x \le M.$$

Formulas (10.12) and (10.14) will be referred to in what follows as the *exponential* model.

Note that pdf p in (10.12) is monotonically decreasing on $[m, M]$, which implies that under the exponential model, among metastases present at primary tumor excision, larger ones occur with smaller probability.

It was proven in [173, 174] that parameters M, a, b are identifiable from pdf p. (Recall that a stochastic model is identifiable if distinct vectors of model parameters produce distinct distributions of model output (see Section 6.5)). Thus, only three combinations (M, a, b), specified in (10.13), of the five biological model parameters $T, \beta, \theta, \rho, \gamma$ (as well as any other triples of parameter combinations obtained from M, a, b through one-to-one transformations) are identifiable.

Known primary tumor size

$$S = N_0 \exp\{\beta(U - T)\} \tag{10.15}$$

represents yet another such parameter combination. Recall that N_0 is the primary tumor size at inception, while T and U are the patient's ages at primary tumor inception and volumetric measurement, respectively. The case $U = W$, applicable to the four RCC patients in question, is more informative, for in this case not only $\rho\gamma$ is identifiable (see (10.13)), but also β/γ, and hence parameter θ as well. In fact, it follows from (10.13) and (10.15) with $U = W$ that

$$\frac{\beta}{\gamma} = \frac{\log \frac{S}{N_0}}{\log M}, \qquad \theta = a\,\frac{\log M}{\log \frac{S}{N_0}}. \tag{10.16}$$

In view of (10.13), parameters M, a, b of the exponential model are *dimensionless*. Furthermore, according to formula (10.12), the estimates of these parameters can equivalently be obtained by maximizing the likelihood based on the dimensionless version $p(x)x$ of the pdf p. Notice that, due to (10.12) and (10.14), the modified likelihood depends only on the *ratios* of M, m and x. Therefore, the estimates of parameters a, b as well as of parameter M expressed in volumetric units are independent of the volume of a single cancer cell and can be obtained from volumetric measurements $x_1, x_2, \ldots, x_n$ alone. On account of (10.13) and (10.16), the same is also true for the estimates of $\rho\gamma$, β/γ and θ; however, converting the estimate of M into the number of cells would require the knowledge of the volume, c, of a single cancer cell.

It follows from the inequalities $M \geq x_n$, $T \geq 0$ and the first formula in (10.13) that parameter γ, the rate of growth of metastases, is bounded away from zero: $\gamma \geq (\log x_n)/W$. Also, a lower limit on the cell cycle duration and hence on the tumor volume doubling time implies that γ and β are both bounded above. Furthermore, the formula for parameter M in (10.13) implies that the same is true for M. Likewise, from (10.15) we derive the following lower bound for β:

$$\beta \geq \frac{\log \frac{S}{N_0}}{U}. \tag{10.17}$$

The upshot of these estimates is that the only biologically relevant special cases and limiting forms of the exponential model are the following ones (see also [139]):

(A) The *instantaneous seeding (IS)* model, where $\rho = 0$ or equivalently $b = \infty$. Letting $b \to \infty$ in (10.12) and (10.14) yields

$$p(x) = \frac{a}{m^{-a} - M^{-a}} x^{-(a+1)} \quad \text{and} \quad G(x) = \frac{m^{-a} - x^{-a}}{m^{-a} - M^{-a}}, \quad m \le x \le M. \tag{10.18}$$

(B) The *long-latency (LL)* model, where $\rho = \infty$ or equivalently $b = 0$. In this case,

$$p(x) = (Cx)^{-1}\left[\left(\frac{M}{x}\right)^a - 1\right], \quad m \le x \le M, \tag{10.19}$$

where

$$C = a^{-1}\left[\left(\frac{M}{m}\right)^a - 1\right] - \log\frac{M}{m}. \tag{10.20}$$

Then the corresponding cdf is given by

$$G(x) = C^{-1}\left\{a^{-1}\left[\left(\frac{M}{m}\right)^a - \left(\frac{M}{x}\right)^a\right] - \log\frac{x}{m}\right\}, \quad m \le x \le M.$$

As a self-consistency check, note that the homogeneous model (10.8), (10.9) can alternatively be obtained by passage to limit as $a \to 0$ in (10.12) and (10.14). The same is true regarding the IS and LL submodels of the homogeneous model (see (10.10) and (10.11)), and the respective submodels of the exponential model specified in (10.18) and (10.19), (10.20).

10.4.3 Gompertzian growth of the primary tumor

The clonal Gompertz growth law (10.7) leads, after some computation, to the following expression for the pdf p specified in (10.2) (see [139]):

$$p(x) = \frac{b}{Cx}\left(\frac{x}{M}\right)^b \int_0^{\log(M/x)} \exp\{bu - k\exp\{-\mu u\}\}du, \quad m \le x \le M, \tag{10.21}$$

and $p(x) = 0$ elsewhere. Here,

$$C = \int_0^{\log(M/m)} \exp\{-k\exp\{-\mu u\}\}\left[1 - \exp\left\{-b\left(\log\frac{M}{m} - u\right)\right\}\right]du, \tag{10.22}$$

where parameters M and b are the same as in (10.13) and

$$k = \frac{\beta\theta}{\lambda}, \quad \mu = \frac{\lambda}{\gamma}. \tag{10.23}$$

A straightforward computation based on (10.21) produces the following formula for the corresponding cdf for $m \leq x \leq M$:

$$G(x) = C^{-1}\left[h(x)\left(\frac{x}{M}\right)^b - h(m)\left(\frac{m}{M}\right)^b + \int_{\log(M/x)}^{\log(M/m)} \exp\{-k\exp\{-\mu u\}\}du\right],$$

where

$$h(x) = \int_0^{\log(M/x)} \exp\{bu - k\exp\{-\mu u\}\}du$$

and C is given by (10.22).

The *Gompertz* model (10.21), (10.22) depends on four dimensionless parameters M, b, k, μ representing various combinations of the original six biological parameters T, β, λ, θ, ρ, γ. Notice that it shares parameters M and b with the exponential model. Also, parameter $a = \beta\theta/\gamma$ of the exponential model can be expressed through parameters (10.23) of the Gompertz model: $a = k\mu$. It was shown in [139] by means of a fairly sophisticated mathematical argument that parameters M, b, k, μ of the Gompertz model are identifiable from the pdf (10.21), (10.22). Although any one-to-one transformation of the parameter space, formed by all admissible parameter vectors (M, b, k, μ) into $\mathbb{R}^4$ produces an equivalent set of four identifiable model parameters, the chosen parameterization seems to be among the most convenient ones for the Gompertz model.

Suppose now that the volume of the primary tumor, S, measured at some age U is also available, as is the case for the four RCC patients analyzed in this chapter. In view of (10.1) and (10.7), equation $\Phi(U - T) = S$ can be represented in the form

$$N_0 \exp\left\{\frac{\beta}{\lambda}[1 - e^{-\lambda(U-T)}]\right\} = S. \tag{10.24}$$

Combining this with the first formula in (10.13) and the second formula in (10.23) yields

$$S = N_0 \exp\left\{\frac{\beta}{\lambda}[1 - \exp\{\lambda(W - U)\}M^{-\mu}]\right\}.$$

In the case $U = W$ this formula takes on a simpler form

$$S = N_0 \exp\left\{\frac{\beta}{\lambda}(1 - M^{-\mu})\right\}. \tag{10.25}$$

Therefore, in this case the ratio β/λ and therefore also parameter $\theta = k\lambda/\beta$ are identifiable.

Taking into account that $T \geq 0$, we find from (10.24) that

$$\frac{\beta}{\lambda}(1 - \exp\{-\lambda U\}) \geq \log \frac{S}{N_0}. \tag{10.26}$$

Since $e^{-x} \geq 1 - x$ for all $x \in \mathbb{R}$, we infer from (10.26) that, just like for the exponential model, under the more general Gompertz model, the net intrinsic rate of primary tumor growth, β, satisfies the same inequality (10.17), so that β is again bounded above and below. Also, because $0 < e^{-x} \leq 1$ for $x \geq 0$, we derive from (10.26) that $\lambda \leq \beta / \log(S/N_0)$, hence λ is bounded above.

Therefore, the only limiting versions of the Gompertz model, to be explored when model parameters are estimated, are the following ones (see also [139, 175]):

(A) The *exponential* model arising when $\lambda \to 0$ (or equivalently $\mu \to 0$) and all its submodels cataloged in Subsection 10.4.2.

(B) The *Gompertz instantaneous seeding (IS)* model arising for $\rho = 0$ (or equivalently $b = \infty$). A straightforward computation based on formulas (10.4) and (10.7) yields

$$p(x) = (Cx)^{-1} \exp\left\{-k\left(\frac{x}{M}\right)^{\mu}\right\}, \quad m \leq x \leq M, \tag{10.27}$$

and 0 otherwise, where

$$C = \int_{m/M}^{1} \exp\{-ku^{\mu}\}\frac{du}{u}. \tag{10.28}$$

The corresponding cdf has the form

$$G(x) = C^{-1} \int_{m/M}^{x/M} \exp\{-ku^{\mu}\}\frac{du}{u}, \quad m \leq x \leq M,$$

where C is specified in (10.28).

(C) The *Gompertz long-latency (LL)* model, where $\rho = \infty$ (or equivalently $b = 0$). In this case, by passage to limit as $b \to 0$ in (10.21), (10.22) one obtains

$$p(x) = (Cx)^{-1} \int_{0}^{\log(M/x)} \exp\{-k \exp\{-\mu u\}\}du, \quad m \leq x \leq M, \tag{10.29}$$

with

$$C = \int_{0}^{\log(M/m)} \exp\{-k \exp\{-\mu u\}\}\left(\log \frac{M}{m} - u\right)du. \tag{10.30}$$

In this case,

$$G(x) = C^{-1}\left[\log\frac{M}{m}\int_{0}^{\log(M/m)}\varphi(u)du - \log\frac{M}{x}\int_{0}^{\log(M/x)}\varphi(u)du - \int_{\log(M/x)}^{\log(M/m)}u\varphi(u)du\right]$$

for $m \leq x \leq M$, where $\varphi(u) = \exp\{-k\exp\{-\mu u\}\}$ and C is defined in (10.30).

The Gompertz IS and LL models depend on three parameters M, k, μ, whose identifiability was established in [139].

10.5 Data analysis

Model parameters were estimated from the data for patients 1–4, see Tables 10.1 and 10.2, by the method of maximum likelihood applied to the parametric models presented in Section 10.4. To this end, the normalized dimensionless negative log-likelihood function

$$L(x_1, x_2, \ldots, x_n) = -\frac{1}{n}\sum_{k=1}^{n}\log[x_k p(x_k)] \tag{10.31}$$

was minimized over relevant parameter spaces. Normalization of function L, i. e., dividing the dimensionless negative log-likelihood represented by the sum in (10.31) by n, enables comparison between different patients. Along with the homogeneous and Gompertz models, function L was also minimized for all their biologically relevant limiting cases—the homogeneous IS and LL submodels, the Gompertz IS and LL submodels and the exponential model and its IS and LL submodels (see Table 10.3 for a summary of all nine nested (sub)models, their biological and identifiable parameters and parameter degenerations producing various submodels).

Table 10.3: Nested models and their limiting cases.
The table is reproduced from Hanin L, Jandrig B, Pavlova L, Seidel K. The natural history of renal cell carcinoma with pulmonary metastases illuminated through mathematical modeling. Math Biosci 2019, 309, 118–130.

Model name	Eq. (10.X) X =	Biological parameters	Identifiable parameters	Model degeneration	
				Biological parameters	Identifiable parameters
Homogeneous	8, 9	T, ρ, γ	M, b	$\theta = 0$	N/A
Homogeneous IS	10	T, γ	M	$\theta = 0, \rho = 0$	$b = \infty$
Homogeneous LL	11	T, γ	M	$\theta = 0, \rho = \infty$	$b = 0$
Gompertz	21, 22	T, $\beta, \lambda, \theta, \rho, \gamma$	M, b, k, μ	N/A	N/A
Gompertz IS	27, 28	T, $\beta, \lambda, \theta, \gamma$	M, k, μ	$\rho = 0$	$b = \infty$
Gompertz LL	29, 30	T, $\beta, \lambda, \theta, \gamma$	M, k, μ	$\rho = \infty$	$b = 0$
Exponential	12, 14	T, $\beta, \theta, \rho, \gamma$	M, a, b	$\lambda = 0$	$k = \infty, \mu = 0$
Exponential IS	18	T, β, θ, γ	M, a	$\lambda = 0, \rho = 0$	$b = \infty, k = \infty, \mu = 0$
Exponential LL	19, 20	T, β, θ, γ	M, a	$\lambda = 0, \rho = \infty$	$b = 0, k = \infty, \mu = 0$

For every data set and each model, a global minimum of function L over the entire relevant parameter space was computed using various Matlab™ optimization routines. To ascertain that the true global minimum was reached, the global profiles for function L, defined in the caption to Figure 10.1, were visually examined. All the profiles displayed one of the following two patterns: (1) those with a unique interior point of global minimum or (2) monotonic pattern leading to model degeneration. Typical examples of such profiles are shown in Figure 10.1.

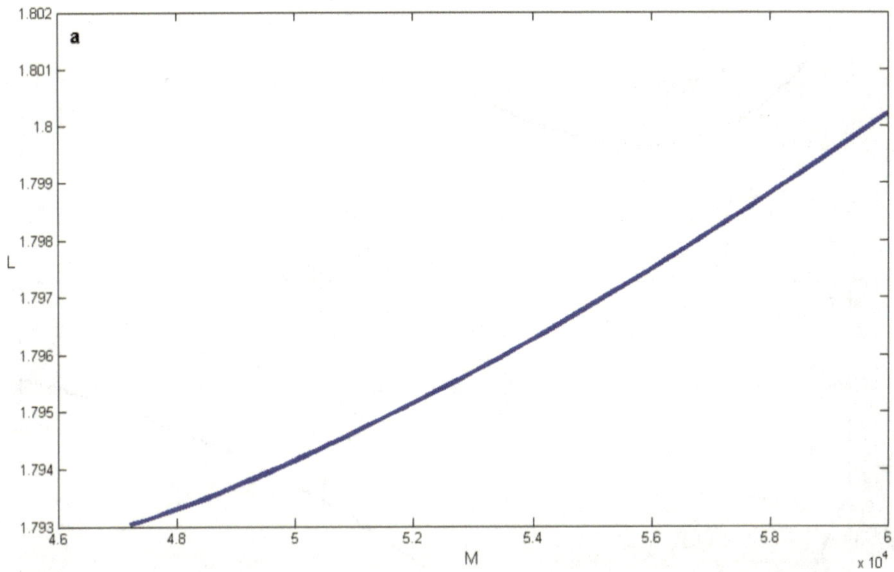

Figure 10.1: Profiles of function ***L*** defined by formula (10.31) in parameters **M**, **k**, $\boldsymbol{\mu}$ of the Gompertz IS model for patient 4. All parameters except one were fixed at their optimal (likelihood-maximizing) values (see Table 10.4), while the parameter of interest varied over its entire domain. Note the monotonic pattern for parameter M in Figure 10.1a and the unique interior points of global minimum of function L for parameters k and μ in Figures 10.1b and 10.1c, respectively. See Sections 10.3–10.5 for context and technical details. The figure was reproduced with permission from Hanin L, Jandrig B, Pavlova L, Seidel K. The natural history of renal cell carcinoma with pulmonary metastases illuminated through mathematical modeling. Math Biosci 2019, 309, 118–30.

Optimization of model parameters required painstaking, laborious numerical work due to the presence, especially in the integrands associated with the Gompertz model, of very small and very large numbers, that prohibited automatic unsupervised computation and necessitated the use of adaptive scaling factors on every step of the optimization process. Their selection was guided by visual examination of the profiles of function L for all relevant parameters with an eye on the stability of outputs.

The results of parameter optimization are shown in Table 10.4. For patients 1 and 2, the Gompertz model degenerated into the exponential IS submodel ($\lambda = \rho = 0$). In this

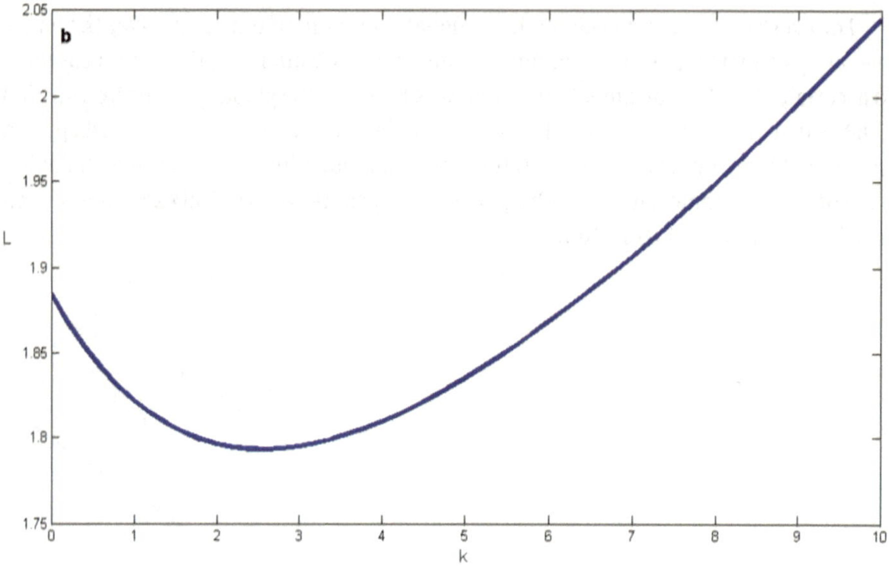

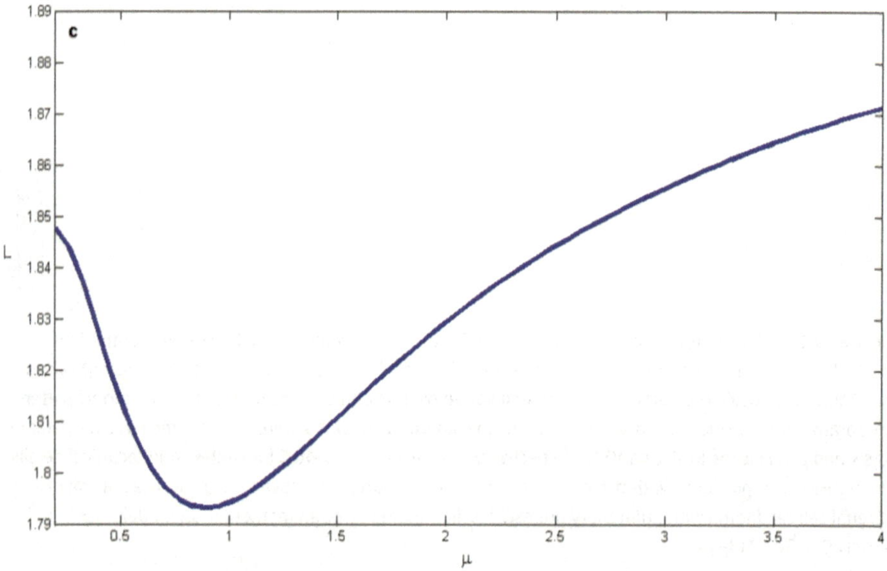

Figure 10.1: (continued).

case, optimization of parameters M and a can essentially be done analytically. In fact, it follows from the first formula in (10.18) that, for any fixed $x \in [m, x_n]$ and $a > 0$, pdf p is a decreasing function of parameter M on $[x_n, \infty)$, so that the likelihood is maximized for $M^* = x_n$, the largest observed volume of metastases. Also, it was shown in [173] that the likelihood-maximizing value, a^*, of parameter a is uniquely determined by the quantity

$$R = \frac{\bar{x} - \log x_1}{\log x_n - \log x_1}, \quad \text{where } \bar{x} = \frac{1}{n}\sum_{k=1}^{n} \log x_k.$$

Specifically, if $R \geq 0.5$, then $a^* = 0$, while, if $R < 0.5$, then a^* is a unique solution of the equation

$$\frac{1}{a\log(x_n/x_1)} - \frac{1}{(x_n/x_1)^a - 1} = R. \tag{10.32}$$

The values of R are 0.3674 for patient 1 and 0.1747 for patient 2. Then the respective values of a^* found from (10.32) turned out to be 0.4410 and 1.0748 (see Table 10.4).

Table 10.4: Results of likelihood maximization and the value of the goodness-of-fit measure K. The table is reproduced from Hanin L, Jandrig B, Pavlova L, Seidel K. The natural history of renal cell carcinoma with pulmonary metastases illuminated through mathematical modeling. Math Biosci 2019, 309, 118–130.

Patient #	Optimal model	Optimal parameters	L	K (mm^3)
1	Exponential IS	$M = x_n = 2,949$ mm^3 [a] $a = 0.4410$	1.2400	145.5
2	Exponential IS	$M = x_n = 12,695$ mm^3 $a = 1.0748$	0.9604	738.4
3	Gompertz IS	$M = x_n = 66,929$ mm^3 $k = 3.01665$ $\mu = 0.1369$	1.8195	689.0
4	Gompertz IS	$M = x_n = 47,223$ mm^3 $k = 2.5518$ $\mu = 0.8916$	1.7930	741.1

[a]Here and elsewhere in this table, the estimated theoretical upper limit, M, of the size of lung metastases is represented in volumetric units.

For patients 3 and 4, by contrast, the Gompertz model experienced only a single degeneration into its IS submodel ($\rho = 0$), and the model parameters were optimized numerically. Interestingly, we found that, in both cases, $M^* = x_n$, similarly to the exponential IS model (10.18) that proved optimal for patients 1 and 2.

An important question is how good is the optimal model's fit to the data for each patient. The latter was quantified by the Kantorovich distance (10.3) between the theoretical and empirical distributions of the volumes of detected metastases (see Table 10.4). The excellent visual fit between the two cdfs is exemplified in Figure 10.2 featuring patient 3, where, for the purpose of better visualization, the normalized volumes x_k/M, $1 \leq k \leq n$, where $M = x_n$, were employed.

The estimates of identifiable model parameters shown in Table 10.4 enable computation of certain unobservable clinically important characteristics of the individual natural history of metastatic cancer. Specifically, for patients 1 and 2, we used (10.16) to compute the ratio β/γ of the rates of growth of primary tumor and lung metastases and

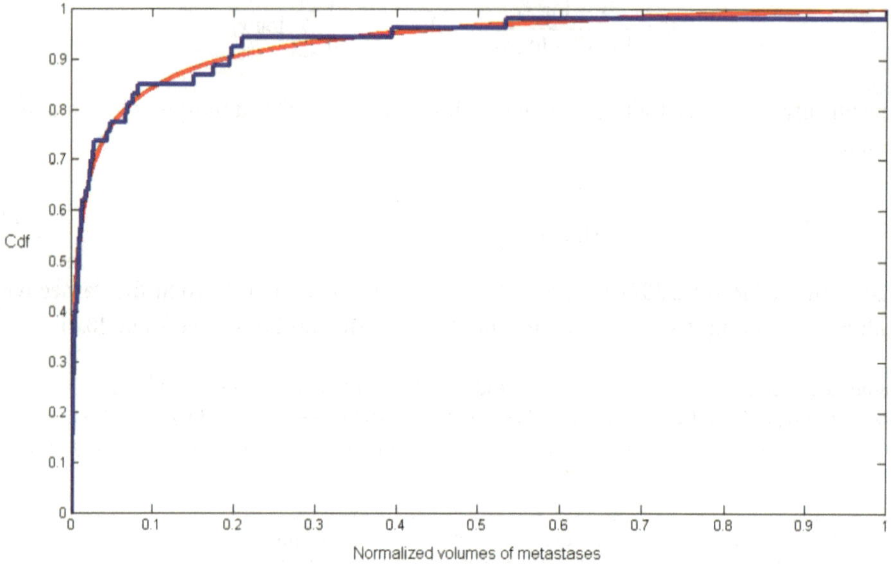

Figure 10.2: Cdfs of the theoretical (continuous red curve) and empirical (step-wise blue curve) distributions for the normalized volumes $\mathbf{x_k/M}$, $\mathbf{1 \leq k \leq n}$, of lung metastases for patient 3. Of note is an excellent fit between the two cdfs. Likelihood-maximizing parameters of the theoretical distribution are given in Table 10.4.
The figure was reproduced with permission from Hanin L, Jandrig B, Pavlova L, Seidel K. The natural history of renal cell carcinoma with pulmonary metastases illuminated through mathematical modeling. Math Biosci 2019, 309, 118–30.

the value of parameter θ characterizing the intensity of metastasis shedding by the primary tumor. In these and other similar computations, the value of parameter M, which was originally estimated in volumetric units (mm^3), had to be converted into the number of cells.

Formulas (10.13) for β/γ and θ involve the unknown size N_0 of the primary tumor at inception expressed in volumetric units. To estimate it, we assumed that primary tumor at inception had spherical shape and that its diameter d falls within the Folkman limit of 1–2 mm for avascular tumors. Accordingly, Table 10.5 contains the estimates of the quantities β/γ and θ computed for these extreme values of d. It is easy to verify that the values of the same quantities for diameters d between 1 and 2 mm fall between the lower and upper estimates given in Table 10.4. Similarly, for patients 3 and 4, we used formulas (10.23) and (10.25) to compute β/γ and θ:

$$\frac{\beta}{\gamma} = \frac{\mu \log \frac{S}{N_0}}{1 - M^{-\mu}} \quad \text{and} \quad \theta = \frac{k(1 - M^{-\mu})}{\mu \log \frac{S}{N_0}}.$$

The lower and upper bounds for these quantities and for the limiting primary tumor volume $S(\infty)$ are also reported in Table 10.5.

Table 10.5: Estimates of clinically important quantities.
The table is reproduced from Hanin L, Jandrig B, Pavlova L, Seidel K. The natural history of renal cell carcinoma with pulmonary metastases illuminated through mathematical modeling. Math Biosci 2019, 309, 118–130.

Patient #	β/γ	θ	$S(\infty)$ (mm^3)
1	0.7112 (d = 1 mm)	0.6201 (d = 1 mm)	N/A
	0.6084 (d = 2 mm)	0.7248 (d = 2 mm)	
2	0.5923 (d = 1 mm)	1.8145 (d = 1 mm)	N/A
	0.4965 (d = 2 mm)	2.1648 (d = 2 mm)	
3	2.1690 (d = 1 mm)	1.3908 (d = 1 mm)	3,978,977 (d = 1 mm)
	1.8722 (d = 2 mm)	1.6113 (d = 2 mm)	3,641,706 (d = 2 mm)
4	9.8750 (d = 1 mm)	0.2584 (d = 1 mm)	33,811 (d = 1 mm)
	8.0209 (d = 2 mm)	0.3181 (d = 2 mm)	33,811 (d = 2 mm)

10.6 Biomedical conclusions

The presented model-based analysis of the four clear-cell RCC patients with pulmonary metastases detected at presentation leads to the following conclusions about the individual natural history of their disease:

1. The model suggests that the most likely scenario for all four patients is almost immediate inception of metastatic cells in the lungs. This means that, according to the model, the combined duration of the migration of metastatic cells from the kidney tumor to blood vessels or lymphatic channels, their free circulation, extravasation, migration within the lungs and single-cell dormancy was negligible compared to the duration of metastatic growth. This picture is consistent with the pattern of aggressive metastatic disease apparent in these clinical cases.
2. Recall that, for all four patients, the optimal value of parameter M, representing the theoretical upper limit for the volume of lung metastases achievable under the model, was equal to the largest volume of detected lung metastases. Combined with the optimality of the instantaneous seeding (IS) model, this means that in all likelihood inception of the largest metastasis in all four patients had occurred very soon after inception of the primary tumor. At that time, the latter had the diameter of about 1–2 mm and was therefore still undetectable. Thus, in accordance with the model, *early detection and surgical treatment of the primary tumor would not have prevented metastatic spread of RCC in all four patients analyzed.*
3. This leads to the following clinically important question: *How large was the largest lung metastasis when the primary tumor became detectable and was this metastasis itself detectable?* For the four RCC patients, the answer to the second question is decidedly negative. In fact, let's look at the patient with the fastest growing metastases in relation to primary tumor, i. e., patient 2 whose ratio β/γ was the smallest one with the estimated value 0.5923 for $d = 1$ mm and 0.4965 for $d = 2$ mm (see Table 10.5). Denote by Y the patient's age at which primary tumor became detectable,

then $N_0 \exp\{\beta(Y - T)\} = m$, so that $Y - T = [\log(m/N_0)]/\beta$. We are interested in the volume, v, of the largest metastasis at age Y. Recall that, under the likelihood-maximizing scenario, inception of such metastasis occurred at the age T of primary tumor inception. Therefore,

$$v = c\exp\{\gamma(Y - T)\} = c\exp\left\{\frac{\gamma}{\beta}\log\frac{m}{N_0}\right\} = c\left(\frac{m}{N_0}\right)^{\gamma/\beta}. \tag{10.33}$$

Apart from constants c, m, N_0, volume v depends on the *identifiable* parameter γ/β, whose values for the four patients are shown in Table 10.5. For patient 2, we find from (10.33) that $v = 0.0167\,\text{mm}^3$ for $d = 1\,\text{mm}$ and $v = 0.0012\,\text{mm}^3$ for $d = 2\,\text{mm}$. Clearly, such a microscopic metastasis is undetectable, and so are all other smaller metastases present at age Y. The same conclusion holds for the other patients as well. Thus, *early primary tumor detection would not have led to discovery of the metastatic disease.*

A similar computation would show that the volume, v_1, of the primary tumor at the time when the largest metastasis would have become detectable is given by the formula

$$v_1 = N_0\left(\frac{m}{c}\right)^{\beta/\gamma}.$$

For patient 2, this is somewhere between $8.8\,\text{cm}^3$ and $14.6\,\text{cm}^3$, and even larger for other patients, i. e., fairly late into the natural course of the disease.

4. Although primary kidney tumors in all four patients failed to completely suppress the growth of pulmonary metastases, they nevertheless could have retarded it. However, the extent of this effect, if present, varied. In fact, while the rate of growth of lung metastases in patients 3 and 4 was about 2–10 times smaller than the net (intrinsic) rate of growth of the primary renal tumor, lung metastases in patients 1 and 2 were growing about 1.4–2 times faster than the primary renal tumor (see Table 10.5). Interestingly, the putative suppressing effect was not proportional to the primary tumor size at diagnosis. In fact, by far the smallest primary kidney tumor in patient 4 had by far the largest metastatic growth suppression ratio β/γ.
5. Unlike the case $W > V$ exemplified by the breast cancer patient examined in Section 9.1, in the case $W = V$, the net (intrinsic) rates of growth of primary tumor and metastases as well as the patient's age, T, of primary tumor inception are inestimable from the volume of the primary tumor and site-specific volumes of metastases.
6. According to the model, the rate, $r(t) = \alpha\Phi^{\theta}(t)$, of metastases shedding off the primary tumor depends critically on parameter θ. Its estimated values, reported in Table 10.5, were found to be fairly large for all four patients, which implies that metastases-producing cells form a relatively fast growing subpopulation within the primary tumor. This is consistent with the fact that by (or about) the time of primary

tumor resection, all patients developed numerous pulmonary metastases. By contrast, for the breast cancer patient from Section 9.1 and 12 prostate cancer patients analyzed in [136], the estimated value of θ was very small, which points to the presence within the primary tumor of a relatively stable subpopulation of metastases-producing cells and thus indirectly validates the empirically proven existence of breast and prostate cancer stem cells [49, 184, 194, 50], compare with the discussion of this subject in Section 9.1. In the case of RCC, the existence of cancer stem cells remains uncertain [195, 196]. For a brief discussion of the subject of cancer stem cells (see Section 3.4).

7. Interestingly, and contrary to what one would expect, the number of detected lung metastases does not increase with θ. For example, the smallest value of θ occurred for patient 4, who developed the largest number, $n = 60$, of detectable lung metastases, to be compared with $n = 15$ for patient 2 with the highest estimated value of θ (see Table 10.5). This may be due to the dependence of the rate of generation of viable metastases on unknown patient-specific coefficients α and q inestimable from the type of data here considered. Another potentially relevant factor is patient-specific inhibition of metastatic growth by primary tumor that could have kept many metastases undetectable. Because the rate of growth, γ, of pulmonary metastases is inestimable, distinguishing between these two possibilities would require collection of a different type of data and formulation of a different model describing the distribution of such a data. One attractive, yet mathematically challenging, candidate would be longitudinal volumetric data on metastases, i. e., the number and volumes of lung metastases surveyed at two or more time points.
8. The assumed value of the Folkman's limiting diameter d for avascular tumors has only a moderate effect on the estimates of identifiable biological parameters β/γ and θ (see Table 10.5). For those patients whose primary tumor growth is best described by the Gompertz model (that is, for patients 3 and 4), the same is also true for the limiting volume, $S(\infty)$, of their primary kidney tumor.
9. To sum up the conclusions 1 and 6, the negligible duration of metastatic latency, combined with relatively large value of θ for all four patients, confirms a particularly aggressive phenotype of their metastatic cancer consistent with the clinical picture of their disease. In particular, this agrees with the presence of numerous lung metastases at, or about, the time of primary diagnosis and the fact that the largest among them have reached considerable size. Recall that the aggressive metastatic phenotype was partially built into the model through the assumptions of concurrency of vascularization and growth of metastases and that exponential metastatic growth kicks in at inception of single-cell metastases. This serves as a demonstration, albeit an implicit one, of the model's self-consistency.

10.7 Comments on the model's adequacy

An important question regarding the amount of trust one can put into these conclusions hinges on model adequacy and reliability of numerical procedures used for parameter estimation. The following four facts appear reassuring in this respect:

(a) Patient 3 was previously analyzed in [139], but the volumes of his pulmonary metastases were measured using a different method. This chapter, therefore, presents an independent statistical and numerical analysis of the modified data set for patient 3. Despite some divergence in quantitative estimates of model parameters, which can be attributed to the differences in the data and model assumptions, the qualitative conclusions from the two analyses are fairly similar. This serves as an indirect validation of the modeling approach and numerical methodology.

(b) Importantly, the model with likelihood-maximizing parameters produced an excellent fit to the data sets for all four patients, as evidenced by Figure 10.2 and the relatively small values of the Kantorovich distance (10.3) between the theoretical and empirical distributions of the volumes of lung metastases reported in Table 10.4. Furthermore, such fit was achieved in spite of the fact that optimal models experienced single or double degeneration (see Table 10.3). Note that the criterion of fit to the data is independent of likelihood maximization, for an inadequate model with likelihood-maximizing parameters may still fit the data poorly.

(c) Optimization of model parameters was done without any calibration. However, the estimated values of all identifiable biological variables fell into plausible ranges and were reasonably consistent among the patients analyzed. For example, the values of parameter $a = \beta\theta/\gamma$ in the two exponential cases (specifically, $a = 0.4410$ and $a = 1.0748$ for patients 1 and 2, respectively) and two Gompertz cases (specifically, $a = k\mu = 0.4130$ and $a = 2.2752$ for patients 3 and 4, respectively) all agree reasonably well with each other. The same consistency between the four patients was also observed for the minimum value of function L (see Table 10.4).

(d) The optimal model for patients 3 and 4 involved Gompertzian growth of the primary kidney tumor with the limiting tumor size $S(\infty) = N_0 \exp\{\beta/\lambda\}$, shown in Table 10.5. Recall that the ratio β/λ is estimable from the data (see formula (10.25)). This enables comparison between the limiting volume of the primary tumor with its observed volume and determination whether at the time of volumetric measurement the growth of the primary tumor was close to saturation. If true, this would corroborate the Gompertz model, while the opposite outcome would point to the possibility that the tumor could still be in the exponential phase of its growth. We found that the ratio of the observed primary tumor volume to the limiting volume was 52–57 %, depending on the assumed value of d, for patient 3 and about 100 % for patient 4. Thus, in both cases, the primary tumor has passed the inflexion point and was well into the saturation phase of its growth (recall from Section 7.3 that Gompertz growth transitions into the saturation phase when the population reaches about 37 % of its limiting size). This serves as an evidence of self-consistency of the Gompertz growth model employed in the foregoing analysis.

10.8 Concluding remarks

This chapter showcased the ability of the phenomenological model developed in Sections 8.1 and 10.2 to generate clinically significant knowledge about unobservable aspects of the natural history of cancer and the effects of treatment in an individual patient (see Section 10.6). Discovered in the process was a surprising utility of the volumes of metastases detected in a single secondary site, such as the lungs, augmented with the volume of the primary tumor at diagnosis or surgery. Two key factors enabled partial reconstruction of the individual natural history of cancer. The first is availability of a closed-form expression for the distribution underlying site-specific sizes of metastases derived through a very general model of metastatic cancer progression under minimal biological and mathematical assumptions (see Sections 8.1 and 8.2). The second is a parsimonious parameterization of the general model based on the assumptions of exponential or Gompertz growth of the primary tumor, power law (9.1) for the rate of seeding of metastases by the primary tumor, exponentially distributed metastases latency times and exponential growth of metastases. Although five model parameters are not fully identifiable from the aforementioned data, their four simple combinations are, and they proved to be informative enough to lead to important biomedical insight.

I close with a few remarks and conclusions related to the methodology and the results of this chapter:

1. The general formula (10.2) for the distribution underlying site-specific sizes of metastases opens up a possibility of exploring a variety of growth laws for primary tumor and metastases, parametric forms for the dependence of metastasis shedding intensity on the size of the primary tumor and distributional forms for the duration of metastatic latency. The results and computational experience suggest that the model should be kept as parsimonious as possible because: (1) the number of identifiable model parameters can be much smaller than the total number of biological parameters; and (2) due to the presence of multiple local extrema of the likelihood function or another criterion used for parameter estimation, its potential flatness around the point of global extremum, and the fact that some functions involved in the model can take extremely small or extremely large values, the increase in model complexity could greatly complicate parameter estimation.
2. Within the model explored in this chapter, neither the patient's age at inception of the primary tumor or of any among the detected metastases nor quantitative characteristics of the growth of the primary tumor and metastases are estimable from the data. However, various quantities that relate the primary tumor and detected metastases to each other, such as the volume of such a metastasis at the time when

the primary tumor reached a detectable size, depend on identifiable parameters alone and thus are computable (see Section 10.6).

3. In all four RCC patients analyzed in this chapter, inception of the largest metastases had occurred long before primary tumor became clinically detectable. Thus, these patients fall into the ambit of the Fisher effect (see Section 4.1). This calls into question applicability to RCC, and thereby the universality, of the following three cornerstones of contemporary oncology: (1) the conventional system of cancer staging; (2) emphasis on early cancer detection and treatment; and (3) the prominent role of surgery as the first line cancer treatment. Combined with the Ehrlich effect (see Section 4.3) and the phenomenon of surgery-induced acceleration of metastasis described in Sections 5.2 and 5.3 and confirmed mathematically in Section 9.2, this lends support to the notion that certain categories of patients with clear-cell RCC should be treated systemically from the outset.
4. Identifiable parameters of the model of individual natural history of cancer designed in this chapter depend on the assumed initial volume N_0 of the primary tumor and metastases at inception. This makes its accurate determination for various types of cancer and metastatic sites a worthwhile endeavor.
5. Plumbing even greater depths of the individual natural history of cancer may become possible with an expanded set of observables. Two possibilities for such an expansion naturally come to mind. The first is collecting longitudinal data on site-specific volumes of metastases at multiple time points. The second is measuring volumes of metastases at multiple secondary sites. Because mathematical models seeking to describe such data share parameters accounting for primary tumor growth and shedding of metastases, the results of such data analyses can be compared with each other and with those obtained for a single metastatic site and single volumetric measurement.

11 How synergistic interaction between mathematics and biology leads to new actionable knowledge of cancer: an example

What is the key to successful mathematical modeling of biomedical processes, where "successful" means leading to important insights, translational knowledge and useful clinical recommendations? As I argued in Chapter 6, it is certainly not the amount of detail built into the model because very detailed models require many explicit or tacit assumptions that may or may not hold in a particular setting and may be empirically untestable. Additionally, such detailed models are very rarely solvable in closed form, which complicates their theoretical analysis. Finally, they depend on numerous unknown parameters causing a researcher to face a difficult dilemma: either prove general results about model behavior that are true for all admissible values of parameters or estimate all the parameters from observations; both options are only rarely feasible.

In this chapter, I focus on the effects of tumor shrinkage on cancer recurrence as an example highlighting three key ingredients of successful mathematical modeling: (1) selecting a biomedical question that allows for a definitive mathematical answer, (2) a synergistic combination of biological and mathematical arguments, and (3) sufficient generality of the mathematical models enabling them to cover a wide range of biomedical possibilities.

This chapter borrowed many ideas and technical results from my article [105].

11.1 Why does cancer often come back with a vengeance?

Published clinical case studies, popular literature on cancer and our personal experience are replete with stories like the following one. A cancer patient undergoes treatment, as a result of which his or her tumor shrinks to an undetectable size and seemingly disappears. Treating oncologists call it a day, declare the patient cancer-free and celebrate him or her as cancer survivor. The celebration, however, proves to be short-lived—in a few months cancer returns with a vengeance. What are the root causes of such an unfortunate outcome? Is this just a strike of bad luck or are there systematic biological reasons behind the ubiquity of the described scenario?

In the grand scheme of things, there are three potential outcomes of cancer treatment:

(a) cure, where cancer is eradicated for all practical purposes;
(b) induction of a stable disease due to a number of nonmutually exclusive mechanisms, such as reaching an equilibrium between cancer cell proliferation and death, competition between cancer and normal cells, resistance of the tumor microenvironment, suppression of tumor growth by the immune system and the dominance

https://doi.org/10.1515/9783111334035-014

of angiogenesis inhibitors over angiogenesis promoters that arrests the tumor in the avascular phase of saturated growth and precludes its spread to distant sites;
(c) treatment failure manifesting in aggressive tumor regrowth and metastasis.

This chapter is mostly focused on the last, and most unfavorable, scenario.

Central to the explanation of aggressive tumor relapse presented here is the heterogeneity of cancer cells, discussed in detail in Section 3.4. One of its many aspects is substantial differences in proliferation rates between various subpopulations of cancer cells forming a residual tumor. As a reminder from Section 7.2, what is meant by the proliferation rate in a homogeneous cell population, is the *net* proliferation rate, i. e., the difference between the rate of cell division (also called the birth rate) and the rate of cell death from all sources (apoptosis, necrosis and autophagy). The resulting net proliferation rate is an outcome of a complex interplay between intrinsic factors, such as functioning of the intracellular molecular and genomic machinery, and external factors, including microenvironmental and systemic interactions.

Some of the factors that most immediately affect proliferative behavior of cancer cells are:
(1) heritable "intrinsic" rates of cell proliferation and death;
(2) competition with other cancer and normal cells for space, nutrients, oxygen, growth factors and other vital resources;
(3) beneficial interactions with other cells and the tumor microenvironment;
(4) interaction with the immune system and acquisition of immune-system evasion capabilities;
(5) spatial position within the cell population. For example, a cell surrounded by other cells receives from them contact inhibition signals that block cell division;
(6) the ability of a cell to migrate, called *motility*;
(7) proximity to blood vessels, which may bestow on cancer cells additional survival and proliferative advantages; and
(8) efficiency in the use of the existing vasculature and induction of neoangiogenesis.

As was described in Section 3.4, when internal and external conditions are unfavorable for cell growth, cycling and division, a cell may become *quiescent*, i. e., enter G_0, the resting phase of the cell cycle, in which it can reside indefinitely. Such cells do not contribute to the net proliferation rate. Because the duration of an uninterrupted cell cycle can only change within narrow limits, an increase in the net proliferation rate of a cell population is mostly due to a decrease in the rate of cell death. Another, and possibly concurrent, reason for such an increase is enhanced asymmetric, and occasionally symmetric, division of cancer stem cells (again, see Section 3.4).

Due to toxicity, unfavorable side effects and the development of resistance (see Section 5.5), every protracted cancer treatment must end or take a break. The treatment leaves in its wake a void formerly occupied by eliminated cancer cells. There are many biological reasons why some cancer cells in a given location may have survived the treatment. For example, some of them may have preexisting or acquired mutations that confer resistance to a particular anticancer agent. In particular, they may owe their survival to a well-developed capability of transporting the agent (e. g., cytotoxic chemotherapy drug) across the cell membrane. Yet another category of cancer cells might have persisted because their spatial position made them inaccessible to the agent or caused them to receive a nonlethal dose.

The overall goal of this chapter is to present a detailed discussion and quantitative analysis of the following phenomenon, which I believe is of paramount importance in cancer treatment. As surviving residual cancer cells fill the void left at the end of treatment or the beginning of a treatment break, *a regrowing tumor will be progressively dominated by increasingly faster proliferating cancer cells*, provided that their fitness is superior, or at least comparable, to that of slower proliferating cancer cells. The emergence and self-selection of subpopulations of increasingly faster proliferating cancer cells is a universally occurring evolutionary process rooted in two basic properties of cancer cells—their heterogeneity and insensitivity to internal and external signals regulating cell cycle, cell division and apoptosis.

I have always regarded this phenomenon as almost self-evident, somewhat akin to the principle of Darwinian selection, and have briefly mentioned it in [158]. Surprisingly, I have never seen it discussed in the literature on cancer. However, it should be mentioned that as an empirical fact, the phenomenon of treatment-induced accelerated tumor repopulation in radiation therapy was recognized long ago [197–199].

Even acting alone, progressive enrichment of a regrowing residual primary or secondary tumor with faster proliferating cells may bring about or accelerate treatment failure, thus reducing patients' disease-free, recurrence-free and overall survival. In reality, however, it acts in concert with other sources of resistance to treatment exacerbating their effects.

It is therefore imperative to identify mechanisms producing faster proliferating cancer cells. Three among them stand out as likely the most significant ones:

(i) Every efficacious protracted local or systemic treatment results in a decrease in cancer cell density, which leads to a greater per cell supply of space, oxygen, nutrients and growth factors as well as diminished competition between surviving cancer cells for these resources. This brings about a drop in death rates of cancer cells.
(ii) One of the hallmarks of cancer cells is their genomic instability, which causes spontaneous emergence of aberrant malignant clones with heritable higher net proliferation rates;
(iii) Due to random biological variation, net proliferation rates of daughter cells may occasionally be higher than those of mother cells.

While mechanism (i) is unidirectional, mechanisms (ii) and (iii) may lead to the emergence of either faster or slower proliferating cells. However, the aforementioned enrichment of the surviving cancer cell population with faster proliferating cells will bring about a gradual overall increase in net proliferation rates within the residual tumor.

11.2 Treatment-induced tumor shrinkage and long-term survival of cancer patients: a consensus rooted in misconception

Comparison of various treatments or the responses of different patients to the same treatment is based on measures of the effect, also termed *endpoints*. One commonly used endpoint is the overall survival, i. e., the duration of a patient's residual lifetime after the end of treatment. Another useful endpoint is recurrence-free survival, i. e., the post-treatment time until cancer recurrence, detected through a medical exam or due to the onset of symptoms. In this chapter, I will also utilize an endpoint defined as the occurrence of the event that a regrowing tumor reaches its pretreatment size, which signifies treatment failure.

A quantitative measure ostensibly predictive of treatment success and widely used in clinical practice for assessment of the results of treatment and planning subsequent interventions is the *tumor-shrinkage factor*, denoted by k. Although its measurement is based, according to the RECIST guidelines [200], on linear dimensions of the tumor, in this chapter I will adopt a simpler and biologically more relevant definition of the tumor-shrinkage factor—the ratio of the posttreatment size of a tumor to its pretreatment size (as a reminder, the size of a cell population is the number of cells). Equivalently, the tumor shrinkage factor can be defined as the ratio of the respective tumor volumes. Note that $0 < k < 1$ and that *smaller* values of k correspond to *greater* extent of tumor shrinkage.

Tumor shrinkage is a convenient surrogate for more biologically meaningful endpoints. In clinical trials of anticancer drugs and other interventions, instead of waiting many months or years until the effect of a treatment on a patient's overall or recurrence-free survival manifests [201], treatments are often evaluated and compared on the basis of tumor shrinkage, which can be readily measured at, or soon after, the end of treatment. For example, one of the reasons (and, in many cases, the sole reason) for regular or accelerated FDA approval granted to the majority (41 out of 71 or 58 %) of oncology drug applications from 1990 through 2002 was "complete or partial response" to treatment. These categories of responses are defined using the following surprisingly lax criteria: Complete response is "*complete disappearance of all tumor and all manifestations of tumor for at least 1 month*", while partial response is "*a 50 % decrease from baseline in the sum of the cross-products of all bidimensionally measurable tumors lasting at least 1 month*" [202].

There is an almost universal agreement among cancer biologists and oncologists that greater tumor shrinkage at the end of treatment or a treatment cycle leads to longer overall and recurrence-free survival of cancer patients. The reason for this conclusion, illustrated in Figure 11.1, looks very convincing. In fact, the smaller the tumor size at the

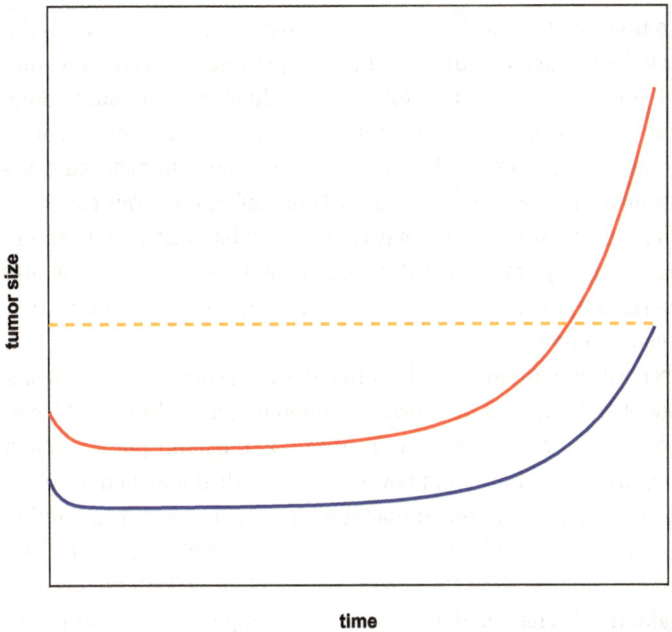

Figure 11.1: Illustration of the widely accepted notion that greater tumor shrinkage at the end of treatment leads to longer survival of cancer patients. Red and blue solid curves describe the dynamics of a residual tumor for two different shrinkage factors according to the same growth law. Dashed line represents a tumor size threshold for a given survival outcome. Notice that greater extent of tumor shrinkage leads to longer survival. The growth curves and the threshold line are not drawn to scale. For further explanation, see Section 11.2.

end of treatment, the deeper the nadir point reached by the size of the residual tumor after the clearance of tumor debris and completion of transient processes of inactivation and recovery of damaged cancer and normal cells and, therefore, the longer the time it will take a regrowing tumor to reach a certain size threshold used to define a specific survival endpoint. This argument, however, rests on an hidden assumption that the dynamics of posttreatment tumor growth is independent of the tumor-shrinkage factor. In the following, we explore this dependence and identify biological and mathematical conditions under which greater tumor shrinkage leads, paradoxically, to a more aggressive growth of the residual tumor. Under these conditions, the exact opposite of the aforementioned consensus belief is true, i. e., that greater tumor shrinkage leads to a shorter patient's survival.

11.3 Problem formulation, basic assumptions and notation

As was explained earlier, progressive enrichment of a regrowing residual tumor with faster proliferating cancer cells is a likely posttreatment scenario. My principal specific aim in this chapter is to investigate how the enrichment phenomenon depends on the tumor-shrinkage factor k. To characterize this dependence quantitatively, I assume that the surviving cancer cell population consists of finitely many homogeneous subpopulations, each evolving independently of other subpopulations according to its own growth law. Some of them may contain cancer cells that are sensitive to the administered treatment; most of these cells have already been eliminated. Other subpopulations comprise resistant cells. Additionally, the residual tumor may contain a stable subpopulation consisting of quiescent cells and/or asymmetrically dividing cancer stem cells. All these subpopulations are characterized by their fractional sizes, or weights, relative to the current total size of the cancer cell population.

Letting N_0 be the pretreatment tumor size, the initial size of the posttreatment residual tumor is kN_0. Denote by p the weight of a certain subpopulation at the end of treatment or the beginning of a treatment break (more precisely, at the nadir point reached shortly thereafter (see Figure 11.1), which from now on won't be distinguished from the end of treatment). Then the initial size of this subpopulation is kpN_0. I will be assuming in what follows that p is independent of k. Denote by $r(t)$ the weight of the fastest growing subpopulation at time t, counted from the end of treatment or a treatment cycle. It will be assumed throughout this chapter that it is *the same* subpopulation that grows faster than other subpopulations for all times $t \geq 0$ of interest. Denote by T the time when the size of the regrowing tumor reaches a certain threshold μN_0, where $\mu > k$ is a preselected coefficient (for example, reaching this threshold with $\mu = 1$ signals treatment failure). Finally, we set $r = r(T)$. To emphasize the dependence of r on k for a fixed μ, I will also write $r = r(k)$.

The next two sections will zero in on the case where the *fastest growing subpopulation* forming the residual tumor expands exponentially (see Section 7.2):

$$n(t) = n_0 e^{\lambda t}, \tag{11.1}$$

where $n(t)$ is the size of this subpopulation at time t, $n_0 = n(0)$ is its initial size and $\lambda > 0$ is the growth rate. The biological mechanism (i) discussed at the end of Section 11.1 suggests that greater tumor shrinkage may cause an increase in λ (or, in other words, that λ may be a decreasing function of k). Also, due to mechanisms (ii) and (iii), λ may also be an increasing function of time. These dependencies are very complex and hard to model on either mechanistic or phenomenological grounds. Therefore, in what follows it will be assumed that growth rate λ is *fixed* (and similar assumptions will be made regarding more sophisticated growth laws employed later in this chapter). Importantly, however, in every case where it will be found that the weight of the fastest growing subpopulation with a fixed growth rate is a decreasing function of k, thus implying shorter patient survival, *even shorter survival would be expected should the growth rate of this subpopulation increase with time and/or the extent of tumor shrinkage.*

A specific research question to be dealt with below is as follows:

– *How does r depend on the tumor-shrinkage factor k?*

In particular,

– *Under what conditions is r a decreasing function of k?*

If such conditions are met, then greater tumor shrinkage at the end of treatment would lead to a larger fractional size of the fastest growing subpopulation of the residual tumor at a specific time point of interest and, accordingly, to shorter patient's survival.

11.4 A proof of principle

To see that greater tumor shrinkage may favor the enrichment of the residual tumor with faster proliferating cells, consider the following simple schematic example. Suppose a surviving cancer cell population consists of a stable subpopulation of constant size and two exponentially growing subpopulations with net growth rates λ and 2λ for some unspecified $\lambda > 0$. Denote by p and q, where $0 < p, q < 1$ and $p + q < 1$, the respective weights of the subpopulation growing at the rate 2λ and the stable subpopulation at the end of treatment, then the initial weight of the other growing subpopulation is $1 - p - q$.

The total size of the residual tumor equals the sum of sizes of all its constituent subpopulations. Then, for the time T when the regrowing tumor will reach a given threshold size μN_0 with $\mu > k$, we have

$$kpN_0e^{2\lambda T} + k(1 - p - q)N_0e^{\lambda T} + kqN_0 = \mu N_0 \tag{11.2}$$

or equivalently, in terms of $x = e^{\lambda T}$,

$$kpx^2 + k(1 - p - q)x + kq - \mu = 0.$$

This equation can be expressed through independent parameters p, q and $a = k/\mu$, where $0 < a < 1$, as follows:

$$apx^2 + a(1 - p - q)x + aq - 1 = 0. \tag{11.3}$$

Solving the quadratic equation (11.3) for its positive root x, we find after a quick algebraic manipulation that

$$x = \frac{2(1 - aq)}{\sqrt{a^2(1 - p - q)^2 + 4ap(1 - aq)} + a(1 - p - q)}. \tag{11.4}$$

At the time T determined by equation (11.2), the weight, r, of the fastest growing subpopulation is $kpN_0e^{2\lambda T}/(\mu N_0) = apx^2$, and in view of (11.3) and (11.4), we find, again after some algebra, that

$$r = 1 - aq - a(1-p-q)x = (1-aq)\frac{\sqrt{1+\theta}-1}{\sqrt{1+\theta}+1}, \tag{11.5}$$

where

$$\theta = \frac{4p(1-aq)}{a(1-p-q)^2}. \tag{11.6}$$

Consider, in particular, the simplest case of a balanced residual cancer population without a stable subpopulation ($p = 0.5$, $q = 0$) with $\mu = 1$ so that $a = k$ (i. e., take a snapshot of the residual tumor at the time when it reaches the pretreatment tumor size). Then $\theta = 8/k$ and

$$r = \frac{\sqrt{1+8/k}-1}{\sqrt{1+8/k}+1}.$$

We now draw a few conclusions from formulas (11.5) and (11.6).

1. Surprisingly, for any given shrinkage coefficient k and threshold parameter $\mu > k$, the weight r of the fastest growing subpopulation at time T when the regrowing tumor reaches a threshold size μN_0 is independent of λ.
2. For fixed initial weights p and q, the weight r is a function of the ratio $a = k/\mu$ alone.
3. Notice that

$$G(\theta) = \frac{\sqrt{1+\theta}-1}{\sqrt{1+\theta}+1} \tag{11.7}$$

(see (11.5)) is an increasing function of θ, while θ given by (11.6) is a decreasing function of $a = k/\mu$. Therefore, for any fixed k, the weight r given by (11.5) is an increasing function of μ for $\mu > k$ or equivalently an increasing function of time T. In particular, since at time $t = 0$ we have $\mu = k$ and $r = p$, we conclude that $r > p$ for every coefficient $\mu > k$. This confirms our earlier biological intuition about the enrichment effect: *The fractional size of the fastest growing subpopulation of the residual tumor increases with time.*
4. It follows from the monotonicity analysis that, for any fixed μ, the weight r is a decreasing function of $k < \mu$. In other words, *greater tumor shrinkage leads to more extensive enrichment of the residual tumor with the fastest proliferating cancer cells.* Heuristically, this is not entirely surprising because greater tumor shrinkage leaves more room for the growth of the residual tumor and provides its fastest growing subpopulation an opportunity to progressively outgrow other subpopulations.
5. Is there any limit to this progressive enrichment? From formula (11.6), $\theta \to \infty$ as $a \to 0$, while in view of formula (11.7) $G(\theta) \to 1$ as $\theta \to \infty$. Therefore, (11.5) implies $r \to 1$ as $k \to 0$ for any given μ. Thus, in the case at issue, we reached the following important conclusion: *The greater the extent of tumor shrinkage, the closer the fastest growing subpopulation comes to completely dominating the residual tumor.*

I now illustrate the dependence of r on k in the case $\mu = 1$. How r depends on k for $p = 0.5$ and $q = 0,\ 0.1,\ 0.2,\ 0.4$ is shown graphically in Figure 11.2 (middle panel). For comparison, Figures 11.2 also shows this dependence for $p = 0.25$, $p = 0.75$ and the cited values of q subject to the condition $p + q < 1$. Figure 11.2 displays a qualitatively similar pattern of the dependence of r on k for different values of q and clearly demonstrates that $r \to 1$ as $k \to 0$.

The latter conclusion is a culmination of our analysis of the particular case investigated in this section. This invites two further questions:

(a) *Does the same effect hold for more general patterns of posttreatment tumor dynamics?*

(b) *What are the biological conditions underpinning this effect?*

These questions will be addressed below in Sections 11.5–11.7.

11.5 Exponentially growing subpopulations with arbitrary growth rates

Suppose the residual tumor consists of a stable subpopulation with a weight q and $n \geq 2$ exponentially growing subpopulations with net growth rates $0 < \lambda_1 < \lambda_2 < \cdots < \lambda_n$ and the initial posttreatment weights $p_1, p_2, \ldots, p_n > 0$ such that $q + p_1 + p_2 + \cdots + p_n = 1$. As before, I assume that the growth rates $\lambda_1, \lambda_2, \ldots, \lambda_n$ and the initial subpopulation weights $p_1, p_2, \ldots, p_n$ are independent of the shrinkage factor k. Our goal is to demonstrate that the just-described effects of tumor shrinkage on the enrichment of the surviving cancer cell population with the fastest proliferating cells hold in this more general case.

Similar to equation (11.2), we have

$$kN_0 q + \sum_{j=1}^{n} kN_0 p_j e^{\lambda_j T} = \mu N_0.$$

Equivalently, setting $x = e^{\lambda_n T}$ and $\gamma_j = \lambda_j/\lambda_n$, $1 \leq j \leq n$, this equation can be represented in the form

$$q + \sum_{j=1}^{n} p_j x^{\gamma_j} = \frac{\mu}{k}. \tag{11.8}$$

Observe that $\gamma_n = 1$ and $0 < \gamma_j < 1$ for $1 \leq j \leq n - 1$. It follows from (11.8) that for any fixed $\mu > 0$, we have $x \to \infty$ as $k \to 0$.

Differentiating (11.8) implicitly in k and solving for dx/dk we find that

$$\frac{dx}{dk} = -\frac{\mu}{k^2 \sum_{j=1}^{n} p_j \gamma_j x^{\gamma_j - 1}} < 0. \tag{11.9}$$

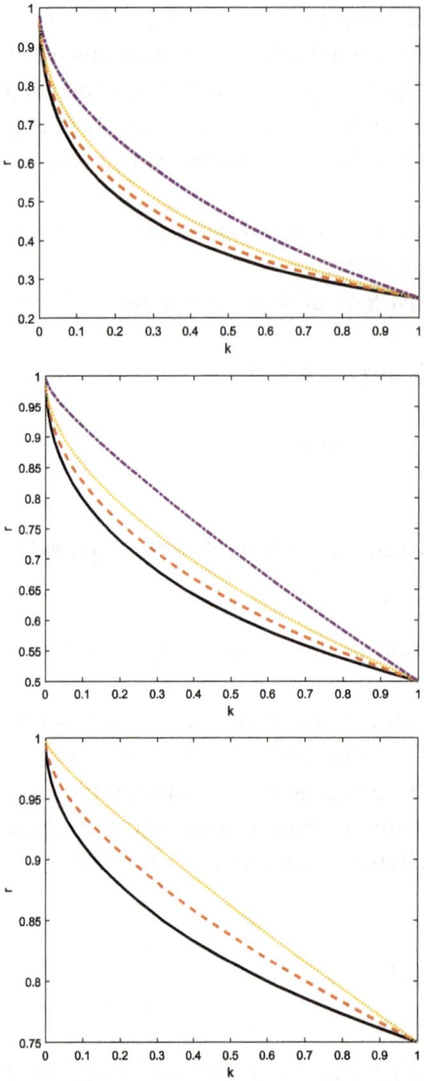

Figure 11.2: The weight **r** of the faster growing subpopulation as a function of tumor shrinkage factor **k** in the case of exponential growth kinetics. The weight r was computed through formulas (11.5) and (11.6) at the time when a regrowing tumor reached its pretreatment size. The residual tumor was assumed to consist of a quiescent subpopulation with weight q and two subpopulations growing exponentially with unspecified net rates λ and 2λ. The following values for the initial post-treatment weight p were assumed in Figure 11.2: p = 0.25 (upper panel), p = 0.5 (middle panel) and p = 0.75 (lower panel). The values adopted for q, assuming $q < 1 - p$, were $q = 0$ (solid line), $q = 0.1$ (dashed line), $q = 0.2$ (dotted line) and $q = 0.4$ (dashed-dotted line). See Section 11.4 for more details.
The figure was reproduced with permission from Hanin L. Paradoxical effects of tumor shrinkage on long-term survival of cancer patients. Front Appl Math Stat 2020, 6, 27.

The weight, r, of the fastest growing subpopulation at time T is given by

$$r = \frac{p_n x}{q + \sum_{j=1}^{n} p_j x^{\gamma_j}}. \tag{11.10}$$

Therefore,

$$\frac{dr}{dx} = p_n \frac{q + \sum_{j=1}^{n-1} p_j (1-\gamma_j) x^{\gamma_j}}{(q + \sum_{j=1}^{n} p_j x^{\gamma_j})^2} > 0. \tag{11.11}$$

Combining the inequalities in (11.9) and (11.11), we conclude that r is a decreasing function of k for any fixed value of μ. Also, it follows from (11.10) that r approaches 1 as $k \to 0$.

Thus, the main conclusions (see items 4 and 5 in the previous section) hold for any number of exponentially growing subpopulations forming a residual tumor.

11.6 A three-compartmental clonal growth model

As the reader recalls from Section 7.2, the exponential growth law (see formula (11.1)), can be derived mathematically from the assumption that cells in a population proliferate and die independently of each other at constant rates. I now introduce a more general growth pattern where, as before, larger tumor shrinkage leads, barring complete tumor ablation or induction of a stable disease, to greater enrichment of the residual tumor with faster proliferating cancer cells. The principal assumption here is that *proliferating clones generated by cancer cells present at the end of treatment or the start of a treatment break do not interact with each other*. By contrast, arbitrary interactions are allowed between cancer cells *within* the same clone.

Specifically, I assume that along with a subpopulation of quiescent cells the residual tumor contains two subpopulations of growing clones—one where clones expand according to a growth law $f(t)$ and another one where clones follow a growth law of the form $g(t) = f(t)h[f(t)]$, where f and h are increasing differentiable functions such that $f(0) = 1$ and $h(1) = 1$. The latter two conditions reflect the fact that each clone starts from a single initiator cell. Additionally, suppose that $\lim_{x\to\infty} h(x) = \infty$ (or in shorthand, $h(\infty) = \infty$). This implies that the second subpopulation grows "much faster" than the first one. Importantly, functions f and h are assumed to be independent of the shrinkage factor k.

This general model can be illustrated with the following three simple and widely used particular examples of growth laws f and g:

A. *Exponential* growth laws, where $f(t) = e^{\lambda t}$ and $g(t) = e^{\gamma\lambda t}$ with $\lambda > 0$ and $\gamma > 1$. Here, $h(x) = x^{\gamma-1}$. The case $\gamma = 2$ was considered in Section 11.4.

B. *Gompertz* growth laws (see Section 7.3), where

$$f(t) = \exp\left\{\frac{\lambda}{\beta}(1 - e^{-\beta t})\right\} \tag{11.12}$$

and

$$g(t) = \exp\left\{\frac{\gamma\lambda}{\beta}(1 - e^{-\beta t})\right\}$$

with $\lambda, \beta > 0$ and $\gamma > 1$. Here again, $h(x) = x^{\gamma-1}$. As was discussed in Section 7.3, coefficients λ and $\gamma\lambda$ represent the intrinsic net per cell growth rates of the clones within the two respective subpopulations, while coefficient $\beta > 0$, assumed the same for both subpopulations, is the growth inhibition coefficient.

C. *Power* growth laws of the form $f(t) = (1 + ct)^a$ and $g(t) = (1 + ct)^b$ with $a, c > 0$ and $b > a$, in which case $h(x) = x^{b/a-1}$. The power law was first used to describe tumor growth in the 1960s [203]; for more recent applications of this law, see [161, 162].

I now proceed to analyze, using the three-compartmental model of independently growing clones formulated here, how the weight of the faster growing subpopulation depends on the shrinkage factor k.

The size of each growing subpopulation follows the clonal growth formula (7.2). Therefore, similar to equation (11.2),

$$kpN_0 g(T) + k(1 - p - q)N_0 f(T) + kqN_0 = \mu N_0, \tag{11.13}$$

where, as before, $\mu > k$ is a *fixed* fractional threshold tumor size attained at a certain time T, while $p, 1 - p - q, q$ are the weights of the three respective subpopulations at the end of treatment. Setting $x = f(T)$ in (11.13) yields

$$apxh(x) + a(1 - p - q)x + aq - 1 = 0, \tag{11.14}$$

compare with (11.3), where, as before, $a = k/\mu$. Note that according to the assumptions on function f, we have $x \geq 1$.

Denote by $\Phi : [1, \infty) \to \mathbb{R}$ the left-hand side of (11.14) viewed as a function of x. It follows from our assumptions that Φ is an increasing function, $\Phi(1) = a - 1 < 0$ and $\Phi(\infty) = \infty$. Therefore, equation (11.14) has a unique solution $x = x(a)$. Differentiating this equation in a and taking into account our assumptions that the weights p, q and function h are independent of k, we obtain

$$pxh(x) + ap\left[h(x) + xh'(x)\right]\frac{dx}{da} + (1 - p - q)x + a(1 - p - q)\frac{dx}{da} + q = 0.$$

Solving this equation for dx/da yields

$$\frac{dx}{da} = -\frac{x[ph(x) + 1 - p - q] + q}{a[ph(x) + pxh'(x) + 1 - p - q]}. \tag{11.15}$$

In view of (11.13) and (11.14), the weight, $r = r(a)$, of the faster growing subpopulation at time T is given by $r = apxh(x) = 1 - aq - a(1 - p - q)x$. Then

$$\frac{dr}{da} = -\left[q + (1 - p - q)\left(x + a\frac{dx}{da}\right)\right].$$

Substituting dx/da with the expression from (11.15) and simplifying the resulting formula, we finally obtain

$$\frac{dr}{da} = -p\,\frac{q[h(x) + xh'(x)] + (1 - p - q)x^2h'(x)}{p[h(x) + xh'(x)] + 1 - p - q} < 0.$$

Therefore, for a fixed μ, we also have $dr/dk < 0$, which means that r is a decreasing function of k.

I now aim to identify the limiting behavior of r as $k \to 0$. In this case, $a \to 0$ as well and therefore, in view of (11.14), $x \to \infty$. From (11.13),

$$r = \frac{kpN_0g(T)}{kpN_0g(T) + k(1 - p - q)N_0f(T) + kqN_0} = \frac{pxh(x)}{pxh(x) + (1 - p - q)x + q},$$

which implies, due to the assumption $h(\infty) = \infty$, that $r \to 1$. Thus, under the general three-compartmental model of independent clonal growth, the progressive enrichment of the residual tumor with faster proliferating cancer cells is qualitatively the same as for exponentially growing subpopulations discussed in Sections 11.4 and 11.5.

11.7 Expansion of interacting clones: Gompertzian growth

I now turn to analyzing the effects of tumor shrinkage on the weight of the fastest growing subpopulation in a more general setting, where cell interaction in a cancer cell population is allowed to happen not only within the clones generated by initiator cells present at the end of treatment or the start of a treatment break but also *between* the clones within the same homogeneous subpopulation. One of the most popular growth laws allowing for such interactions is the Gompertz law (see Section 7.3).

Consider a cell population growing according to the Gompertz law. The reader is reminded that the size, $y(t)$, of such a population satisfies the following ODE:

$$y' = \lambda y - \beta y \log y, \quad y(0) = N_0. \tag{11.16}$$

Here, as before, $\lambda > 0$ represents the intrinsic net per cell proliferation rate, and $\beta > 0$ is the growth inhibition coefficient. Recall that the solution to equation (11.16) has the form

$$y(t) = N_0^{\exp\{-\beta t\}} \exp\left\{\frac{\lambda}{\beta}(1 - \exp\{-\beta t\})\right\}, \tag{11.17}$$

compare with formula (11.12) corresponding to the case $N_0 = 1$. The limiting size of the population as $t \to \infty$ is $K = \exp\{\lambda/\beta\}$. The Gompertz growth law (11.17) can alternatively be represented through parameters K and β (see Section 7.3) as

$$y(t) = K\left(\frac{N_0}{K}\right)^{\exp\{-\beta t\}}. \tag{11.18}$$

Our assumptions are as follows. Suppose the residual tumor consists of two non-interacting subpopulations, S_1 and S_2, whose growth is governed by Gompertz laws with respective kinetic parameters λ_1, β and λ_2, β with $\lambda_2 > \lambda_1$, so that S_2 grows faster than S_1 in the sense that for the same subpopulation size, the rate of growth of S_2 is larger than that of S_1 (see (11.16)). As before, let p denote the weight of the faster growing subpopulation at the end of treatment (cycle) and

$$K_1 = \exp\left\{\frac{\lambda_1}{\beta}\right\}, \quad K_2 = \exp\left\{\frac{\lambda_2}{\beta}\right\}$$

be the respective carrying capacities. We assume that there is no stable subpopulation.

For the time T, when the total population reaches a given size M, where $kN_0 < M < K_1 + K_2$, set

$$z = \exp\{-\beta T\}. \tag{11.19}$$

Using formula (11.17), we obtain

$$[k(1-p)N_0]^z \exp\left\{\frac{\lambda_1}{\beta}(1-z)\right\} + (kpN_0)^z \exp\left\{\frac{\lambda_2}{\beta}(1-z)\right\} = M$$

or equivalently

$$K_1\left[\frac{k(1-p)N_0}{K_1}\right]^z + K_2\left(\frac{kpN_0}{K_2}\right)^z = M. \tag{11.20}$$

Therefore, the time T entering this equation through relationship (11.19) is a decreasing function of the tumor-shrinkage coefficient k.

Denote by y_1 and y_2 the respective sizes of subpopulations S_1 and S_2 at time T. Notice that the weight, $r(k) = y_2/M = y_2/(y_1 + y_2)$, of subpopulation S_2 has the same pattern of monotonicity in k as the ratio y_2/y_1. Moreover, the same is also true for the ratio u_2/u_1 of the subpopulation sizes scaled to their carrying capacities, where, from (11.18) and (11.19),

$$\frac{u_2}{u_1} = \left[\frac{\frac{kN_0 p}{K_2}}{\frac{kN_0(1-p)}{K_1}}\right]^z = \left(\frac{\frac{p}{K_2}}{\frac{1-p}{K_1}}\right)^z. \tag{11.21}$$

Interestingly, the ratio u_2/u_1 depends on k only through variable z (or equivalently, time T).

This leads to the following conclusions. If at the end of treatment (cycle), subpopulation S_2 had a larger weight relative to its carrying capacity, i. e., if

$$\frac{p}{K_2} > \frac{1-p}{K_1}, \tag{11.22}$$

then (11.21) implies that, under the stated assumptions, for any admissible threshold, M, for the total population size and any pretreatment tumor size N_0, greater tumor shrinkage followed by tumor repopulation will favor expansion of the slower growing subpopulation S_1. Conversely, if at the end of treatment, subpopulation S_1 constituted a larger fraction of the residual tumor, relative to its carrying capacity, than the faster growing subpopulation S_2, then greater tumor shrinkage will favor expansion of subpopulation S_2 at the expense of S_1. Notice a stark contrast with the case of noninteracting clones discussed in Sections 11.4–11.6, where more extensive tumor shrinkage was found to confer a blanket advantage on the faster growing subpopulation.

To illustrate the complex dependence of the weight of the faster growing subpopulation on the shrinkage factor for a fixed total population size in the case of Gompertzian growth, I selected the following values of model parameters: (i) $K_1 = 10^{13}$ cells and $K_2 = 2 \cdot 10^{13}$ cells, which implies that λ_2 is 2.3 % larger than λ_1; (ii) $N_0 = 10^9$ or 10^{10} cells (i. e., about 1 or 10 cm^3, respectively); (iii) the survival endpoint was defined as reaching the total tumor size of $M = 10^{12}$ cells (or about 1,000 cm^3), assumed lethal; and (iv) for the initial posttreatment weight, p, of the faster growing subpopulation, we chose two values: $p = 0.5$ and $p = 0.8$ (notice that the latter satisfies the inequality in (11.22), while the former does not). With these parameters, the weight, $r(k)$, of the faster growing subpopulation is given by

$$r(k) = \frac{2}{\left[\frac{2(1-p)}{p}\right]^z + 2}, \tag{11.23}$$

where z is related to k through (11.20). The results shown in Figure 11.3 for the two selected values of N_0 confirm the aforementioned dependence of the monotonicity pattern of $r(k)$ on the relationship between p/K_2 and $(1-p)/K_1$ specified in (11.22). It follows from equation (11.20) that z approaches 0 as $k \to 0$, and from (11.23) we conclude that the limiting value of $r(k)$ as $k \to 0$ is 2/3, which is clearly seen in Figure 11.3.

In conclusion, we found in Sections 11.4–11.6 that under the assumption of independent clonal expansion, the weight of the fastest growing subpopulation is invariably a decreasing function of the tumor-shrinkage coefficient k. In this section, we discovered an unexpected barrier to the universality of this phenomenon. Specifically, even in the simple case of two independently evolving Gompertz subpopulations with distinct intrinsic growth rates that share the same growth inhibition coefficient, greater tumor

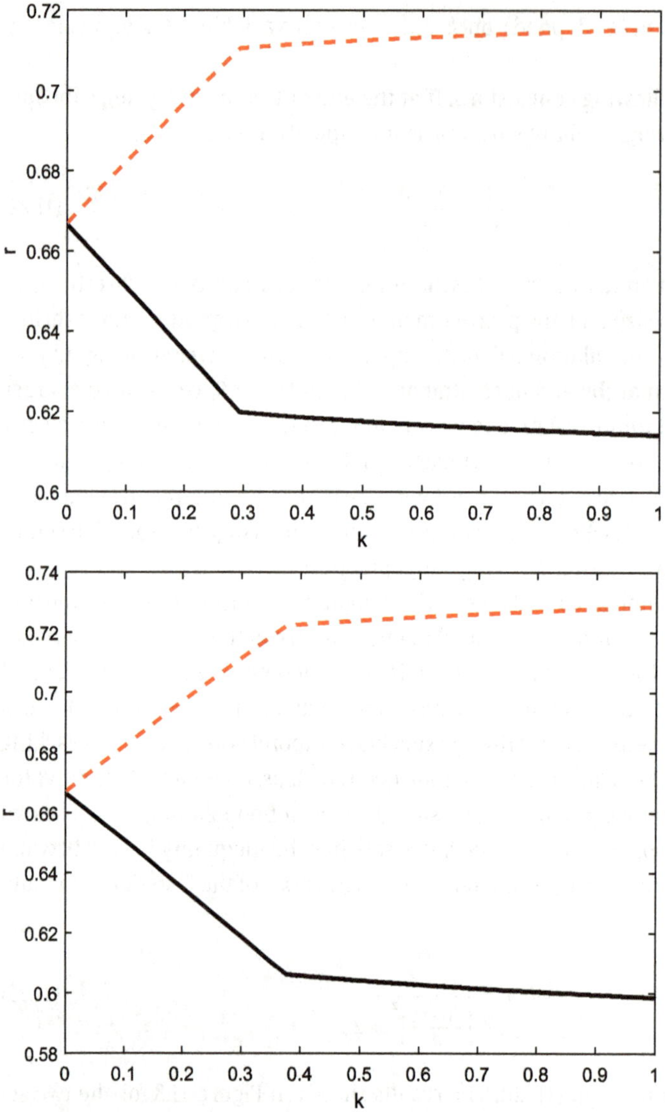

Figure 11.3: The weight **r** of the faster growing subpopulation as a function of tumor shrinkage factor **k** in the case of Gompertzian kinetics. The two surviving subpopulations of cancer cells were assumed to grow independently according to Gompertz laws with the same unspecified growth inhibition coefficient β and carrying capacities $K_1 = 10^{13}$ cells and $K_2 = 2 \cdot 10^{13}$ cells. The initial pretreatment tumor size is $N_0 = 10^9$ cells in the upper panel and $N_0 = 10^{10}$ cells in the lower panel of the figure. The weight r of the faster growing subpopulation was computed at the time when the regrowing residual tumor reached a total size $M = 10^{12}$ cells, assumed lethal. For the initial posttreatment weight p of the faster growing subpopulation, the following two values were selected: $p = 0.5$ and $p = 0.8$. The respective plots for r are the lower (solid) curves and the upper (dashed) curves. For background and relevant equations, see Section 11.7.
The figure was reproduced with permission from Hanin L. Paradoxical effects of tumor shrinkage on long-term survival of cancer patients. Front Appl Math Stat 2020, 6, 27.

shrinkage leads to preferential expansion of either faster or slower growing subpopulation depending on the ratio of the initial weight of the subpopulation to its carrying capacity (see (11.22) and Figure 11.3). Sample computations show that this relationship becomes more complex for two independent Gompertzian subpopulations with *distinct* growth inhibition coefficients, in which case the pattern of preferential expansion as function of k depends not only on the kinetic parameters but may also change with time (or the end point-defining size threshold M). Even more complex patterns can be expected when the residual tumor consists of two or more *interacting* subpopulations. In this case, greater tumor shrinkage may be expected to bestow greater or lesser advantage on faster growing subpopulations depending on their kinetic parameters, the initial composition of the residual tumor, the tumor-shrinkage coefficient and time.

11.8 A summary and discussion of findings

This chapter brought into focus the enrichment of a recurrent residual tumor posttreatment with faster proliferating cancer cells. This universally occurring phenomenon is due to the fact that with the passage of time faster proliferating cells tend to occupy an increasingly larger space left after treatment-induced elimination of sensitive cancer cells, compared to their slower proliferating counterparts. The enrichment process is also happening, although perhaps to a lesser degree, during treatment.

The enrichment is accompanied by a gradual increase in net proliferation rates of certain subpopulations and lineages within the residual tumor. This is due to three mechanisms: (a) continuous generation of faster proliferating mutants due to genomic instability of cancer cells; (b) random emergence of offspring with the ability to proliferate faster than their mother cell; and (c) a drop in cancer cell density following treatment, which leads to a greater per cell supply of space, oxygen, nutrients and growth factors and diminished competition between cancer cells for these resources and thereby to a decrease in their death rates. Observe that mechanisms (a) and (b) are genetic in nature, while (c) operates on the population level. Furthermore, if faster proliferating subpopulations and lineages have superior or comparable fitness compared to their slower proliferating counterparts, then over time they will take over the growing residual tumor.

It is well-known (see Section 3.5) that tumor latency time from the emergence of the first malignant clonogenic cell to tumor detection comprises many years or even decades. Yet in a considerable fraction of clinical cases, treatment-induced tumor shrinkage to undetectable size is followed by an aggressive tumor recurrence within just a few months. Enrichment of the regrowing tumor with faster proliferating cells offers a natural explanation for this observation. It also explains why sequential tumor recurrences following unsuccessful treatment cycles tend to occur increasingly faster. In essence, treatment breaks act as a filter that gradually replaces slower proliferating cancer cells with faster proliferating ones, unless the treatment had a curative effect or induced a stable disease. Such filtering makes the success of subsequent treatments, or cycles of the same treatment, increasingly unlikely. Additionally, tumor shrinkage occurs mostly at the expense of sensitive cancer cells, while leaving resistant cells essentially intact. The emergence of faster proliferating resistant subpopulations narrows treatment options, necessitates dose escalation with an attendant increase in the risks and severity of adverse side effects and often leads to treatment failure.

In Sections 11.4–11.7, I investigated, by means of mathematical modeling of population dynamics, the effects of treatment-induced tumor shrinkage on long-term survival of cancer patients and questioned a widely accepted notion that greater tumor shrinkage leads to longer recurrence-free and overall survival. My general premise was that the residual tumor consists of a quiescent subpopulation and a number of independently growing subpopulations, each expanding in accordance with its own fixed growth law. The quantity of interest was the fractional size (or weight) r of the fastest growing subpopulation, where it was assumed additionally that the weights of the residual subpopulations at the end of treatment are independent of tumor-shrinkage factor k. The main finding was that if the clones spawned by the surviving cancer cells evolve *independently*, then r is a decreasing function of k, or, in other words, that more extensive tumor shrinkage entails increasingly greater dominance of the fastest proliferating cancer cells within the residual tumor. This undoubtedly predicts shorter recurrence-free and overall survival. The same conclusion is even more assured if one takes into account the abovementioned drift of net proliferation rates of subpopulations comprising the residual tumor to the right.

Thus, the lack of interaction between the clones generated by surviving cancer cells present at the end of treatment (cycle) emerges as a critical condition that brings about the paradoxical effect of tumor shrinkage on a patient's recurrence-free and overall survival. Conversely, in the presence of a significant interaction between the clones the monotonicity pattern of the dependence of r on k is not guaranteed and can even be reversed, as was discovered in Section 11.7 in the case of Gompertz growth.

Are there biological scenarios under which independent propagation of clones generated by surviving cancer cells is likely to occur? First, surviving cancer cells that have preexisting or acquired migration capability will tend to spread over a larger volume; the resulting spatial separation of the initiator cells will reduce interaction between their clones. Second, such separation of clones can also be due to anatomic reasons; for example, primary colon tumors grow through the expansion of clones anatomically sequestered in crypts and the involvement of new crypts in the carcinogenic process through crypt fission [204]. Third, many cancers form deposits on nutrient- and oxygen-rich surfaces of blood vessels. When cancer cells on such a surface spawn their clones, the presence of a spatial dimension orthogonal to the surface reduces inter-clone competition for space, which would tend to make the growth of such clones independent as long as contact inhibition and competition for essential chemicals remain insignificant. Finally, extensive treatment-induced tumor shrinkage rarifies the surviving cancer cell population, thus creating physical conditions for independent propagation of clones generated by the surviving initiator cells, at least in the initial stages of tumor repopulation.

In summary, somewhat paradoxically and contrary to the commonly held belief that greater tumor shrinkage is universally beneficial for long-term survival, it can be expected that, in a significant fraction of patients, increased tumor shrinkage is actually a predictor of treatment failure and will entail shorter survival. Furthermore, this conclusion is likely to hold across a variety of local and systemic treatments, types of solid cancer and stages of the disease. Thus, tumor shrinkage may be a poor surrogate for long-term survival endpoints in clinical trials of anticancer drugs and other interventions.

11.9 Connection to statistical methodology

One would expect that the utility of tumor shrinkage as a predictor of long-term survival of cancer patients can be confirmed through statistical analysis, or meta-analysis, of data resulting from observational studies or clinical trials. Although scores of such studies have been conducted, analysis of their results produced controversial conclusions (see, e. g., [205–210]). This can be attributed to a number of nonmutually exclusive factors:

(1) Observations on tumor shrinkage and long-term survival for the same cancer patient are separated, as a rule, by a long duration of time, typically ranging from a few months to many years or even decades [201]. Quite often, various health-related events and interventions occur over this period of time, which may significantly affect the association of interest.
(2) Short- and long-term responses of cancer patients to treatment are very heterogeneous. Whereas some patients fail to positively respond to treatment, responses of others may fall anywhere between partial and complete. Additionally, the treatment may produce detrimental side effects ranging from minor and transient to permanent and life-threatening, which also affects long-term survival in many essential ways. This results in distributional heterogeneity of individual survival responses in any group of patients, which may preclude rigorous statistical analyses and have dramatic effects on their outcomes; this important subject will be thoroughly discussed in Chapters 12 and 13 (see also [9, 11]).
(3) Effects on long-term survival of progressive enrichment of a recurrent primary tumor with increasingly faster proliferating cancer cells can be confounded by acceleration of metastases induced by treatment of the primary tumor (see Sections 5.2–5.4), which would make separation of these two phenomena by statistical means a difficult task. Furthermore, the results of this chapter and arguments made

in Sections 5.2–5.4 suggest that reduction in patient overall survival caused by either mechanism is expected to be more pronounced for greater primary tumor shrinkage.
(4) Statistical methods utilized to ascertain an association between short-term response to treatment including tumor shrinkage and its long-term benefits are predicated on various untestable assumptions. For example, the Cox proportional hazards model, widely used for establishing such an association, depends on the empirically untestable, and most likely unrealistic, assumption that (unobservable) individual hazard functions of cancer patients in a queried population for the long-term outcome of interest are proportional.
(5) Finally, rigorously filling the gap between the real goal of establishing a cause-and-effect relationship between tumor shrinkage and improvement in long-term survival of cancer patients on the one hand and confirming a statistical association between them on the other hand is a daunting task [157].

11.10 Clinical considerations and recommendations

Cancer cells killed by treatment never produce offspring. This simple observation, as we know, is the ultimate reason behind the MTD (maximum tolerated dose) approach to cancer therapy. Two major factors traditionally challenge the dominant role of MTD in clinical oncology: (1) toxicity of chemotherapy drugs, radiation and other agents, which increases with the dose; and (2) emergence or survival and subsequent proliferation of resistant cancer cells facilitated by massive elimination of sensitive cells (see Section 5.5), which renders the administered treatment ineffective regardless of the dose. This chapter adds another important factor to this list. In fact, although not always stated explicitly, the goal of MTD treatment is to maximize tumor shrinkage. As was demonstrated in this chapter, if a treatment fails to eliminate or stabilize the disease, the residual resistant tumor would be likely to grow more aggressively posttreatment than the original one, and the more aggressively the larger the extent of tumor shrinkage.

To overcome some of these challenges, alternative "smart" approaches have been devised [211, 212] seeking to constrain proliferation of resistant tumor cells through competition with sensitive cancer cells and normal cells in the tumor microenvironment. Keeping these competitors alive requires capping the dose of the administered agent or its intermittent delivery.

To be sure, the choice between the MTD and "smart" lines of attack on cancer is a delicate one. One the one hand, resistant cells pose a greater threat to a patient's survival than sensitive ones, and constraining proliferation of resistant cells through competition seems to be a reasonable approach conducive to improvement in the patient's overall survival. On the other hand, cancer cells usually become resistant to treatment through acquisition of new functions (for example, the ability to degrade the treating agent or transport it across the cell membrane) or enhancement of the existing ones, which requires extra energy and material resources. As a result, resistant cells tend to be less fit than sensitive ones [213]. Therefore, the residual tumor posttreatment is more likely to be progressively enriched with faster proliferating sensitive cells than resistant ones, which would favor a subsequent round of more aggressive therapy against sensitive cells. Thus, employing adaptive combinations of the two treatment strategies like the ones advocated in [212] appears promising.

Progressive enrichment of the residual tumor with faster proliferating cells has a universal prerequisite—interruption or termination of treatment, usually due to severe side effects and/or emergence of resistance. One therapy type which does not necessitate such interruption is *metronomic treatment*, i. e., protracted delivery of low doses of chemotherapy or other anticancer agents. Such a therapy directly contravenes the MTD principle and therefore can potentially avoid or diminish its adverse effects including the enrichment phenomenon. For a more detailed discussion of metronomic treatment, the reader is referred to Section 5.6. Results of this chapter suggest that metronomic therapies deserve a much greater attention than they have gained so far.

Many patients whose tumor shrunk to undetectable levels as a result of anticancer therapy are declared “cancer-free” and put on a laxer follow-up schedule than patients whose treatment did not result in such a dramatic reduction of tumor burden. Quite often, tumor recurrence in such highly responsive patients is detected through the onset of symptoms rather than in the course of a prescheduled medical exam. The findings of this chapter suggest a recommendation that cancer patients with extensive tumor shrinkage should be followed up, at least initially, as frequently as other cancer patients, and perhaps even more so. It is expected that the proposed management of this well-defined group of patients will require relatively few additional resources.

On the diagnostic side, timely detection of rapid recurrence in cancer patients whose treatment resulted in extensive tumor shrinkage requires development of highly sensitive biomarkers that would reliably differentiate between fast and moderately growing or indolent tumors before they become visible on CT, PET, MRI and other diagnostic images.

Part IV: **Methodological barriers to winning the War on Cancer**

12 How statistical orthodoxy has ruined and discredited science

This chapter represents a far-reaching extension and elaboration of the ideas developed in [9, 11]. Article [11] can be consulted for additional technical details pertaining to some of the mathematical arguments presented in Sections 12.9–12.11.

12.1 The pivotal role of statistics in biomedical sciences

If there is a mathematical science on which cancer research and treatment depend most directly and critically, it is statistics. In particular, statistics plays an important part in the testing of treatments against cancer and other diseases. Such testing is conducted through large-scale controlled experiments on human subjects called *clinical trials*. The methodological essence of clinical trials, the causes for their failure to meet public expectations and the major pitfalls of statistical analysis of trial data are discussed in detail in Chapter 13 (see also [9]). The discussion in Chapter 13 relies heavily on the findings of this chapter.

Statistics has been employed in biology, medicine and social sciences for at least 300 years. In the past, this was mostly limited to calculating various descriptive summary measures such as the sample mean, median and standard deviation and the use of probability and statistics for computing age and income distributions, mortality tables and designing other practical tools in demography, economics and the insurance business. The dependence of biomedical sciences on statistical methods has greatly increased with the advent of molecular biology and genetics. This was chiefly due to a transition from directly observable and easily countable macroscopic events and objects to ultramicroscopic ones that can only be counted, measured or classified indirectly. For example, the number of cells or molecules with certain properties is commonly estimated by measuring the intensity of a signal emitted by fluorescent or radioactive label bound to these cells or molecules. Such changes in methods and technology of data generation necessitated a shift from descriptive statistics to statistical inference.

The stakes of getting applications of statistics in biomedical sciences right are very high indeed. When applied rigorously and honestly and confirmed by basic science, the methods of statistical inference can advance medical knowledge and save countless lives, as is the case with the discovery that smoking dramatically increases the risk of lung cancer [214]. To the contrary, this chapter will amply demonstrate that a cavalier approach to statistics, misuse of statistical methodology and its expedient deployment to rationalize predetermined conclusions may result in public health disasters.

It is important to make a distinction between mathematical (or theoretical) statistics and applied statistics. Like all mathematical sciences, mathematical statistics is based on theorems consisting of assumptions and conclusions. The validity of the arguments by

https://doi.org/10.1515/9783111334035-016

which the conclusions are derived from the assumptions is there for anyone to verify. In applied statistics, the methods and tests resulting from these theorems are employed to generate new knowledge based on empirical data. Two questions, often neglected in practice, lie at the heart of establishing the validity of applied statistical inference: (1) *Are the assumptions underlying a statistical analysis met?* and (2) *How sensitive are the outcomes of the statistical analysis to violation of these assumptions?* These two questions are among the principal focal points in this chapter.

In this chapter, I investigate how and why applied statistics has in many ways lost its way and propose a few recommendations on how to put it back on track. My starting point is a sweeping transformation of the culture and social fabric of scientific research that came about during a few decades following WWII.

12.2 Academic climate change

Dozens of millions of research articles in the experimental sciences have been published since the inauguration of the first research journals in the 17th century. But are their results and conclusions actually true? Since time immemorial, experimental sciences have used a universal criterion to answer this question, i. e., independent replication of experiments. Even just a few decades ago, when a major experimental discovery was published or announced through personal communication, researchers, driven by curiosity and healthy competition, used to rush to their labs to replicate and further study the phenomenon. However, beginning somewhere in the 1960s or 1970s, this mechanism of advancement of science through self-purification started to gradually break down. This change was brought about by powerful, yet acting slowly and mostly behind the scenes, political and social processes.

During WWII, scientists played a crucial role in the war effort. They designed aircraft and ballistic missiles, advanced naval warfare, developed nuclear weapons, encoded and decoded secret communications, optimized military logistics and created powerful computers. The ensuing arms and space races and a rapid succession of discoveries in microelectronics and molecular biology have led to an acute realization that science and technology offer enormous benefits to the society and are a key to military, economic and quality-of-life superiority. This ushered in an unprecedented administrative and financial involvement of government and industry in science at universities and research labs. As a result, science became more regulated, competitive and crowded. Former ivory towers housing otherworldly researchers with arcane academic pursuits have gradually transformed into busy crossroads of social forces vying for success and influence.

This caused slow but cumulatively dramatic changes in the climate governing both science and the institutions of research and higher education where it is created. Four among these changes stand out:

(1) Scientific research became a mass profession promising a relatively comfortable life, decent salary and some level of job security, which brought about a decline in the average quality of research;
(2) Formerly largely self-governed by faculty, universities and colleges increasingly found themselves under the rule of professional administrators who tend to run their academic institutions as corporations;
(3) Science's once universal goal of finding out the truth about the natural world and human society increasingly became mixed with motives extraneous to science, such as financial gain and political power, and more recently, achieving desirable ideological and social engineering aims and outcomes;
(4) While in the past scientific publication was mostly a natural product of the creative impulse and the desire to share new knowledge with others, in the new hypercompetitive academic world, publishing has acquired an existential quality of *sine qua non* of academic survival, a phenomenon commonly referred to as the "publish or perish" mentality.

To become competent in subjects as complex as cancer and its treatment and eventually develop a vision of their own, fledgling scientists and physicians have to go through many years, and often for as long as two decades, of study, training and practice. Brought up academically within a certain paradigm or school of thought, they initially view their subject through the eyes of their professors, academic and clinical advisors and mentors who teach them, suggest subjects and problems to study, approaches to take and literature to read. These senior faculty shepherd their disciples through coursework, theses and academic or medical degrees. To give them a leg-up in the fiercely competitive academic environment, they help them publish and otherwise disseminate their work and secure jobs, internships, fellowships and research awards. They also support their academic protégés financially by putting them on research grants, write recommendation letters and usher them into close-knit networks of colleagues. Biomedical and clinical scientists often have to rely on such support well into their thirties and beyond. This puts on maturing researchers and physicians a pressing moral obligation to be grateful, collegial and loyal to the group that has propelled them to a prominent place in their academic or professional community.

Now, imagine an up-and-coming researcher or clinician becoming convinced that the theories inculcated in him or her during the earlier years are incomplete, more limited in scope than previously thought or outright wrong. A researcher who puts pursuit of truth and patients' well-being first and makes such findings public would rankle a lot of colleagues and be branded an ingrate, renegade and traitor, which will incur incalculable damage to his or her career. In today's parlance, the researcher would likely be canceled. Such researchers would also have to somehow distance themselves from, disown or retract their own previous work published in numerous papers, often with multiple coauthors. At that stage of their careers, scientists and physicians have so much to lose that very, very few would dare to risk it. And even when they reach full independence and themselves acquire a senior status, they have to reckon with their former gurus serving as editors of prestigious journals, holding key positions in major funding agencies and dictating medical guidelines and recommendations. What I have described is not just a hypothetical scenario. For an example of what befalls those who dare to challenge the dominant orthodoxy, one would only have to look at the story, poignantly narrated by Clifton Leaf in [5, pp. 22–28], of John Bailar III, a senior scientist and proven leader in the field of cancer research.

12.3 Replication crisis: signs of trouble

The last three decades have brought to light an ever-growing alarm over poor replicability of results in experimental sciences (see e. g. [215, 216]), commonly referred to as the *replication crisis*. This triggered a comprehensive study of this phenomenon commissioned by the US National Academies of Science, Engineering and Medicine [217]. The committee consisted of 146 leading scientists and NSF program officers who additionally interviewed dozens of experts. The committee report expressed concern about the low rate of replicability of scientific findings and formulated numerous recommendations [217].

The report distinguishes between a more narrow concept of *reproducibility* and a broader and more open-ended notion of *replicability*. A research finding is reproducible if an independent repetition of the original study by a different research team, that used the same data or data-generating protocols, the same research methodology and the same computational procedures, produced results that are identical or very close to the original ones. Thus, barring fraud and technical or computational errors, irreproducibility typically results from (1) insufficient standardization of research protocols; (2) inadequate reporting of experimental procedures and data, research methods and statistical tools; and (3) failure to provide details of the software and computational code used for data processing and analysis. By contrast, replicability refers to obtaining similar quantitative results and reaching identical conclusions when some of the following alterations are made: (1) Different datasets are collected for the same research objects, subjects or population; (2) data are collected for other similar objects, subjects or populations; (3) alternative statistical methods are used for data processing; and (4) different computational tools are employed. Clearly, the broader the range of replicability, the higher the reliability and scientific value of the research finding. Although this distinction between reproducibility and replicability is by no means standard across experimental sciences, it is made in this book. However, to simplify the terminology, I will be assuming that the term "replicability" includes reproducibility as a particular case.

Although vitally important, replication studies are relatively rare, for a number of reasons. Firstly, only a small fraction of research papers report experimental procedures, datasets, statistical methodology and computational tools in sufficient detail to be faithfully reproduced. Secondly, many researchers, especially those working in the private sector, view the data they generate as proprietary or have a contractual obligation to do so. And thirdly, replication studies have low priority due to academic requirements of novelty and significance of results that figure prominently in matters of hiring, promotion, tenure and research funding.

But even if replication studies were highly desirable and technically feasible, vetting the body of published research would be an insurmountable task given the sheer volume of publications. In spite of this, it is a common occasion that different individual scientists or research groups investigate the same research question, with or without an explicit purpose of replicating or validating previous work. Analyzing these occurrences has led to a conclusion that a substantial proportion of research findings in experimental sciences, mostly biomedical and social, are irreplicable. As one striking example, a meta-analysis study [218] found that out of 26 of the most highly cited reports of controlled randomized clinical trials that appeared in top medical journals, claimed positive effects of medical interventions and were later retested on larger groups of patients, nine studies (35 %) were either refuted or their claims of effect were found to be greatly exaggerated. As yet another example, an effort to reproduce 100 prominent results in the field of experimental psychology revealed that replication effects were on average half the magnitude of the original effects and that overall only 39 % of effects were subjectively rated to have replicated the original result [219].

Replicability of a research finding and its truth value are interrelated in a complex and subject area-specific manner. In physics and chemistry with their immutable laws, replicability of experimental results, broadly construed, is an empirical criterion of truth. In biomedical and social sciences, where no such laws have ever been discovered, the degree of separation between the replicability and validity of scientific results is much greater than in the physical sciences. A typical research finding in experimental biomedical and social sciences is a quantitative statement about biological objects, subjects or populations, or their response to a defined condition or intervention. Because of substantial inter-subject, and potentially intra-subject, variation, these statements are often formulated in statistical terms. As a result, a replicable finding may occasionally be false; however, a finding that fails several replication attempts is most likely erroneous. An additional factor of the essence in social sciences is the subjects' beliefs and information available to them as well as the body of empirically untestable general ideas permeating a given field. This dilutes the concept of objective truth even further and widens the epistemological divergence between replicability and validity of scientific knowledge.

Thus, the replication crisis goes hand in hand with a much graver phenomenon—*accumulation of false knowledge*. Because nowadays researchers typically cannot independently verify all the scientific facts and theories they rely upon in their work, they take many of them for granted. This may potentially lead to propagation of false knowledge, especially if scientists don't carefully read and critically analyze all the literature that was cited in, or has otherwise contributed to, their studies. Sometimes they realize on their own that the results they have published are false, which in an ideal world would not be a big deal given that science is nothing more than a path from ignorance to knowledge. But, in the real world, retraction of such publications or public admission of their falsehood are embarrassing and damaging to egos, reputations and careers, which makes such occurrences relatively rare. If wrong scientific findings are foundational for a specific field of knowledge, the field may get contaminated with false knowledge in its entirety. False knowledge propagates through publications, citation and research presentations and is transmitted from teachers and mentors to their students and disciples. As one would expect, generation and dissemination of false knowledge is a major driver of the widespread and growing public distrust of science [12].

Like other empirical sciences, cancer research is not impervious to false knowledge, and in this book I have discussed a number of instances where theories of cancer and cancer treatment practices are based on dubious ideas or those with vastly overstated generality.

Most importantly for the subject of this chapter, empirical sciences are increasingly dependent on statistical inference, which, as I show in the next section, complicates replication and validation of research findings and thus makes their truth value more uncertain.

12.4 Why the use of statistical methods limits replicability

The idea that certain aspects of statistical methodology are implicated in the irreplicability and falsity of scientific findings is not new by any means. However, most authors who have written on this subject largely attributed the replication crisis to widespread overuse, misuse, abuse, misinterpretation and inappropriate dichotomization of *p*-values as well as to the use of null hypotheses beyond their intended purpose, misinterpretation of confidence intervals and failure to adequately account for multiple hypothesis testing [220–226]. Thus, the identified main culprit was not statistical methods per se but rather their misunderstanding and misuse by scientists who employed them.

The subject of *p*-values will be extensively discussed in this chapter and the next one. Recall that *p*-value is a quantitative measure of the agreement between the data and the null hypothesis mediated by a test statistic with known distribution under the null hypothesis. Specifically, *p*-value is the probability that the test statistic takes a value more extreme (in the one- or two-sided sense) than its value computed for the data in question under the null hypothesis [148, p. 474].

Implicit in statistical methodology is the assumption that the phenomenon of interest involves random variation or chance. The observed or measured quantity may be random due to its intrinsic variation or it may vary among objects or subjects sampled from a given population. Additionally, the measurements may involve random error or noise. Therefore, replication studies other than strict reproducibility ones cannot even in principle be expected to generate exactly the same quantitative outcome as the original study. In theory, if all the assumptions behind a statistical method are satisfied and all approximation errors are properly accounted for, then due to the effects of averaging, application of the *same* statistical methodology to *different* sufficiently large datasets drawn from the same population should produce similar quantitative results and thereby lead to replicable conclusions. As I argue in this chapter, *these conditions are almost never met in biomedical and social sciences*. Furthermore, replicability is still in greater doubt when a replication attempt employs a *different* statistical method (including different methods of parameter estimation), even if applied to the same data set. Ditto for other methodological alterations such as the selection of different null and alternative hypotheses, the use of different test statistics under a given null hypothesis and choosing different thresholds including those for statistical significance and power.

It is widely believed that reproducibility of a scientific finding is a matter of keeping and following a complete digital footprint of the computations that produced the original result. Unfortunately, this is not always the case, and the most notable example is estimation of model parameters from data through the use of extremal principles, e. g., by maximizing the likelihood, minimizing the ordinary or weighted least squares criterion or optimizing other objective functions. (As noted aptly by my colleague Michael Retsky, introduced in Section 5.6, such problems are somewhat akin to looking for the deepest lake in Wisconsin). My own experience with this type of problems suggests that even for simple models depending on as few as five or six parameters, unsupervised computation based on standard optimization algorithms may routinely produce wrong results. The reasons are many including: (1) multiplicity of local extrema; (2) flatness of the objective function around the point of global extremum; (3) the occurrence of very small or very large numbers, which requires one to adaptively design scaling factors; (4) location of the global extremum on the boundary of the parameter space; (5) the presence of sharp narrow peaks of the objective function that can be missed by optimization algorithms; and (6) the occurrence, accumulation and propagation of errors due to finite-digit computer arithmetic. Thus, correct estimation of model parameters is somewhat of an art form depending critically on numerical intuition developed through many years of computational experience. Also, transparency with the algorithm and code alone won't necessarily guarantee reproducibility, let alone replicability. An example demonstrating how estimation of model parameters can be bedeviled by numerical intricacies was presented in Section 9.1.

12.5 Irreplicability and false knowledge: the role of bias

What are the root causes of high prevalence of false and irreplicable research findings in biomedical and social sciences? In a pioneering article titled "Why Most Published Research Findings are False" [227], John Ioannidis sought to explain this phenomenon.

He assumed the following model of scientific discovery: Several groups of investigators independently study a number of research questions by performing statistical analysis of the empirical data. Each research finding has a prior probability to be true; however, this probability is modulated by random effects of statistical analysis with certain rates of false positive and false negative discoveries. A key model parameter is "bias," defined as the probability to report as true a finding that was found by a research team to be false. The model leads to a Bayes-type formula for the probability of false discovery as a function of model parameters. Sample computations based on this formula have led the author of [227] to the conclusion encapsulated in the title of his paper.

Since the publication of [227], the most common explanation for falsity and irreplicability in science has been bias. It can result, among many other sources, from data fabrication and tampering; fraudulent misrepresentation of research findings; conscious or unwitting manipulation of experimental design and data analysis procedures including selection of data subsets, explanatory variables, endpoints and statistical methods that produce more favorable outcomes; the human tendency to confirm preconceived notions and expectations, known as *confirmation bias*; other cognitive biases [228]; and selective publication of the most impressive results, termed *publication bias*. Among many social factors that enable widespread bias are the pervasive "publish or perish" mentality, warped incentives and performance criteria for scientists employed in academia, industry and government, and the dominant climate in research journals, funding agencies and professional societies [229].

Thus, bias in its various forms is a manifestation of human fallibility and frailty modulated by the social environment in which scientists operate. However, many areas of science such as mathematics, computer science, physics, chemistry and engineering are much less susceptible to accumulation of false knowledge and systematic irreplicability. The reason is, of course, three-fold: (1) they have a more well-defined criterion of truth than biomedical and social sciences; (2) they are less dependent on statistical methodology; and (3) when employing the latter, they are more fastidious about it.

In the rest of this chapter, I show how *statistical methodology itself* and the way it is applied in experimental sciences make generation of false and irreplicable results unavoidable. Thus, although bias is a sufficient cause for the replication/validity crisis in science, it is not a necessary one.

12.6 The iid assumption: a theoretical perspective

Scientists commonly recognize, of course, that the assumptions they make, or fail to explicitly make (see Section 6.1), cannot be exactly met in the real world. However, they believe that the effects of their violation are negligible. In Sections 12.6–12.9, we eye the most important assumption underlying applications of statistics in science and far beyond, along with dramatic consequences of its violation.

Virtually all applications of statistics are based on, or are eventually reduced to, the assumption that the set of observations, say $x_1, x_2, \dots, x_n$, is a *random sample* from a probability distribution. Informally, this means that the observed values result from independent replications of the same random experiment, just like a sequence of "heads" and "tails" represents outcomes of successive flips of a coin or a sequence of natural numbers 1 through 6 results from repeated rolls of a die. The exact meaning of the "random sample" assumption is as follows: There exists a sample space S with a probability measure on it and *jointly stochastically independent* (i) and *identically distributed* (id) random variables $X_1, X_2, \dots, X_n$ on S, such that $X_1(s) = x_1, X_2(s) = x_2, \dots, X_n(s) = x_n$ for some point s in S. In biomedical and social sciences, random variables $X_1, X_2, \dots, X_n$ are often called *response variables*.

Critically, the iid assumption cannot be verified empirically, for each response variable is represented in the data set by a *single* value. An essential and almost universal feature of applications of statistics in empirical sciences is that even if $x_1, x_2, \dots, x_n$ is a random sample from some distribution, the latter is *unknown*.

Beyond the iid premise, most statistical methods and tests fail; even measures as simple as the sample mean lose their inferential significance. Thus, the most basic assumption underlying statistical inference from data is necessarily and invariably taken on faith.

The strength of one's faith in the iid assumption is setting-specific. For example, in cell biology, preexisting or emerging genetic differences among cells, variation in their spatial position within a cell population, their distinct functional states (e. g., proliferating vs. quiescent or stem vs. differentiated) and interaction between cells all make the iid assumption unrealistic. For multicellular organisms, the possibilities for violation of the iid assumption are vastly more abundant, even more so for humans with enormous variety of their biological and psychological traits. As one example, when observations are made on a pathological condition in a group of subjects, substantial differences in susceptibility of the subjects to this condition and its severity will make the underlying response variables non-iid.

Additionally, if some of the subjects are identical twins, siblings or more generally have a common ancestor, they may have inherited common genetic traits resulting in a shared predisposition to a specific disease, which could result in stochastic dependence between their response variables. One specific example is the well-known increase in cancer risk in individuals with a family history of cancer. The same can be said in the case where some subjects in a group were exposed to similar environmental, professional or lifestyle hazards. Finally, when sampling from a small population (e. g., when studying a rare disease or a rarely occurring combination of attributes), the mere fact of sampling from it without replacement makes observations stochastically dependent.

In experimental sciences, departure from the iid assumption is almost universally disregarded, likely based on the belief that the deviations are "small" and therefore inconsequential. A fundamental question, then, is how to quantify these deviations and assess their impact on the outcomes of statistical analysis. This question is taken up in the next section.

Importantly, an outcome of a statistical analysis is in the final count an output value of a certain data processing algorithm, that is, just a function of observations whose value is unaffected by the validity of the random sample or any other assumption about the process of data generation. Thus, no red flags signaling their violation will ever appear in the process of data analysis, unless the validity of the underlying assumptions is deliberately questioned and investigated.

Determining whether a given set of observations is or isn't a random sample can be quite subtle, as illustrated by the following example motivated by the study of metastatic cancer progression in Chapters 8–10.

Example 12.1. Let $x_1, x_2, \ldots, x_n$ be the volumes of metastases detected in a particular cancer patient in a given distant site at a certain moment in time. Is this a random sample?

Focusing on the data-generating process, let us assume for simplicity that metastases shed off a primary tumor and bound for the site of interest evolve independently, survive with the same probability, grow according to the same deterministic law and become detectable when their volumes reach a fixed threshold, as was done in the model presented in Section 8.1. Then, neglecting metastatic dormancy, one concludes that the volumes of detected metastases at the time of survey are a nonrandom transformation of their random shedding times. Because the rate of shedding is, generally speaking, time-dependent (e. g., it may depend on the current size of the primary tumor), the observed volumes of metastases cannot result from independent replications of *the same* random experiment. Thus, they don't form a random sample from any probability distribution even under the stated simplifying assumptions. Consequently, conventional summary statistics such as sample mean, median and standard deviation, although readily computable, are inferentially meaningless, a fact commonly neglected in volumetric studies of metastases. However, as was shown in Section 8.2 (see Theorem 8.2), violation of the random sample property can be mitigated under the assumption that metastases shedding events follow a Poisson process.

12.7 Quantification of deviations from the iid assumption

One of the central questions addressed in this chapter is this: *How do deviations from the iid and other assumptions affect the outcomes of statistical analyses?* Examples of such outcomes are a point estimate and confidence interval for a parameter of interest such as the population mean or variance; p-value and statistical power; estimate of the sample size; the correlation coefficient and the coefficient of determination in regression analysis, etc. In particular, in the setting of hypothesis testing, the question is how much a deviation from the assumptions modifies the distribution of the test statistic under the null or alternative hypothesis. The distributions of the commonly used test statistics, such as the standard Gaussian, Student's t and chi-squared distributions, depend in very essential ways on the iid assumption. Absent this, one cannot fully rely on these standard distributions anymore.

Assessment of the effects of deviations from the iid or any other assumption on the outcome of a statistical analysis requires quantification of these deviations. I begin with quantification of stochastic dependence between random variables, and hence also, as a particular case, between random events. A simple and universally used measure of dependence between two random variables is their covariance or its normalized version, the correlation coefficient. This measure, however, is grossly inadequate because: (1) zero correlation does not imply independence; and (2) a collection of pairwise independent random variables is not necessarily jointly independent, which is an essential requirement for the iid property. Thus, even designing a practicable quantitative measure of the deviation from joint independence represents a considerable mathematical challenge.

Along with a possible lack of independence, a statistical analysis is bound to encounter a more consequential violation of the equidistribution (id) assumption. As with stochastic dependence, to assess a deviation from the id assumption, one has to somehow quantify the distance (viewed as a measure of proximity) between probability distributions. This can be done by employing one of the well-known probability metrics such as the total variation, Kolmogorov–Smirnov, Kantorovich (or Wasserstein), Cramér–von Mises, Lévy and other distance functions [230]. To simplify our terminology, we define the distance between random variables as the distance between their distributions.

One of the most widely used probability metrics is the Kolmogorov–Smirnov distance d_{KS} defined by

$$d_{KS}(X, Y) = \sup\{|F_X(x) - F_Y(x)| : x \in \mathbb{R}\}, \tag{12.1}$$

where $F_X(x) = \Pr(X \leq x)$, $x \in \mathbb{R}$, is the cumulative distribution function (cdf) of random variable X. The importance of the KS distance stems from the fact that if the KS distance between two random variables is small, then the probabilities that these random variables take values from any given interval are uniformly close to each other. In fact, if $I = (a, b]$, then it follows from $\Pr(X \in I) = F_X(b) - F_X(a)$ that

$$|\Pr(X \in I) - \Pr(X \in I)| \leq 2d_{KS}(X, Y).$$

Due to continuity properties of the probability measure, the same is also true for intervals of the form $I = (a, b)$, $[a, b)$ and $[a, b]$.

Because distributions of individual response variables are typically unknown and inestimable from the data, so are pairwise distances between them. Suppose, however, for the purpose of our argument, that response variables are jointly independent and that the maximum value of a selected distance d for all pairs of underlying random variables is, or does not exceed, some positive number ε. Let y be an outcome of a statistical analysis. Let y_0 and y_1 be the values of y computed under the iid assumption and without it, respectively. A question of both theoretical and practical importance is as follows: *How sensitive is the deviation* $|y_1 - y_0|$ *to the departure from the id assumption, as measured by* ε*? In particular, is it true that* $|y_1 - y_0| \to 0$ *as* $\varepsilon \to 0$*?* Mathematically, such sensitivity is characterized by the maximum absolute deviation, $\delta(\varepsilon)$, of the outcome of interest as a function of ε. To ascertain robustness, i. e., that $\delta(\varepsilon) \to 0$ as $\varepsilon \to 0$, one has to design a tight and relatively simple upper bound for $\delta(\varepsilon)$ that still has the same "continuity at zero" property, while to show the lack of robustness, one needs to construct a simple lower bound without this property. With a few exceptions, obtaining such bounds goes beyond the reach of contemporary probability theory.

Scientists commonly believe that δ is small if ε is. That this can be patently false is demonstrated in Section 12.9.

12.8 Averaging under and beyond the iid assumption

Suppose $X_1, X_2, \ldots, X_n$ are random variables with finite expected value μ. Then, for their average

$$\bar{X}_n = \frac{X_1 + X_2 + \cdots + X_n}{n}$$

one also has

$$\mathbb{E}\bar{X}_n = \mu, \tag{12.2}$$

where $\mathbb{E}$ stands for the expected value. According to the (strong) *Law of Large Numbers* (LLN) [148, Section 10.5], which is one of the most basic results in probability, if $\{X_m, m = 1, 2, 3 \ldots\}$ is an infinite sequence of iid random variables with finite expected value μ, then

$$\bar{X}_n \to \mu \quad \text{as } n \to \infty \tag{12.3}$$

almost surely, i. e., with probability 1. This means by definition that the set of points s in the underlying sample space S such that

$$\bar{X}_n(s) = \frac{X_1(s) + X_2(s) + \cdots + X_n(s)}{n} \to \mu \quad \text{as } n \to \infty$$

has probability 1. The combined validity of relations (12.2) and (12.3) is also reflected by saying that the sample mean

$$\bar{x}_n = \frac{x_1 + x_2 + \cdots + x_n}{n}$$

of observations $\{x_m, m = 1, 2, 3 \ldots\}$ is a *(strongly) consistent unbiased estimator* of μ. A useful heuristic interpretation of (12.3) is that fluctuations of averaged iid random variables around their expected value asymptotically cancel out.

In the case where random variables $\{X_m, m = 1, 2, 3 \ldots\}$ are indicator functions of a sequence of independent random events $\{A_m, m = 1, 2, 3 \ldots\}$ occurring with the same probability p, relation (12.3) amounts to stating that the observed frequency, r/n, of the occurrence of the events A_m in a sequence of n trials converges to p as $n \to \infty$, which constitutes the all-important frequentist interpretation of probability.

Thus, almost miraculously, the LLN allows one to estimate empirically an unknown (and often unobservable), yet important and desirable for both theoretical and practical purposes, quantity μ (or p) based on a sufficiently large number of observations. This is why the LLN forms one of the cornerstones of statistical inference.

But what about a much more realistic, at least in biomedical and social sciences, situation where independent random variables $\{X_m, m = 1, 2, 3 \ldots\}$ (e. g., patients' response variables) have distinct distributions? For simplicity, let's consider a particular case, where among the distributions of these random variables there are only a finite number, $N \geq 2$, of distinct distributions with finite expected values $\mu_1, \mu_2, \ldots, \mu_N$ occurring with relative frequencies (or weights) $p_1, p_2, \ldots, p_N$ such that $p_1 + p_2 + \cdots + p_N = 1$. Note that typically the number, N, of distinct distributions is unknown, and so are their weights p_k and expected values μ_k, $1 \leq k \leq N$. Although mathematically the LLN (12.3) is still valid with

$$\mu = p_1\mu_1 + p_1\mu_1 + \cdots + p_N\mu_N,$$

its practicality is greatly diminished since one cannot extract any knowledge about N, the expected values μ_k and their weights p_k from the estimated value of μ alone. Therefore, distributional heterogeneity severely limits the utility of averaging.

12.9 Averaging: the lack of robustness

Let $x_1, x_2, \ldots, x_n$ be observations generated by random variables $X_1, X_2, \ldots, X_n$. Suppose these random variables are iid with a nominal distribution P and finite expected value μ. Since in practice the distribution of random variables X_m, $m = 1, 2, \ldots, n$, is unknown and unobservable, the true distribution of some or all of them may be different from P. The following example examines the effect of such a misspecification on $\mathbb{E}\bar{X}_n$.

Example 12.2. Suppose that for some $p \in (0, 1]$ the fraction $1 - p$ of random variables $X_1, X_2, \ldots, X_n$ have the distribution P, while the variables in the remaining fraction p have a different distribution Q, which is a mixture of P and some other probability distribution T : $Q = (1 - \varepsilon)P + \varepsilon T$ for some $\varepsilon \in (0, 1]$. How large is the deviation of the expected value $\mathbb{E}\bar{X}_n$ from μ under such perturbation?

It is readily verified using formula (12.1) that $d_{KS}(P,Q) \leq \varepsilon$ for any distribution T, so that Q can be thought of as a "small" perturbation of P. Let's now choose $T = T(\varepsilon)$ in such a way that its expected value, $\rho(\varepsilon)$, satisfies the relation $\varepsilon\rho(\varepsilon) \to \infty$ as $\varepsilon \to 0$ (examples of such distribution T include exponential distribution $\mathrm{Exp}(\varepsilon^{\theta})$ and uniform distribution $U(0, \varepsilon^{-\theta})$ for any $\theta > 1$). Then, for $\nu = \mathbb{E}\bar{X}_n$ we have

$$\nu = (1-p)\mu + p[(1-\varepsilon)\mu + \varepsilon\rho(\varepsilon)] = \mu + p\varepsilon[\rho(\varepsilon) - \mu].$$

Therefore, for any fixed p, no matter how small, $\nu - \mu \to \infty$ as $\varepsilon \to 0$. In particular, this holds true for $p = 1$, i. e., when the presumed distribution P of all response variables is misspecified and their distribution actually equals Q.

Thus, *arbitrarily small deviations from the id assumption, as measured by the KS distance, can bring about arbitrarily large deviations in the expected value.* Observe that this result is independent of the sample size n and therefore holds for arbitrarily long sequences of observations and response variables.

Combining Example 12.2 with the LLN leads to a conclusion that the difference between sample means with and without misspecification of the distribution P can almost surely be made arbitrarily large for sufficiently large n and sufficiently small ε. In particular, even a minor deviation from the distribution P (resulting, e. g., from assuming normality or any other convenient distributional form) may have a devastating effect on the estimation of its expected value. Because sample means are ubiquitous in statistical analyses, the lack of robustness to small perturbations of the underlying distribution P will likely translate into high sensitivity of the outcomes of these analyses to such perturbations.

To reiterate what was stated in Section 12.7, establishing the robustness of a statistical analysis depends critically on the availability of a tight, readily computable upper bound for $\delta(\varepsilon)$, the maximum deviation of the outcome of the analysis, such that the bound tends to zero as $\varepsilon \to 0$. Example 12.2 shows that selection of an appropriate probability metric d is essential for obtaining such upper bounds. If the latter is beyond reach for all suitable probability metrics or if available bounds do not have the above "continuity at zero" property or are too conservative to be practical, there is no guarantee that even a methodologically sound and unbiased statistical analysis won't produce a false and/or irreplicable outcome.

12.10 Samples of random size

Yet another reason why the volumes of detected metastases in Example 12.1 do not form a random sample is that their number, n, is random. This is so because many aspects of the life trajectory of a metastasis, such as its shedding time, survival, duration of the latency time and the time from inception to detection in the site of interest, all depend on chance [176].

Although a tacit assumption of fixed sample size is almost universal in empirical studies, it is quite often violated in practice. Samples of random size arise when reaching a predetermined number of observations proves impossible or impractical due to limited resources, constraints on the observation time or difficulty recruiting the requisite number of study participants. Another systematic source of random sample size is the researchers' natural inclination to collect observations that are as representative of the phenomenon under study as possible. Finally, random sample size results from study designs that require a sufficiently large number of events of interest randomly occurring in tested subjects rather than the number of subjects. In the last two examples, sample size is not only random but also stochastically dependent on observations.

Importantly, samples of random size cannot be handled with standard statistical tools because even the most foundational results in probability that form the bedrock of statistical inference such as the LLN lead to erroneous conclusions if applied to samples of random size. Given next are two examples of a spectacular failure of the LLN.

To formulate a natural extension of the classic LLN to random sample size, consider a sequence $\{N_n : n \geq 1\}$ of positive integer-valued random variables (sample sizes).

Definition. Sequences $\{X_n\}$ of random variables with the same finite expected value μ and $\{N_n\}$ satisfy the LLN if

$$Y_n = \frac{X_1 + X_2 + \cdots + X_{N_n}}{N_n} \to \mu \quad \text{as } n \to \infty \tag{12.4}$$

in probability (or almost surely in the case of strong LLN).

Clearly, if $N_n = n$ with probability 1 for all n, then (12.4) is identical to (12.3). Observe that in this case, for every natural number m, we have $\Pr(1 \leq N_n \leq m) = 1$ if $n \leq m$ and 0 otherwise, so that $\Pr(1 \leq N_n \leq m) \to 0$ as $n \to \infty$. The latter relation means that the probability mass of random variables N_n eventually "escapes to infinity."

Consider now a sequence of random variables $\{N_n\}$, not necessarily independent, for which the probability mass does not escape to infinity in the sense that, for some natural number m and $p \in (0,1)$,

$$\Pr(1 \leq N_n \leq m) \geq p \quad \text{for all } n. \tag{12.5}$$

Example 12.3. Let $\{X_n : n \geq 1\}$ be iid random variables with a finite expected value μ and a distribution P other than the unit mass at μ. Suppose that, for each $n \geq 1$, random variables N_n and X_k, $1 \leq k \leq n$, are stochastically independent and that condition (12.5) is satisfied with some $p \in (0,1)$. Then the sequence of random variables Y_n defined in (12.4) does not converge to μ in probability, hence also almost surely.

For a proof of this statement in the case $\mu = 0$, which can always be assumed without loss of generality, the reader is referred to [11, Section 4].

The next example addresses the situation where, for each n, random sample size N_n and random variables $X_1, X_2, \ldots, X_n$ are stochastically dependent.

Example 12.4. Let, as in Example 12.3, $\{X_n : n \geq 1\}$ be iid random variables with a finite expected value μ and a distribution P other than the unit mass at μ. Define random variables N_n as follows: $N_1 = 1$ with probability 1 and for $n \geq 2$ set $N_n = 1$ if $X_1 \geq \mu$ and $N_n = n$ if $X_1 < \mu$. Then the generalized LLN property (12.4) fails.

In fact, let $q = \Pr(X_1 \geq \mu)$, then $0 < q < 1$. Observe as an aside that $\mathbb{E}N_n = q + (1-q)n \to \infty$ as $n \to \infty$. Note that $Y_1 = X_1$, while for $n \geq 2$ we have $Y_n = X_1$ with probability q and $Y_n = \bar{X}_n$ with probability $1-q$. Therefore, according to the standard LLN, the almost sure limit in (12.4) equals X_1 with probability q and μ with probability $1-q$, i. e., is a nonconstant random variable rather than μ.

Finally, the Central Limit Theorem (CLT) [148, Section 10.6], another fundamental theorem in probability and a source of most asymptotic results in statistics, generally fails [231] beyond a few special cases, e. g., when the sample size has Poisson distribution [232, p. 4699]. Note also that an example somewhat similar to Example 12.4 was designed in [231] to show that the CLT may fail when random variables $\{X_n\}$ and random sample sizes $\{N_n\}$ are stochastically dependent.

12.11 Effects of the Gaussian approximation on statistical significance and *p*-values

Scientists employing statistical methods certainly realize that approximations they make generate errors. However, many of them believe that the errors are negligible. In this section, I focus on the ubiquitous Gaussian approximation and show that this belief is unfounded. Results of this section constitute another major source of false and irreplicable research findings in experimental sciences.

The Gaussian approximation arises from the CLT, which approximates the distribution of the normalized sum of iid random variables by the standard Gaussian distribution [148, Section 10.6]. Specifically, if $\{X_n : n \geq 1\}$ are iid random variables with a finite expected value μ and finite standard deviation $\sigma > 0$, then, in accordance with the CLT, for random variables

$$Z_n = \sqrt{n}\,\frac{\bar{X}_n - \mu}{\sigma}, \tag{12.6}$$

one has $d_{KS}(Z_n, Z) \to 0$ as $n \to \infty$, where Z is a random variable with the standard Gaussian distribution $N(0,1)$. It follows from (12.6) that, for each n, random variable $\bar{X}_n$ can be approximated in the KS distance by the Gaussian random variable $\mu + \sigma Z/\sqrt{n}$. Such a replacement leads to many standard test statistics including Z-statistic, the Student's t statistic and chi-squared statistic widely used in data analysis.

What are the effects of the error resulting from the Gaussian approximation? The following example is the first step in a demonstration that this error can have drastic consequences for p-values and statistical significance of research findings.

Example 12.5. Let $X_1, X_2, \ldots, X_n$ be a random sample from a continuous (but not necessarily absolutely continuous) probability distribution P with an unknown expected value μ, known variance $\sigma^2 > 0$ and a finite third absolute central moment $\beta = \mathbb{E}|X - \mu|^3$, where X is a random variable with the distribution P. How does one compute the p-value for a null hypothesis $\mu = \mu_0$ from a sample of observations $x_1, x_2, \ldots, x_n$ using the one-sided Z-test?

According to the CLT, under the null hypothesis, the distribution of random variable

$$Z_n = \sqrt{n}\,\frac{\bar{X}_n - \mu_0}{\sigma}$$

can be approximated in the KS metric by the standard Gaussian distribution represented by a random variable Z. Denote by

$$z_n = \sqrt{n}\,\frac{\bar{x}_n - \mu_0}{\sigma}$$

the empirical analog of Z_n, called the *Z-statistic*. Let π_n be the *true* one-sided p-value, that is, $\Pr(Z_n \geq z_n)$ if $z_n \geq 0$ and $\Pr(Z_n \leq z_n)$ if $z_n < 0$. Because the distribution of the random variable Z_n is unknown, it is a common practice to compute the *approximate* one-sided p-value, p_n, based on the standard Gaussian approximation to the distribution of Z_n. Thus, p_n is given by the probability $\Pr(Z \geq z_n)$ if $z_n \geq 0$, and $\Pr(Z \leq z_n)$ if $z_n < 0$. This provides the answer to the question posed in Example 12.5.

How large is the maximum value, Δ_n, of the error $|\pi_n - p_n|$ in p-value determination, with respect to data variation? Here is the answer: $\Delta_n = d_{KS}(Z_n, Z)$ (see my article [11, Section 5] for a detailed proof). Note also that the error for the two-sided p-value satisfies the inequality $\Delta_n \leq 2d_{KS}(Z_n, Z)$, but the equality is generally not guaranteed.

Let $\delta_n = d_{KS}(Z_n, Z)$ be the error resulting from the CLT-based standard Gaussian approximation. The fact that, for the one-sided Z-test, $\Delta_n = \delta_n$ has important implications for p-values and the nominal statistical significance level, α, when Z-statistic is used to test the null hypothesis that $\mu = \mu_0$ based on a random sample of size n.

A key to understanding this relationship is the following important result, called the Berry–Esseen theorem, which provides an estimate for the error in the CLT [233–236]:

$$\delta_n \leq \frac{0.5C}{\sqrt{n}}, \quad \text{where } C = \frac{\beta}{\sigma^3} \geq 1.$$

Importantly, this is not true if the coefficient 0.5 is replaced with 0.4. Specifically, it was shown in [234] that $\delta_n > 0.4C/\sqrt{n}$ for a discrete distribution P with two probability masses (and therefore also for infinitely many other distributions including continuous ones). Since $C \geq 1$, for any such distribution, one also has $\delta_n > 0.4/\sqrt{n}$. This implies that there exist infinitely many discrete and continuous probability distribution P for which the inequality

$$|\pi_n - p_n| > 0.4/\sqrt{n} \tag{12.7}$$

holds for some, and actually infinitely many, random samples of size n drawn from P.

Relation (12.7) sheds light on the range of significance levels α that can be used in the one-sided Z-test. Recall that the standard practice is to reject the null hypothesis if $p_n \leq \alpha$. This inequality is a surrogate for the inequality of interest $\pi_n \leq \alpha$, which is typically very hard or impossible to verify directly. Of course, one should only consider those *admissible* values α that, for any distribution P, *both* inequalities $\pi_n \leq \alpha$ and $p_n \leq \alpha$ hold for at least one random sample drawn from P. Because π_n, $p_n \geq 0$ and, for some distributions P and random samples drawn from P, inequality (12.7) holds, any significance level $\alpha \leq 0.4/\sqrt{n}$ is inadmissible. In other words, every significance level α admissible for the one-sided Z-test must satisfy the inequality $\alpha > 0.4/\sqrt{n}$.

Applying this inequality to $\alpha = 0.05$, we conclude that this standard significance level is admissible for the one-sided Z-test only for sample sizes $n \geq 65$ ($n \geq 257$ for the two-sided test), and these are just conservative lower bounds based on the smallest possible value $C = 1$, which occurs only for discrete distributions with two equal probability masses of 0.5!

In a recent article [237], 72 distinguished statistical scientists advocated a blanket reduction of the nominal significance threshold to $\alpha = 0.005$. In the case of Z-test, this is feasible only if $n \geq 6,401$ ($n \geq 25,601$ for the two-sided test). Clearly, sample sizes in the majority of empirical studies do not meet these requirements.

Lower bounds, L_n, for the maximum error, Δ_n, in p-value computation for a fixed sample size n can, at least in principle, be obtained for other statistical tests that use the CLT-based Gaussian approximation. As just shown, every such L_n also serves as a lower bound for the nominal significance level α and therefore leads to a lower bound for the sample size given α. The argument made implies that, for any such test, significance levels $\alpha \leq L_n$ are inadmissible. The same is also true for p-values p_n such that $p_n \leq L_n$. In fact, this inequality implies, due to $|\pi_n - p_n| > L_n$, that, for certain random samples, the true p-value π_n satisfies the inequality $\pi_n - p_n > L_n$. Such a divergence between the true and empirical p-values renders pursuit of sufficiently small p-values p_n for a fixed sample size n meaningless.

12.12 A nontechnical summary of main findings

I realize that Sections 12.4–12.11 are quite technical. Therefore, this section contains, for the reader's convenience, a nontechnical discussion of the material of these sections along with a compendium of the main ideas and results in the foregoing part of this chapter.

The last 30 years have brought the scientific community and the society at large to a slow, yet cumulatively shocking, realization that a large fraction of published research findings in biomedical and social sciences are irreplicable and that, perforce, many of them are false. The replication crisis is commonly explained by reference to the liabilities of human nature manifesting in fraud, cognitive biases and conflicts of interest. Additionally, it is attributed to the dysfunction of various social institutions, which engenders misplaced research incentives, outdated educational practices, bureaucratic inertia and inefficiency and institutional corruption. Although human and social factors undoubtedly play an important part in science, the notion that they are the principal cause of the replication crisis has a major flaw—it cannot explain why the replication crisis has left mathematics, physics, chemistry, computer science, geology, engineering and other hard sciences relatively unscathed. This chapter propounds a different rationale for the replication crisis and false knowledge generation—intrinsic flaws of the methodology of applied statistics.

The main findings on this front can be summed up as follows:

1. A major source of false and irreplicable experimental findings is various empirically untestable assumptions. The most important among them is the stochastic independence and distributional homogeneity of data-generating random variables, collectively called the *iid assumption*. Many scientists are unaware of the iid assumption, others take it for granted or believe that its violations are minor and therefore inconsequential. Contrary to this belief, it is well-known among probabilists and mathematical statisticians (and rigorously shown by means of an example in Section 12.9) that arbitrarily small deviations from the id (i. e., distributional homogeneity) assumption can cause arbitrarily large deviations in the outcomes of statistical analysis.
2. Another significant source of false and irreplicable results is the use of various approximations, most notably the CLT-based Gaussian approximation, without heeding the associated errors. As was shown in Section 12.11, using the one-sided Z-test as a case in point, employing statistical significance levels and pursuing p-values smaller than $L_n = 0.4/n^{1/2}$, where n is the sample size, is meaningless because the error in p-value determination due to the Gaussian approximation may exceed L_n, and therefore the p-value itself. The same is true for many other statistical tests, although for them the critical value L_n is much harder to quantify.
3. Applied statisticians commonly ignore the fact that, in many settings, sample size is random and, furthermore, can be stochastically dependent on the data. This affects both the truth value and replicability of research findings because most statistical methods and tools break down when applied to samples of random size. As was shown in Section 12.10, even such foundational principle in probability and statistics as the Law of Large Numbers (LLN) fails for random sample size.

4. A popular belief that, with the data and code used to process it at hand, the original results will be exactly reproducible by another research team, is not always true. As was argued in Section 12.5, computer code is just a tip of the computational iceberg, while many other critical components of the numerical work can be an open-ended process that is hard or impossible to formalize.
5. False and irreplicable results may also originate from using a wrong methodology, e. g., applying stochastic models to essentially deterministic processes or vice versa.
6. Finally, yet another cause of replication/validity crisis is the use of non-identifiable mathematical models (see Section 6.5). Although parameters of such models are even in principle inestimable from the data, running statistical or general-purpose optimization software on a dataset in order to estimate model parameters would generate an output that might look like a legitimate solution.

12.13 The p-value crisis and beyond: a bigger picture

The generation of false and irreplicable scientific findings strikes at the very heart of science, undermining its goal and public mission of uncovering the truth about the natural world and human society and the credibility of this arguably most important human endeavor. To see how susceptible statistics has become to this destructive trend, one need not look any further than the phenomenon of undue elevation of p-values. That such a marginally important statistical measure has become, despite numerous objections and warnings issued over the last century, the single most important maker or breaker of scientific research in biomedical and social sciences and an arbiter of its scientific significance is nothing short of scandalous. As one example, a massive meta-analysis study [238] found that, among almost two million biomedical papers published between 1990 and 2015, 96 % appealed to the $p < 0.05$ criterion to claim significance of their findings. Thus, p-values, especially the magic $p < 0.05$ criterion, have become a de facto filter of empirical knowledge employed by scientists, journals that publish their work and agencies that fund it. In reality, p-values have little to do with the validity or importance of scientific findings, and the glaring discrepancy between their publicly accepted and real value has invited misuse, abuse and misinterpretation of p-values on a massive scale, and outright fraud.

The p-value crisis largely came about as a result of uncritical adoption of Sir Ronald Fisher's views on hypothesis testing, statistical significance and p-values and their facile synthesis with an alternative philosophy of statistical hypothesis testing developed by Jerzy Neyman and Eagon Pearson. An historical background on how and why this happened and evolved into a cult-like orthodoxy is vividly described in [239].

Researchers have considerable freedom in selection of null hypotheses. For example, in the setting of clinical trials (see the next chapter), when effects of an experimental intervention are compared to those of a control treatment, one can use either the *weak null hypothesis* that responses in the two arms of the trial have equal expected values or the *strong null hypothesis* that they are equidistributed, or anything in between. Likewise, there are plenty of test statistics to choose from for any given null hypothesis. All researchers have to do is to look for a null hypothesis and a statistical test for which the data happens to satisfy the $p < 0.05$ or another arbitrary criterion and call it a day, a practice fittingly called "p-hacking." This is one of the many ways which pried the door of applied statistics wide open to bias and manipulation, all under official cover of statistical guidelines.

Playing fast and loose with statistics engendered growing distrust of statistical methods by scientists including, in extreme cases, their rejection in toto. That is the choice made by several of my colleagues.

Belatedly, the American Statistical Association (ASA) issued in 2016 a formal position statement on p-values [225] followed in 2019 by an editorial and a broad discussion in *The American Statistician* of how to transition to the world beyond $p < 0.05$ [226]. The 43 contributions to [226] showed no clear consensus regarding the path forward.

The p-value crisis is but one symptom of many problems with the methodology of applied statistics. A particularly glaring among them is a cavalier attitude to errors resulting from various assumptions and approximations. It is a basic tenet of engineering that the design for, say, a load-bearing structure will not be commissioned or certified unless it can withstand a load far exceeding the one that would occur under the most unfavorable conditions of operation. Nor would a numerical method be considered satisfactory without hard estimates for the effects of systematic and round-off errors. In contrast to this sound precautionary ethos, scientific researchers and practitioners often blindly accept the results of statistical analysis based on empirically untestable assumptions and various approximations without paying heed to the magnitude of associated errors. This is particularly troubling given that statistical methods are often used for making critical policy decisions in healthcare, food and drug safety, environmental protection and other vital areas.

12.14 Statistics vs. science and medicine

The stark opposition between deterministic and stochastic description of biomedical phenomena discussed in Section 6.4 creates a considerable tension between the philosophical views of statisticians and scientists. In the realm of physiology, this tension was forcefully conveyed in the classic book [240] by Claude Bernard (1813–1878), a renowned French physiologist and a founder of modern medicine who introduced the concept of homeostasis. It is therefore instructive to briefly state and juxtapose the two epistemological positions.

Statisticians, on the one hand, believe that an individual observation is a fluke similar to an outcome of a single flip of a coin and that true scientific knowledge can only be gained by inference drawn from many observations and using averaging to filter out random variation. In applications to medicine, statisticians tend to dismiss a single observation on an individual patient as insignificant and anecdotal, aiming instead for large sample sizes.

Biomedical scientists and physicians, on the other hand, propound that what they see in an individual observation is *what is*, i. e., a manifestation of natural laws, with the usual caveats about measurement errors and the involvement of chance. In many experimental situations, they regard averaging multiple observations as inappropriate information compression that distorts the knowledge gleaned from individual data. The statisticians' insistence on averaging is one cause, among many, of the growing distrust of statistics by an increasing number of biomedical scientists and medical doctors [8].

The philosophy of statistics also collides head-on with the time-tested tradition of medicine. Since time immemorial, the purpose of medicine has been to treat an individual patient, while alleviating suffering and minimizing harm to the patient's health. The idea of averaging responses of several patients to the same treatment, which is central in clinical trials (see Subsection 13.6.2), had likely never crossed the minds of medical doctors in the past and even if it had, would probably be discarded as inane. More recently, molecular biology and genetics have put the idea that the course of the same disease and response to identical treatments vary greatly between patients on a solid scientific foundation. Nowadays, the millenia-old physicians' emphasis on a single patient came to be known under a new name of "personalized medicine." This clearly redundant term was coined in opposition to "population medicine" or, to use a more conventional name, "evidence-based medicine," i. e., a body of treatment recommendations based on statistical analyses, and meta-analyses, of clinical trials (see Chapter 13).

As many practicing oncologists would probably testify, there are as many cancers as there are patients. When it comes to cancer (as well as many other systemic and potentially life-threatening conditions, including cardiovascular, metabolic, autoimmune and neurodegenerative diseases), the personalized perspective is not only a more factual and scientifically grounded view than its population alternative but also an ethical imperative. Cancer treatment may produce debilitating side effects and at times even greater pain and suffering than the disease itself, which compels the patient to grapple with an excruciatingly difficult choice between the length and quality of the residual lifetime. What is ideally required from a treating physician is to not only give professional advice and render medical service but also to form a sacred personal bond with the patient and assist him or her in making critical life and death decisions. Those who honestly believe that the experience of such a patient is somehow insignificant and anecdotal disqualify themselves from such a partnership. This aspect of the medical profession is where evidence-based medicine and its statistical underpinnings fall woefully short [13]. That is also one of the principal reasons why this book was written with an individual cancer patient in mind.

12.15 How to put the application of statistics in sciences back on track?

While many aforementioned social, psychological and cognitive sources of irreplicability and false knowledge generation are hard to detect and mitigate, their methodological and educational roots are more tractable and amenable to change. What can be done, then, to mitigate the crisis and the resulting reputational damage beyond improving the design of empirical studies, avoiding conflicts of interest, and enforcing standardization and adequate reporting of experimental protocols, data and computer codes?

What is urgently needed is a radical change in the culture of applied statistical research. One direction such a change might take is ensuring tighter integration of applied statistics with mathematical statistics and probability theory. As a system of knowledge, statistics holds a special place among the mathematical sciences in that understanding and correct application of even the most basic tools of inferential statistics requires extensive technical knowledge of advanced probability as well as many areas of mathematics on which it critically depends such as real, complex and functional analysis and, most importantly, measure theory and Lebesgue integration. Only a fraction of applied statisticians and very few scientists using statistics in their work are able to draw with confidence from this theoretical edifice.

Another avenue of change is deeper integration of any particular statistical analysis with the scientific field to which statistical methods are applied. Too often, statistical data analysis is done ritualistically—ignoring scientific meaning of the data and the process by which the data was generated, and most significantly, omitting verification that the assumptions underlying statistical methods are met. Because many of these assumptions are empirically untestable, their validation requires keen understanding of a scientific problem in question from both subject-specific and formal mathematical viewpoints; however, to be successful, the synthesis of these two perspectives must take place in the same head!

Combining creative use of the theoretical arsenal with additional features built into a particular empirical setting will boost relevance and credibility of statistics. In particular, this could lead to an extension of statistical methods beyond standard assumptions and approximations and to rigorous estimation of associated errors. This would not only enrich statistical methodology but also generate better and more replicable research outcomes and make statistical analysis of a particular scientific problem a unique and exciting endeavor. However, if in spite of all the effort, the challenges are too daunting or if the error estimates prove too conservative to be practical, there is nothing wrong about dropping inferential statistical analysis altogether. Paradoxically, rigorous application of statistical methods is rarely attempted. All too often, the practice of statistics devolves into mindless application of standard statistical methods and tests and computation of p-values and confidence intervals unmoored from their mathematical roots and only loosely related to the scientific problem in question.

Another part of the solution would need to come from an overhaul of the criteria for hiring, evaluation and promotion of researchers in academia, government and industry. The most important scientific problems nowadays are highly interdisciplinary. Drawing on my experience reading, refereeing and editing hundreds of papers on mathematical modeling and statistical analysis in cancer research and other biomedical fields, I have seen firsthand how promising projects produced dubious results and wrong conclusions only because no one on the research team had understood all the aspects of the problem the team sought to address. A typical project aiming at quantitative understanding of cancer requires someone on the research team who deeply understands mathematics, statistics, biology, medicine and often other relevant fields such a physics, pharmacology or medical imaging. Absent this, the truth could fall through the cracks of partial knowledge. There are only a handful of people in the world with such a combined expertise, if at all. That is why senior researchers should be judged not only by the quality and quantity of their publications and the strength of their funding record but also by the breadth and depth of their knowledge.

Growing such Renaissance-type scholars requires the rethinking of graduate education. Creative use of mathematical and statistical methods, their extension beyond conventional premises and assessment of robustness to errors presumes the highest level of mathematical proficiency including intimate knowledge of theory and proofs. This calls for more dual and triple masters and Ph.D. programs that would graduate scientists who are equally well-trained in mathematics, statistics and a broadly defined subject area.

Another direction of reform is revamping undergraduate statistics education. For anyone trained in mathematics or mathematical statistics, reading textbooks in introductory or applied statistics is a painful experience caused by their ritualistic style, dogmatism and lack of rigor. Students would also benefit greatly from learning the history of statistics, which has been almost completely banished from the textbooks and classroom lectures. If it were taught, they would know that many valid criticisms of the concepts of p-value and null hypothesis testing were repeatedly brought forward over the last century [239].

Finally, drastic changes should occur on the interface between science and society. In particular, research journals and funding agencies should focus on the quality of submissions and not on whether all boxes including those related to statistical analysis are checked. All too often, statistical analysis is used as a convenient cover for poor data quality, dubious methodology and trivial results.

13 Clinical trials: gold standard of evidence-based medicine or ineffective and costly ritual?

More than on anything else, the survival and quality of life of cancer patients depends on effective and safe drugs and other anticancer interventions, diagnostic procedures and medical devices. Given that nowadays the road from bench to bedside is mandated to run through clinical trials, it is not surprising that over several recent decades clinical trials in the US and Europe have gradually become an enormous, multi-billion dollar a year public–private enterprise whose linchpin position in health care has endowed it with an exclusive status of "too big to fail." Scientists, medical doctors, healthcare administrators, patient advocacy groups and journalists alike have carefully crafted a public image of clinical trials as an agent of progress and innovation and purportedly the only way to make science-based healthcare decisions in which patients and their families should place their faith. They spared no effort assuring the public that randomized controlled clinical trials are the gold standard of evidence-based medicine. In this chapter, I investigate this claim from various angles. My main focus is on the methodology of clinical trials including their design, planning and execution and especially on statistical analysis of trial data. Evaluation of clinical trials conducted in this chapter was blueprinted in [9].

My investigation starts where it logically should—with the *raison d'être* of clinical trials.

13.1 Clinical trials: the whys and wherefores

Modern molecular biology and genomics have brought about prodigious progress in understanding microscopic mechanisms of life and disease. This has resulted in uncovering endless layers of complexity in structure, function and the regulation of normal and pathological processes in the human body. Paradoxically, the benefit derived by patients from the rapid advancement of biomedical sciences has been so far relatively modest, especially for patients suffering from chronic systemic conditions such as cancer and neurodegenerative, inflammatory, autoimmune and metabolic diseases [5, Ch. 11]. The principal reason is an enormous gap between our understanding of life's molecular machinery and our ability to explain the behavior of living organisms as a whole and to predict their responses to various interventions. This is where clinical trials come in to fill the gap through large-scale clinical experiments where curative, survival and palliative benefits of drugs and other countermeasures as well as the efficacy of various treatment regimens are tested and compared on large groups of patients.

The greatest challenge faced by clinical trials is an enormous variation in the responses of patients to any given intervention ranging from complete to partial to nonexistent. Additionally, patients may experience deleterious side effects of treatment any-

https://doi.org/10.1515/9783111334035-017

where from transient and minor to permanent and life-threatening. That is why clinical trials of a new drug typically include two preliminary phases—phase I, which probes the safety of various doses of the drug in animals and a few healthy human volunteers, and phase II, which tests the efficacy and potential side effects of the agent within the range of doses found safe in phase I, along with the methods and schedules of the agent's delivery, on a small group of patients.

One of the more dramatic manifestations of the gap between the relatively well-understood molecular biology, biochemistry and pharmacology of drug action on the microscopic scale and systemic clinical effects of drugs administered to human subjects is unexpected catastrophic events in phase I and II clinical trials. For example, a phase I trial of a drug BIA 10-2474 aimed at treating anxiety, motor disorders and chronic pain that was conducted in 2015 in Rennes, France, unexpectedly led to the death of one volunteer and irreversible brain damage in five others [241]. In a phase I trial conducted in 2006 in London, a monoclonal antibody TGN1412 intended for treating autoimmune diseases and leukemia caused multiple organ failure in six healthy volunteers [242]. As yet another example, fialuridine, an antiviral agent tested in 1993 by the NIH for treatment of hepatitis B in a phase II clinical trial, resulted in the death of five human volunteers due to severe hepatic toxicity and lactic acidosis [243]. Remarkably, the dose given to volunteers in the London trial was 500 times smaller than the one found to be safe in animals [244].

13.2 The normative essence of clinical trials

The principal emphasis in this chapter is on phase III clinical trials. These are protracted large-scale controlled experiments involving hundreds or even thousands of patients afflicted with a specific disease or condition. The main goal of a phase III clinical trial is to make an empirical comparison of the efficacy of a new treatment (or a new indication or regimen of an established treatment) with a standard treatment or a placebo. In addition, all the side effects and adverse events are carefully recorded, monitored and treated if necessary.

The philosophy and methodology of clinical trials has gradually evolved since the mid- 18th century and is based on the following principles.

1. *Clinical trials are controlled studies.* One of the main deficiencies of medical investigations predating the clinical trials era was that they lacked controls, i. e., observations on a group of similar untreated or conventionally treated subjects. Controls provide a baseline level of effect with which the effect of the proposed intervention can be compared. To ensure steady progress, clinical trials of new agents should ideally use the best available or standard treatment as control. Clinical trials may have several treatment arms, which enables comparison between multiple agents or delivery regimens of the same agent. Many clinical trials are placebo-controlled, which makes it possible to evaluate the net effect of an experimental treatment over

that of placebo (in other words, over the effect of a patient's belief that the treatment works (see Section 13.5)).

2. *Clinical trials are medical experiments.* Another major shortcoming of observational medical studies is that they involve too many variables, which frequently leads to great difficulties in establishing a causal link between a proposed treatment and the observed clinical effects. By contrast, to ensure scientific validity and replicability of clinical trials, they are executed as *medical experiments* with the aim of tightly controlling all sources of variation, except treatment. In particular, in an effort to achieve greater uniformity in clinical and demographic characteristics of trial participants, they are recruited using strict entry criteria. The idea is that this will facilitate attribution of the difference between the observed effects in the arms of a trial to the difference in administered treatments.
3. *Clinical trials are prospective studies.* Yet another common pitfall of many past and present observational studies is that their goals, design and methods of data analysis are set up after the data had been collected. This may lead to biases in data analysis resulting in overfitting the collected data, which reduces generalizability and replicability of the results and conclusions. Clinical trials are, in contrast, strictly prospective. This means that their goals, endpoints, design and statistical methods are selected and agreed upon in advance before any data is collected. Examples of such endpoints in the case of anticancer interventions are overall, disease-free and metastasis-free survival. Some clinical trials are focused on secondary endpoints such as the quality of life, as measured by the patients' functionality and levels of discomfort and pain.
4. *Randomization.* Groups of trial participants receiving one of the compared treatments are called *arms* of the trial. To minimize the degree of heterogeneity in demographic, clinical and other relevant characteristics of trial participants *between* the arms of a trial, recruited subjects are assigned, when feasible and ethically justifiable, to these arms at random. This also eliminates a potential investigator bias in assigning patients to treatments.
5. *Blinding.* To avoid or at least reduce the possibility of conscious or subconscious biases and prevent data manipulation that may skew the outcomes of a clinical trial, many categories of researchers involved in the trial may be blinded to the assignment of subjects to compared treatments. When feasible the same is done with trial participants, which may reduce their drop-out rates from the trial arms viewed by patients as inferior and achieve greater uniformity in the magnitude of placebo effects across the trial's arms. To make patient blinding more effective, some placebo-controlled clinical trials utilize *active placebos* that mimic side effects of experimental drugs.

Clinical trials fall into a variety of categories [1]. Some trials test a single drug used as monotherapy, others a combination of drugs. *Umbrella trials* compare many interventions against the same disease, while *basket trials* test the same drug against many diseases, e. g., different types or subtypes of cancer sharing the same molecular feature, mechanism or vulnerability targeted by the drug. In *adaptive trials*, agents are selected from an assortment of treatment options in an ongoing manner to achieve the best outcomes for a recruited cohort of patients. Finally, one of the aims of clinical trials is to identify responders to a given treatment and analyze their demographic, clinical and molecular profiles, which may serve as a stepping stone to subsequent more narrowly focused clinical trials.

The experimental and control arms of a trial are compared by averaging a certain measure of effect (also termed a *response variable*) over all subjects in each of the two arms of the trial. The difference between the averages represents the net effect of the experimental treatment over that of control. A typical measure of effect in cancer-related clinical trials is either an indicator of the occurrence of a certain event of interest (response to treatment, cure, recurrence of the disease, death, etc.) or the value of some clinical variable (e. g., overall, disease-free or metastasis-free survival, count of some type of blood cells, concentration of a certain cancer marker such as PSA in the case of prostate cancer, and the like). The normalized difference between the above averages often serves as the test statistic employed for analyzing clinical trial data. The same statistic can also be used on the planning stage of a clinical trial to determine the minimum number of trial participants to be recruited or the minimum number of events of interest to be observed.

On the statistical side, clinical trials are designed in such a way that the null hypothesis of equal performance of the compared treatments can be rejected with sufficiently low probability, called the *significance level* and usually taken to be 5 % or 1 %, if they in fact perform equally, and with high enough probability, termed *statistical power* and typically assumed to be 80 % or 90 %, if the alternative hypothesis that the experimental treatment performs better than the control by a given margin is true. After the trial's completion, statistical analysis of its results is conducted to determine the actual significance level and power, compute p-values, assess incidence and severity of side effects, evaluate performance of the compared treatments vis-a-vis secondary endpoints, perform subgroup analyses, etc.

Testing of a medication in a clinical trial, its approval, licensing and release to the market is not the end of the story. The medication continues to be monitored to assess its real-world effectiveness, track its long-term performance, detect rare side effects that could have been missed in smaller phase I–III trials, study interactions with other medications and look for new indications. Such large-scale postapproval surveillance of a medication is often called a *phase IV trial*.

Funding for clinical trials is provided by national governments, research foundations, universities and industry including pharmaceutical, biotechnology and medical device companies. When acting in this capacity, they are called "sponsors" in the clinical trials parlance. As one example, about 40 % of clinical trials of anticancer drugs in the US are funded by the National Cancer Institute (NCI). Large-scale clinical trials involve extensive planning, logistical and administrative effort. This incentivizes sponsors to hire private contract research organizations (CROs) to conduct clinical trials.

13.3 An historical note

The first clinical trial in history was conducted by the Royal Navy surgeon James Lind from May 20 through June 16, 1747. The task in front of him was to mitigate or cure scurvy, a debilitating disease that has killed more British sailors than naval battles and shipwrecks combined. The expectation at the time was that about 50 % of sailors would die of scurvy on any major sea trip. The cause of the disease—vitamin C deficiency—was only discovered in the 1920s–1930s. Although pieces of empirical evidence that vitamin C-containing citrus fruits and their juices can prevent and treat scurvy started to emerge as early as in the late 15th century and were used to the benefit of Spanish and Portuguese, and later French, British and Dutch, sailors and travelers, it was dismissed by medical doctors as anecdotal and going against medical theories of the time. A definitive formal proof of the curative effect of citrus fruits was needed, and it came in the form of the Lind's clinical trial.

Lind selected six pairs of sick sailors who served with him on HMS *Salisbury* and treated each pair with one of the following supplements, atop their regular diet: cider, a mixture of sulfuric acid and alcohol, vinegar, seawater, oranges and lemons, and nutmeg. After six days of treatment the two sailors who were given oranges and lemons got so well by then that they returned to their duties. The condition of other sailors had not improved. Thus, in modern terminology, James Lind conducted a 6-arm small-scale controlled nonrandomized clinical trial.

In 1753 James Lind published a book on scurvy [245], where he reiterated his flawed theory that scurvy is caused by faulty digestion rather than dietary deficiency [246]. In line with this theory and the 18th century conception of human biology and medicine in general, he only mentioned in passing his ground-breaking discovery and did not make a forceful recommendation to use citrus fruits and juices to combat scurvy [246]. Such a recommendation was adopted by the Royal Navy only 42 years later. Nonetheless, to commemorate Lind's methodological breakthrough, May 20 is celebrated as the global Clinical Trials Day.

13.4 The reality of clinical trials

The reality of phase III clinical trials is a world apart from the plaid image laid out in Section 13.2. In this section, I document various aspects of their shocking inefficiency and identify factors and forces that cause clinical trials to fall short of public expectations. In Section 13.6, I will bring to the fore fundamental problems with the statistical methodology employed in clinical trials.

13.4.1 The practical inefficiency of clinical trials

Unlike Lind's clinical trial of 1747 that was completed within less than a month, the duration of modern phase III clinical trials from conception of an idea to filing an application for FDA approval lies typically in the range of 6–10 years, while FDA's regular or expedited approval takes an additional 1–2 years [5, Ch. 11]. Given that the 5-year survival rate for adults diagnosed with many common cancers including pancreatic, brain, liver and oesophageal cancers is less than 20 % (e. g., one can look up cancer survival rates in the UK in [247]), the vast majority of such cancer patients won't benefit from ongoing clinical trials, with the exception, potentially, of those in which they are enrolled. The long duration of clinical trials for treatments against such aggressive cancers makes these trials a logistical nightmare.

Apart from the inherent complexity and a legitimate need to meet ethical and legal requirements associated with the informed consent of recruited patients, their privacy and security of their data, the unreasonable length of clinical trials is also due to an exorbitant amount of paperwork and bureaucratic red tape. For example, planning of clinical trials consists of hundreds of review, decision and approval steps spanning several years [5, Ch. 11]. The planning stage is especially daunting for clinical trials run at many locations. Such multicenter trials additionally require tight coordination and standardization of subject recruitment and treatment.

As an inevitable upshot of the inefficiency of operation and enormous costs, about 60 % of phase III clinical trials are abandoned before completion [5, Ch. 11]. Such a waste of untold human, material and financial resources denies potentially useful treatments an opportunity to enter the market, hinders patient enrollment and makes participants justifiably feel that they are used as guinea pigs (sometimes literally [248]) and that their taking part in clinical trials will only benefit future generations. The popularity of clinical trials in the Western world has reached such a low point that only about 3–5 % of eligible candidates agree to enroll [5, Ch. 11], which makes recruitment of the requisite number of trial participants a formidable task and further increases the rate of trial failure. That is why many US and European clinical trials are conducted in Asia and Latin America, where the supply of willing patients is ample, operational costs are relatively low, regulation is lax and oversight is fairly lenient.

In any scientific experiment, success is never guaranteed. So too, many clinical trials fail to reach their stated objectives or are closed due to an unacceptably high rate and severity of adverse events. This decreases the proportion of clinical trials reaching the stage of FDA approval of their tested agents even further. Finally, an appreciable fraction of drugs and other interventions are filtered out by the FDA's gatekeepers. All told, only about 10 % of treatments tested through clinical trials secure FDA approval [249].

The appalling inefficiency of clinical trials has engendered strong public and legislative pressure on the FDA, which caused it to adopt surrogate criteria of treatment efficacy as sufficient grounds for approval (for a discussion of surrogate endpoints in clinical trials, see, e. g., [8, p. 100–101]). In the case of anticancer drugs and other interventions, the improvement in overall survival, the true measure of treatment efficacy requiring many years to manifest, is often substituted with disease-free, progression-free or recurrence-free survival whose observation requires a shorter time frame. Furthermore, these and similar measures rooted in the clinical course of the disease are being gradually replaced with a more expedient and scientifically questionable criterion of the extent of tumor shrinkage (somewhat elusively called *tumor response*), which can be measured immediately, or shortly after, the end of treatment (see [202, 201] and Section 11.2 for more details). As was shown in Chapter 11 through a combination of mathematical and biological arguments, extensive tumor shrinkage in a fraction of cancer patients may actually entail, somewhat paradoxically, shorter overall survival and serve as a predictor of treatment failure.

All in all, phase III clinical trials are lengthy, wasteful and inefficient—an anachronistic mismatch to the fast pace of scientific discovery and the dire need to counter growing cancer incidence, documented in Section 2.1, with new effective treatments. Unsurprisingly, doubts about practical utility of clinical trials are expressed both in research publications [250] and those intended for a wider audience [5, Ch. 11].

13.4.2 Low quality and poor safety of the approved treatments

Despite ostensibly rigorous methodology of clinical trials, strict oversight of their execution and FDA's austere gate keeping, it is just a matter of fact that the efficacy of many FDA-approved drugs and other interventions is very low. For example, as Nicholas Schork reported in his highly cited *Nature* article published in 2015 [1], ten top-selling drugs on the American market fail to improve health conditions in 75 % to 96 % of patients who take them. Thus, lingering questions remain as to whether even some highly prescribed drugs actually work. Why does this happen?

One reason is rooted in the methodology of clinical trials. It is in essence a flip side of the requirement that, in order to rigorously assess the efficacy of a treatment relative to a comparator, clinical trials should control as many variables and sources of uncertainty as possible and practicable. As a result of this primary focus on efficacy and filtering out unrelated comorbidities and other confounding factors, trial participants generally tend to be younger, healthier, less medicated, and diagnosed at a less advanced stage of the disease than the general population targeted by the treatment (see e. g. [5, Ch. 11] and [251]). Therefore, a sample of recruited trial participants is not, and cannot be, representative of the patient population for which the treatment is designed [8, p. 90–96]. Naturally, the treatment performs worse, and potentially much worse, in the real world than in the sanitized environment of clinical trials. Another factor contributing to the same effect is that patients are removed from clinical trials due to death from the disease in question or unrelated causes, or drop out due to exacerbation of their disease or the occurrence of severe side effects caused by the administered treatment. To summarize, prescription medications are *expected* to be less effective and safe than suggested in the FDA applications and stated in public medication profiles and promotion materials sent out by manufacturers to prescribing physicians.

The second, and perhaps much graver, reason for the perception of clinical trials as not meeting public expectations is an epidemic of side effects caused by prescription medications. As one example, a careful analysis of the reported adverse drug reactions that have occurred in the US in 2011 revealed that properly prescribed and administered medications caused about 128,000 deaths in the US population [250]. This makes prescription medications the 4th most common cause of death in the US after cardiovascular diseases (including heart attacks and strokes), cancer and medical errors [252]. Regarding the latter, in 2013, medical errors caused about 251 thousand deaths, next to cancer standing at 585 thousand and cardiovascular diseases at 611 thousand [252]. Note that the foregoing mortality figure for medications' side effects does not account for (perhaps an almost equal number [253] of) deaths caused by overdose, self-prescribing, neglect of contraindications and largely unknown but potentially significant harmful drug interactions. Combining these two components might even propel prescribed medicines to the third leading cause of death in the US and Europe, according to the prominent Danish epidemiologist and biostatistician Peter Gøtzsche, a former director of the Nordic Cochrane Center (see [253] and [7, p. 1]).

13.4.3 Where are the new breakthrough drugs?

Developing a new drug usually takes many years and dozens of millions of dollars in investment. Combine this with a decade or more required for drug testing through clinical trials and the approval process, high risks of failure at either trial or approval stage, the 20-year term of patent expiration from the filing date adopted in the US, availability of new drug candidates developed by universities, the NIH and small private biotechnology start-ups, and finally the fact that primary fiduciary obligation of pharmaceutical and other biomedical companies is to their shareholders rather than patients—and you have a compelling explanation why major drug companies prefer to play it safe rather than run a risk and invest into new classes of drugs. In this context, "playing safe" means making minor modifications to an already existing drug that has been proven to treat or alleviate a particular condition (such modifications are aptly called "me-too" drugs) or repurposing an existing drug to treat a different condition. Additionally, risks of private drug sponsors are not limited to the loss of investment. The news that a clinical trial for a drug has failed or its approval has been denied promptly reaches investors, which results in a substantial hit to the price of the sponsor's stock.

How bad the risk aversion by private sponsors has really become can be illustrated by the following statistics. Of the 78 drugs approved by the FDA in 2002, only 17 contained new active ingredients, and only seven of these were classified by the FDA as improvements over older drugs. The remaining 71 drugs were variations of old drugs or deemed no better than those already on the market, i. e., were typical me-too drugs [254]. As another example showing that this phenomenon is not limited to the US, it was reported that, among 946 new drugs or new indications for known drugs that have entered the French market between 2002 and 2011, only two can be called breakthrough drugs, 13 offered a significant clinical advantage over existing drugs, 76 were merely clinically superior to the existing drugs, while 148 drugs were found to be more harmful than beneficial (see [5, Ch. 11] and [250]). In summary, the healthcare industry has managed to turn IP protection laws into a source of windfall revenues rewarding pseudo-innovation even more than breakthrough discoveries [250, 254].

Just as the biomedical industry prefers a risk-minimizing approach to innovation, so too the contemporary academic environment of biomedical research discourages scientific inquiries driven by bold new ideas, penetrating intuition and revolutionary insights under the pretext that they are not empirically tested or "hypothesis-driven" [5, Ch. 11]. As a result, novel highly effective drugs are a very rare exception. One of the most recent ones is Gleevec, a popular brand name for imatinib, an inhibitor of tyrosine kinases that was synthesized in the late 1990s and promptly approved by the FDA in 2001. Gleevec revolutionized the treatment of several types of cancers, most notably Philadelphia chromosome-positive chronic myelogenous leukemia (CML). Although generally not a cure for CML, Gleevec radically increased the overall survival of CML patients, thus largely converting a fatal, aggressive cancer of blood cells into a manageable chronic condition.

One consequence of the slow pace of innovation is that old revolutionary drugs dominate the market for decades. In the realm of cancer chemotherapy, many very old agents are still among the principal workhorses. For example, methotrexate (an antifolate that inhibits synthesis of DNA and RNA in fast-proliferating cancer cells) has been used as anticancer agent since 1947, while cisplatin (a platinum-based inhibitor of DNA replication) was identified in 1845 and approved by the FDA as a chemotherapy drug against ovarian and testicular cancers in 1978.

13.4.4 The corrupting influence of the biomedical industry

Because private sponsors have a keen financial interest in seeing their agents through clinical trials and approval, they take every step to make this happen, sometimes crossing over into the realm of unethical. It is important to realize how much leeway private sponsors running clinical trials and CROs doing so on their behalf have in shaping outcomes of a clinical trial: They select a target population of patients, set up trial entry criteria, and choose both a treatment and a comparator as well as their dose regimens [13]. In particular, by comparing their product to a placebo, rather than the best available treatment, they set the efficacy bar so low that even a marginally effective treatment would be viewed as superior and potentially approved by the FDA [254]. It was found that commercially funded trials are at least 2.5 times more likely to favor the sponsor's product than publicly funded ones [250]. One particularly striking manifestation of this bias in clinical trials was reported in [255], where among three specific psychiatric drugs A, B and C, drug A was found to be more effective than B, B more effective than C, and C more effective than A!

An in-depth look at various instances of deliberate bias and institutional corruption in clinical trials conducted or sponsored by industry was taken by Peter Gøetzsche in his remarkable book [7]. He documented numerous cases of withholding and falsifying data, selective reporting, suppressing information on adverse side effects, post hoc changes of endpoints, manipulation of patient inclusion criteria and study duration, and intentional handicapping of comparators as well as an assortment of other unethical profit-driven activities. This has led to numerous major public health calamities. As one example, concealment and fabrication of trial data on the cardiovascular side effects of COX-2 inhibitor Vioxx (rofecoxib), manufactured by Merck and marketed primarily as a NSAID painkiller, has caused, in the US alone, as the FDA itself admitted, between 88,000 and 140,000 heart attacks from 1999 to 2004 [256] with the estimated case-fatality rate of 44 %. Based on his extensive study, Gøetzsche concluded that in the hands of Big Pharma clinical trials have become nothing more than marketing tools in disguise [253, 7].

One of the devices employed by pharmaceutical companies is aggressive advertising of their new (or not so new) drugs on TV, radio and social media. They also work hard to establish “trial-journal pipelines,” whereby they publish favorable results of clinical trials in multiple research outlets in order to give their drugs greater visibility, bump up the citation index and make sure the results are prominently featured in meta-analyses; all the while, negative results are kept unpublished [250]. They even resort to a legal but unethical practice of ghostwriting by publishing articles, abstracts and comments expressing favorable opinions about the company’s products written by hired pens under the name of known biomedical authorities, called “opinion leaders.”

An especially egregious case of a massive ghostwriting campaign in support of hormone-replacement therapy (HRT) in premenopausal and menopausal women was documented in [257, 258] (see also [8, Ch. 1–3]). This aggressive advertising effort paid off. For example, it was estimated that the use of HRT drugs in Western counties between 1970 and 2019 was about 600 million woman-years [259]. Although HRT has been administered to patients since 1960s, its harms came to light only in the early 2000s. As one example, a large randomized clinical trial aimed at quantifying net “benefits” of HRT revealed that HRT actually increased the incidence of invasive breast cancer by 24 % [260], as a result of which the study was stopped early. Likewise, HRT amplifies the risk of endometrial cancer [261].

Yet another avenue used by pharmaceutical companies to promote their drugs is forging special relationships with medical doctors who write prescriptions for these drugs [7, 254]. Sales representatives frequently visit physicians to promote the company’s products, and this is often the only way medical doctors who are busy treating their patients learn about these products. Some companies pay medical doctors for supplying participants to ongoing clinical trials. They also organize free “seminars” for medical doctors educating them about new drugs in the company's portfolio. Quite often these seminars are held in luxurious locations and include lavish entertainment.

Big Pharma companies are keen on strengthening their ties with, and influence on, the FDA, which approves their drugs and grants them exclusive marketing rights. Many high-ranking pharma executives have switched to serving the FDA, while senior FDA officers (including Robert Califf, the 22nd and 25th FDA Commissioner, and Scott Gottlieb, the 23rd FDA Commissioner) were sitting on multiple corporate boards before and/or after their stint at the FDA. This symbiotic relationship has been enhanced through the legislative process. In response to public outcry over long approval times by the FDA, the US Congress introduced in 1992 the law on "user fees," i. e., payments to the FDA made by healthcare companies and intended to accelerate consideration of their products. While addressing a legitimate concern, putting the FDA on sponsors' payroll represents a classic conflict of interest.

The extent of influence of biomedical industry on the standards of FDA drug approval is staggering. For example, out of 161 FDA approvals of drugs against solid tumors in adults issued between 2017 and 2021, 58 (or 36 %) were based on single-arm trials [262], thus reneging on three basic principles of clinical trials—control, randomization and blinding. Furthermore, these trials used a weak and controversial endpoint of *tumor response rate*, defined as the fraction of patients whose tumor shrinkage posttreatment, as measured by the sum of two major tumor diameters, was at least 30 % [262], compare with the discussion of this subject in Section 11.2. Additionally, among the same 161 drug approvals, only 27 % were supported by unequivocal evidence of overall survival benefit [263].

13.5 The placebo conundrum

In the world of clinical trials priding itself on objectivity, the ubiquitous use of placebo as control strikes one as paradoxical. Placebo is a dummy medication that is unlikely to have any specific biological effect or is positively known to have no such effect. In spite of this, many randomized clinical trials of anticancer agents, where patients had been blinded to their allocation to either active treatment or a placebo arm, have reported improvements as high as 10–20 % in various subjective, yet important to the patient, measures of effect in the placebo arm of the trials [264]. Typical examples of such measures are the level of pain (estimated by patients either directly or indirectly as a decrease in the use of painkillers), functional activity reported by patients or physicians and the severity of symptoms caused by cancer. Furthermore, in some trials of anticancer agents [264] and in numerous trials of interventions against other diseases [265], these indicators of improvement were found to be superior to those in the active treatment arm. By contrast, placebo effects are fairly small when the endpoint is objective tumor response as measured by tumor shrinkage [262, 264]. As was mentioned previously, due to the low efficacy of many anticancer agents, a considerable fraction of drugs are aimed at improving the quality of life of cancer patients rather than curing the disease or halting its progression.

One would think that placebo effects in cancer patients are due to spontaneous tumor regression or the organism's adaptation to cancer resulting in symptomatic relief. This is true only to some extent. Results of several nonblinded clinical trials, where control patients knowingly received palliative care (alternatively called *best supportive care*, BSC) alone, suggest that improvements caused by spontaneous changes in the natural history of the disease or potentially by the placebo effect of BSC occur at a lower rate than in comparable single- or double-blinded placebo-controlled trials [264]. Thus, the question arises as to how one can explain the "real" placebo effect.

I would attribute it to two related but nonmutually exclusive factors. The first is the patient's belief that he or she receives an active treatment. Of course, for such a belief to manifest, the patient should indeed be convinced that what he or she receives is an active treatment. To make this happen in a typical randomized placebo-controlled trial, two drastic measures are taken. First, patients, and oftentimes trial personnel, are blinded to the patients' allocation to either active treatment or the placebo arm of the trial. Second, every effort is made to make placebo indistinguishable in appearance from the active treatment, including the following arrangements: (1) placebo pills are made to have the same size, color and taste as their active counterparts; (2) if active treatment is delivered through intravenous, subcutaneous or intramuscular injections, then the same delivery route is chosen for placebo; and (3) if active treatment has known frequently occurring side effects then, when possible and practical, ingredients are added to the placebo to mimic these effects (and thus to make it an *active placebo*). Note that the last two measures are questionable from an ethical standpoint. Interestingly, there is some evidence that a fraction of patients given inactive placebo tend to experience some side effects of the active treatment they don't receive (but probably know about) [264].

The second factor that might explain why placebo works is due to the patient's perception of being in "good hands" and treated with empathy and curative intention. Such perception is directly related to the trust a patient places in the treating physician, which may be elicited by the physician's demeanor, reputation and the amount and quality of attention given to the patient, and can be triggered by the treatment ritual [266].

Whatever the reasons behind the placebo effect, it consists of objective clinical manifestations of a subjective belief and is thus a psychosomatic phenomenon. Although the mind-body interface is poorly understood and viewed with suspicion by traditional medicine, it is well-known that the patient's mental state may trigger production and release of pain-reducing opioids, neurotransmitters that modify bodily functions, and hormones and other molecular signals stimulating or suppressing the immune system.

Although the placebo effect is well-documented, gauging its net magnitude is challenging because of the confounding factor of palliative care (or BSC), which carries its own placebo effect and is provided, or at least promised, to patients in both the placebo and active treatment arms of a trial. Estimating the net effect of BSC would require comparison with outcomes derived from clinical trials where patients receive no treatment at all. Due to ethical requirements and problems with patient recruitment, such trials are very hard to come by.

Given the difficulties with defining and quantifying the placebo effect, the question arises as to why control by placebo is so common in clinical trials, as opposed to control by the best available or standard treatment, which would be more conducive to maintaining steady progress in medicine. I cannot think of any reason other than the desire of the sponsors of clinical trials to play it safe and have a low-efficacy, yet widely accepted, benchmark with which to compare their agents.

13.6 The flawed statistical methodology of clinical trials

In Section 13.4, I reviewed a few biomedical, logistical, economic and regulatory aspects of the severe underperformance of clinical trials and their capture by vested interests. Now we turn our attention to problems with statistical methodology employed in phase III clinical trials for planning and drawing conclusions from trial data.

Inherent in clinical trials are four principal sources of variation: (1) sampling of trial participants from a relevant patient population; (2) intra-subject (individual) variation in the effects of compared interventions; (3) inter-subject variation in these effects; and (4) random assignment of trial participants to treatments.

As was argued in Subsection 13.4.2, sampling of patients from a targeted population is decidedly nonrandom, which makes the sample of trial participants nonrepresentative of the population. This has two consequences. First, the lack of representativity (also known as "external validity" [8]) is a barrier to extrapolating trial findings to the general population. Second, it may potentially lead to divergence of quantitative results between different trials for the same experimental treatment (note that sometimes hundreds of such trials are conducted, many of them concurrently!). Some quantitative divergence is, of course, expected due to chance and differences in demographic, clinical and genetic characteristics of trial participants (compare with Section 12.5). However, it is not uncommon that even qualitative conclusions from trials for the same or similar agents contradict each other (see, e. g., [8, p. 206–215]), suggesting that outcomes of such trials are grossly irreplicable (for a thorough discussion of replicability, see Sections 12.3–12.5).

Nonrepresentative sampling cannot be mitigated by even the best trial design and statistical methodology and is thus not a subject of our further discussion. Our focus in what follows, therefore, will be on the other three aforementioned sources of variation.

13.6.1 Intra-subject variation: the determinism vs. chance dilemma revisited

An important empirical fact central to the subject of clinical trials is that the responses of different subjects to the same treatment display a wide variation. But how conclusive is scientific evidence for the involvement of variation and chance in *individual* responses, beyond the relatively trivial matter of measurement errors? In the general setting of biomedical sciences, the determinism vs. chance dilemma was discussed in Section 6.4. The question in front of us concerns the aspects of this dilemma pertaining to clinical trials.

On the one hand, drawing from repeated casual experience with drugs such as an analgesic, antipyretic or blood-pressure medication, one can safely state that in many cases a fixed single dose of a drug has a well-defined, reproducible, patient-specific effect in terms of both magnitude and timing. Thus, in many settings, the effect of a drug on an individual patient can be viewed as deterministic, unless one is interested in more subtle sources of variation such as timing of drug administration relative to food intake, interaction with other agents present in the patient's system and so on. Then, why wouldn't the same be true for a new drug tested in a clinical trial? On the other hand, as was pointed out in Section 6.4, in many situations patients' individual responses can justifiably be viewed as stochastic.

Of note, treating individual response variables as deterministic does not preclude computation of the p-value of trial data in the setting of patient-blinded randomized clinical trials. In fact, under the (strong) null hypothesis that the effects of the two compared interventions in the two arms of the trial are equidistributed, the values of individual response variables would be the same regardless of the particular assignment of patients to the trial arms. This observation enables computation of the p-value by the permutation test [267].

Thus, contrary to the common practice in clinical trials, the choice between viewing individual effects of treatment as deterministic or stochastic should follow the preponderance of scientific evidence regarding the course of the disease, the mechanism of drug action and the response elicited by treatment. If such evidence cuts both ways, the two approaches could be pursued competitively.

13.6.2 The pitfalls of averaging

On the quantitative side, a key idea in clinical trials and evidence-based medicine more broadly, is the comparison of averages of the observed individual response variables over all subjects in a given arm of a clinical trial (or over a subset of subjects sharing a certain combination of attributes). Representing the value, x_i, of the response variable for the i-th subject as the sum of a central measure, μ, characterizing the effect of a treatment for a notional population these subjects represent, and the individual deviation, ε_i, from μ, we have $x_i = \mu + \varepsilon_i, 1 \leq i \leq n$. The power of averaging lies in the assumption of essential cancellation of individual deviations,

$$\bar{\varepsilon}_n = \frac{\varepsilon_1 + \varepsilon_2 + \cdots + \varepsilon_n}{n} \simeq 0,$$

or equivalently

$$\bar{x}_n = \frac{x_1 + x_2 + \cdots + x_n}{n} \simeq \mu. \tag{13.1}$$

The cancellation assumption thus amounts to positing that the population response μ can be estimated, or approximated, by averaging individual responses. Relation (13.1) will be referred to as the *averaging principle.*

Individual responses to a treatment are typically, and perhaps justifiably, thought of as independent random variables. If in addition they have the same distribution with a common expected value μ (or, more realistically, distributions close to identical with similar expected values), then relation (13.1) is essentially the Law of Large Numbers (see, e. g., [148, Section 10.5] and Section 12.8 in this book). However, as emphasized in the beginning of Section 13.1, the observed responses of different patients to a given treatment usually vary very widely, with some patients manifesting a complete response, others being nonresponsive and the rest falling somewhere in between. Therefore, the expected values of individual response variables may be far from identical, and so may their distributions. Thus, the assumption of distributional homogeneity, let alone identity, is highly unrealistic. Furthermore, if individual response variables are viewed as nonrandom quantities, a possibility entertained and substantiated in Sections 6.4 and 13.6.1, then interpretation of μ in formula (13.1) as a population-based measure of treatment effect is indefensible on either theoretical or empirical grounds. Thus, the validity of the averaging principle in the setting of clinical trials is uncertain.

The principal use of averages in clinical trials is for making comparisons between treatments. The seemingly appealing idea that the best treatment is the one that works best on average may be true in the case of distributionally homogeneous responses. But, as a general comparison principle, it produces fallacies. One of them, illustrating an extreme effect of the heterogeneity of responses to treatment, is described next.

As a simple schematic example, consider three competing drugs, A, B and C, compared on a population of patients. Suppose the efficacy of drug A is 2 units on a certain scale on one half of the population and 0 on the other half, and let drug B have efficacy of 2 on the latter half of the population and 0 on the former. Suppose also that drug C has efficacy of 1.1 across the board. Then, drug C is superior to A and B on average, but for each particular patient, it is almost twice less efficacious than the better of the drugs A or B. This leads to a perplexing conclusion: *The treatment that is best on average is not the best one even for a single patient in the population!*

To enable comparison of treatments based on average responses, trialists have to minimize heterogeneity in the anticipated arm-specific individual responses at the planning stage of the trial. Two measures can be taken to achieve this end: (1) to use all the available prior biomedical information about the targeted disease and the mechanisms by which response to treatment is elicited and expressed; and (2) to adopt strict trial entrance criteria. Implementation of there measures, however, may still fall short of ensuring sufficient homogeneity of responses to treatment, as the following clinical example demonstrates.

13.6.3 The heterogeneity curse: an example

To see how unreasonable is the reliance on the homogeneity of arm-specific responses to a treatment administered to patients in a clinical trial, consider a hypothetical randomized clinical trial that compares overall survival, disease-free survival or metastasis-free survival of stage I–III breast cancer patients under two treatment plans involving surgery and various combinations, doses and regimens of adjuvant treatments such as cytotoxic chemotherapy, external beam radiation and hormonal therapy.

What are the leading factors that determine individual survival outcomes? The single most important among them is the perioperative presence or absence of viable subclinical metastases. Such metastases can be in three distinct states: (1) solitary cancer cells that were released into the bloodstream during surgery or were already present at the time of surgery as circulating tumor cells or quiescent cancer cells lodged at various secondary sites; (2) dormant or slowly growing avascular micrometastases; and (3) aggressively growing vascular metastases that at the time of the most recent medical exam have not yet reached detectable size. If the patient was metastases-free at the time of surgery then, barring primary tumor recurrence, she would be cured. If only state 1 and 2 metastases were present shortly after surgery, then the outcome would depend critically on how long the state of metastatic dormancy will be maintained (for an extensive discussion of metastatic dormancy, see Section 3.6). Finally, the presence of state 3 metastases doesn't bode well for the patient, but the duration of overall survival depends on the efficacy of the systemic components of the administered treatment.

Whether or not metastases will escape from dormancy in a particular patient depends on many factors. Perhaps the most influential among them is the magnitude of long-term and transient effects of surgery and radiotherapy, discussed at length in Sections 5.2–5.4. Another highly significant prognostic factor is the intrinsic aggressiveness of the disease; however, its reliable assessment at early stages of breast cancer has proven so far to be elusive. Additional factors include concentrations of circulating angiogenesis promoters and inhibitors, immunogenicity of the particular kind of breast cancer and the strength of the patient's immune response. Exacerbation of the disease can also be triggered by intercurrent sporadic events such as surgery unrelated to breast cancer, trauma, infection and radiation. Thus, the most critical determinants of the survival outcome of treatment are largely unobservable and unpredictable, and may vary greatly among patients assigned to a given arm of a trial.

The aforementioned determinants of treatment outcomes represent "known unknowns." It is also quite possible that lurking among important predictive factors are "unknown unknowns" still waiting to be discovered.

In practice, the noted unobservable prognostic factors are replaced by less informative observable clinical variables such as (1) age at trial entry; (2) stage and histological grade of the disease; (3) localization and size of the primary tumor; (4) whether or not the tumor has invaded surrounding tissues; (5) the extent of nodal involvement; (6) estrogen receptor, progesterone receptor and human epidermal growth factor receptor 2

(HER2) status; (7) the presence of specific mutations in BRCA1 or BRCA2 tumor suppressor genes; (8) menopausal status; (9) family history of breast cancer; and (10) individual history of other malignancies. Even this rough and incomplete set of clinical variables creates a large number of categories of women in each arm of the trial with potentially very different responses to treatment.

Importantly, randomization won't eliminate the observable and hidden heterogeneity between participants of a clinical trial; it will only reduce the difference in the extent of heterogeneity between the arms of the trial. Additionally, randomization can elevate those unobservable aspects of the heterogeneity in individual responses that owe their significance to the difference in treatments. For example, in the context of the example considered in this subsection, consider a two-arm clinical trial populated by early-stage breast cancer patients comparing surgery plus adjuvant systemic treatment vs. systemic treatment alone. If, say, 30 % of trial participants had subclinical metastases at the start of treatment, then about the same proportion would hold for both arms created by randomization, thus recreating the initial heterogeneity in each arm of the trial. Additionally, as was explained in Section 5.2 and 5.3, surgery will accelerate metastasis in a fraction of metastasis-bearing patients allocated to the surgery arm of the trial, which will cause the hidden heterogeneity to manifest in survival responses of patients in this arm of the trial.

Thus, inter-subject heterogeneity is inherent in clinical trials, as opposed to in vitro experiments with cell lines or lab studies on syngeneic animals. Individual responses of patients in both arms of a trial cannot even approximately be viewed as distributionally homogeneous, let alone iid. The impact of this heterogeneity on the outcomes of statistical analysis of clinical trials is discussed in the next section.

Theoretically, distributional heterogeneity of responses in a clinical trial could be reduced through stratification of trial participants in accordance with their observable clinical variables and comparing treatment effects between the arms of the trial for each individual stratum separately. However, the following two impediments are likely to undermine the feasibility of this approach. First, due to the large number of strata, the sample size of many individual strata will be small, leaving the restricted comparisons underpowered. Second, the presence of hidden variation of the type discussed in this subsection might still cause substantial heterogeneity of the responses within each individual stratum.

13.6.4 Violation of assumptions in statistical analysis of clinical trials

Recall from Section 12.6 that the most fundamental assumption underlying any statistical inference from data including clinical trials is the iid assumption, i. e., that observation-generating random variables are jointly stochastically independent and share the same distribution. What was said in Section 12.6 about possible reasons for violation of the independence assumption applies in equal measure to clinical trials.

Another source of stochastic dependence between individual response variables in clinical trials is a commonly practiced prerandomization run-in period during which all trial participants receive either the same active treatment or a placebo (see [268] and [8, p. 94–95]).

As I have argued theoretically in Section 12.6 and by means of a clinical example in the previous subsection, along with a possible lack of independence, statistical analysis of clinical trials is bound to encounter a much more consequential violation of the equidistribution (id) assumption. This is chiefly due to the devastating discovery of the lack of robustness, made in Section 12.9 (see also [11]), i. e., that arbitrarily small deviations from the id assumption as measured by the KS distance may lead to arbitrarily large deviations in the outcomes of statistical analysis including, importantly, the average arm-specific response to treatment. Because these averages are the building blocks used to compute test statistics that generate the p-value and statistical power of a clinical trial, the aforementioned lack of robustness will likely translate into high sensitivity of the p-value and power to such perturbations. The same applies to computation of such basic trial design parameters as sample size and trial stopping time.

In most clinical trials, including those for cancer treatments, individual response variables are represented by a single observation that cannot be replicated (think, for example, about the duration of overall or cancer-free survival). This renders the iid assumption in the setting of such clinical trials empirically untestable.

An assumption widely used in statistical analysis of clinical trials is that arm-specific averages of individual response variables have a Gaussian distribution, which is a consequence of the CLT-based Gaussian approximation. As shown in Sections 12.11 and [11], the error resulting from this approximation sets up a lower limit on statistical significance and p-value, thus making pursuit of their coveted small values for a fixed trial sample size meaningless.

13.6.5 Sample size in clinical trials: fixed or random?

In most clinical trial designs, the number of trial participants (the sample size) is planned in advance with the goal to reach predetermined levels of statistical significance and power. The target sample size is achieved through ongoing recruitment of consenting eligible patients. In statistical analysis of trial data, the sample size is commonly assumed to be fixed. However, in reality it is often random due to patient drop-out resulting from the lack of treatment benefit, severe side effects, premature death or other reasons. This leads to a difficult dilemma: either to ignore the drop-outs and perform the so-called "intent-to-treat" analysis with the fixed initial sample size under intractable informative data censoring or to deal with a random number of patients followed through the entire trial duration. Random sample size is also encountered in clinical trials where reaching a predetermined number of participants is impossible or impractical due to insufficient supply of eligible participants, limited resources or time constraints. Additionally, random sample size arises in clinical trials planned around the occurrence of a sufficient number of events of interest, which is achieved through ongoing recruitment of subjects until the requisite number of events is observed. Finally, some variation in the number of subjects in a given arm of a clinical trial can be due to randomization. To reduce such variation, block randomization or more advanced schemes are employed [269, 270].

It was shown in Section 12.10 that randomness of the sample size can have severe consequences for outcomes of statistical analysis including potential violation of the LLN and CLT. Furthermore, if recruitment of new subjects is influenced by their expected responses or the previously known responses of other trial participants, the response variables and the random sample size would be stochastically dependent. In this case, as results of Section 12.10 demonstrate, standard tools of statistical inference including the LLN and CLT cannot be deployed with confidence.

That averages of individual response variables over a random number of clinical trial participants occur naturally can be illustrated as follows. Suppose the target population contains some (typically unknown) number, N, of subpopulations, each characterized by distinct distributionally homogeneous responses to a given treatment. Let M be the random number of these subpopulations represented in an n-subject arm of a clinical trial as a result of recruitment and randomization of trial participants. Let also n_j, $1 \leq j \leq M$, be the random numbers of representatives of these subpopulations allocated to the given arm of the trial and $w_j = n_j/n$ be their fractional sizes, or weights. Then the average response for the arm in question is given by the formula

$$\bar{x}_n = \sum_{j=1}^{M} w_j \bar{x}_{n_j},$$

where

$$\bar{x}_{n_j} = \frac{x_1 + x_2 + \cdots + x_{n_j}}{n_j}, \quad 1 \leq j \leq M,$$

are the average responses over the random number of arm-specific representatives.

13.7 Individual case studies: an alternative to clinical trials

There is one case where the aforementioned problems arising from distributional heterogeneity and stochastic dependence of response variables of trial participants are nonexistent, namely, when the sample of trial participants consists of just one subject. A great advantage of such individual case studies is that gaining extensive knowledge of the disease and the effects of treatment in a single subject is feasible both clinically and financially, and that, in this case, inference from generated data is not confounded by inter-subject variation [1]. If one believes that biomedical processes are governed by natural laws and have causes, mechanisms and effects, then studying a single subject thoroughly should be very informative. It can be expected that doing so for many individual patients will reveal over time all the major types, subtypes and characteristics of the disease and eventually enable reliable prediction of effects and side effects of medical interventions in any new patient.

Methodological differences between clinical trials and single-patient studies go far beyond the sample size. Statistical analysis of data generated by clinical trials is driven by large sample sizes and artificial thresholds for statistical significance and power detached from the biology of the disease and mechanisms of the action of administered agents. By contrast, individual case studies generate new knowledge through a detailed, open-ended, science-driven inquiry into a smaller number of patients with ongoing integration of the acquired knowledge. Thus, sample size reemerges in single-patient studies but in a more meaningful way motivated by the fullness of knowledge of the disease and response to its treatments. In essence, single-patient studies is, and has always been, a method by which medical doctors learn their trade and advance medicine.

Individual case studies conducted on pairs of closely matching patients in terms of demographic and clinical characteristics of their disease enable comparison between two treatments, one of which can serve as the control. Moreover, if both treatments were administered to the *same* patient sequentially and the first one was ineffective and did not change significantly the course of the disease and the patient's overall health, then in such a *crossover design* the patient would serve as the best-matching self-control.

13.8 Discussion, conclusions and recommendations

Clinical trials are extolled as a gold standard of evidence-based medicine and an engine of medical and public health innovation. By elevating randomized controlled clinical trials, the evidence-based medicine movement has beguiled medical researchers and physicians by pseudo-certainty of statistical measures, demoted knowledge arising from observational studies and downgraded clinical experience and intuition [271]. In the process, it has also ignored unique, un-averagable needs of the patient [13].

I demonstrated in this chapter that clinical trials fall far short of their declared lofty status in many significant ways. Firstly, the promise of clinical trials was undercut by the bureaucratic inefficiency of academic and healthcare institutions, the stifling influence of overcautious incrementalism that has taken over large swaths of biomedical research community and major funding agencies, and by the capture of clinical trials by the biomedical industry. Secondly, on the methodological side, clinical trials are compromised by statistical orthodoxy. Scientists who design clinical trials and analyze their outcomes conveniently ignore the possibility that individual response variables may be essentially deterministic, which in many cases is supported by scientific evidence. They are also oblivious to the presence of substantial inter-subject heterogeneity within each arm of a trial, of considerable errors resulting from the widely used Gaussian approximation, and of the potential randomness of the trial's sample size. All these factors may render conventional statistical methods dubious.

On the grand scheme of things, clinical trials are plagued by three major internal contradictions reflective of a considerable divergence between the trials' goals and methodology:

(a) The main purpose of a clinical trial is to empirically assess the comparative efficacy of an experimental treatment on a population of patients. However, to be legitimately called a clinical experiment, the trial has to minimize the confounding effects of potentially important demographic and clinical variables such as age, sex, race, stage of the disease, presence of various comorbidities, interaction with other medications prescribed to trial participants, etc. This generally makes the cohort of recruited subjects more homogeneous than the targeted population; in other words, not representative of the latter. This causes the efficacy of the experimental treatment estimated from the trial data to be more optimistic, and perhaps dramatically so, compared to what it would be in the real world.

(b) While the goals of a clinical trial are formulated in medical terms, the trial design and analysis of trial data are mostly driven by statistical concepts such as sample size, null hypothesis, test statistic, significance, p-value, statistic power, risk and odds ratios and their confidence intervals, and the like. An upshot of such a mismatch is that the results of randomized controlled trials are often "statistically but not clinically significant" [13] (compare with Section 1.4).

(c) As Sir Austin Bradford Hill emphasized in his classic work [157], in studies where the differential effect of a treatment over a comparator is uniformly very large (as exemplified by James Lind's trial (see Section 13.3)), formal statistical analysis is unnecessary. It is the case of small differential effects or those of variable size and sign that ostensibly calls for carefully designed large-scale controlled randomized clinical trials and rigorous statistical analysis of their outcomes. Paradoxically, as was shown in this chapter, this is precisely the situation where clinical conclusions can be greatly affected by violation of basic assumptions underpinning statistical analysis of trial data and errors resulting from the Gaussian approximation, randomization and large sample size notwithstanding. As was argued in [8, p. 22–23], increasing the sample size of a trial with small comparative effects is an exercise in waste and futility.

Under the assumption of stochastic individual responses, a key condition that makes or breaks statistical analysis of clinical trials is that of distributional homogeneity of individual response variables. If this condition is seriously violated, then the average response over a trial arm may prove to be a poor preference function for the selection of the best intervention, while the normalized difference between the arm-specific average responses may fail to be a useful test statistic under the null and alternative hypotheses because its distribution may deviate considerably from their assumed standard distributions. As an historical note, the idea that indiscriminate use of averages in biology and medicine may lead to obfuscation of scientific truth was passionately argued more than 150 years ago by the great Claude Bernard (compare with Section 12.14). He also insisted that the duty of a scientist is to find the unique immediate cause behind every health-related event in an individual patient, thus siding unequivocally with the deterministic paradigm [240, p. 137].

A larger degree of distributional homogeneity of individual response variables can potentially be achieved by tightening the subject recruitment criteria based on demographic and clinical characteristics including genomic, molecular, histological and other markers of the disease. Nonetheless, it is quite possible that despite all the effort, responses of trial participants will still be very heterogeneous due to the presence of clinically significant unobservable differences in the state of their disease of the kind described in Subsection 13.6.3. In this situation, a reasonable alternative would be to treat each individual subject's disease and response to treatment as a separate clinical case.

In a nutshell, what I have demonstrated in this chapter is that statistical inference from even a properly randomized, reliably blinded, perfectly executed and faithfully reported controlled clinical trial may still generate false and irreplicable results [9]. Additionally, this methodological challenge is aggravated by various biases and conflicts of interest involved in funding, planning, analyzing and reporting clinical trials.

From its early beginnings, medicine has been "personalized" in that physicians were primarily focused on treating individual patients, one at a time, and their interventions were tailored to the unique patient's condition and course of the disease. Gradual accumulation of medical and biological knowledge has led to a general notion of a disease as a pathological process that may occur in any predisposed or exposed individual and has common etiology, symptoms and natural progression. This led to the search for treatments against diseases as such that would work for any affected patient. This approach has enjoyed a good deal of success with many acute and some chronic diseases, especially those caused by a single internal or external factor, and was a potent formative force behind modern medicine. Unsurprisingly, the impersonal approach to practicing medicine won the accolades of being "scientific," "objective" and "the only one." Accordingly, modern clinical trials lay emphasis on average population effects, large sample sizes and statistical methods, which has been enthusiastically elevated to a new healthcare paradigm known under the name of "evidence-based medicine." Time and clinical practice have revealed, however, that many chronic, systemic diseases of complex multifactorial origin accounting for the bulk of death toll, including cancer in the first place, largely resist the population approach. One conclusion of this chapter is that vis-a-vis such diseases, time has come to expand the original principles of personalized medicine to drug development and other medical innovations including clinical trials. Due to scientific and technological breakthroughs in molecular biology and genomics combined with increased computational power and modern information technology, such expansion may bring about greater diagnostic accuracy and therapeutic efficacy than in the past [1].

Restoring the value and integrity of clinical trials requires: (1) resisting statistical orthodoxy and creatively using a multitude of statistical methods, while occasionally openly admitting that these methods are inapplicable or have failed; (2) validating, whenever possible, all the assumptions underlying statistical analysis; (3) closely coordinating statistical analysis with biomedical research, which provides statistical methods with both context and means for external validation; and (4) using advanced mathematical and computational methods to estimate errors resulting from violation of various assumptions and the use of the Gaussian and other approximations.

Each clinical trial should be treated as a unique scientific project that brings the full arsenal of scientific knowledge to bear on testing an experimental treatment against the targeted disease. This requires close collaboration between basic biomedical scientists, medical doctors, statisticians and mathematicians.

I conclude with a few specific recommendations informed by the analysis undertaken in this chapter:

1. Clinical trials should be publicly funded and conducted by biomedical researchers and medical doctors with no relationship to industry and no undeclared conflicts of interest.
2. No healthcare decision informed by the outcomes of a clinical trial with small or variable absolute or relative effects should be based on statistical evidence alone.
3. Scientific and health care benefits of clinical trials should be compared to those of state-of-the-art controlled individual case studies incurring comparable costs.
4. Trials should be populated in such a way that the anticipated individual responses to the compared treatments are as homogeneous as possible, given all the available prior knowledge.
5. The results of statistical analysis of a randomized clinical trial should be compared with those based on deterministic individual responses and permutation-based p-values, unless there is strong scientific evidence that individual responses are stochastic.
6. In those cases where statistical analysis of clinical trials is based on a Gaussian approximation-dependent test statistic, the use of sample size-independent levels of statistical significance and the pursuit of small p-values for a fixed sample size should be abandoned.

14 Epilogue: summary, path forward and advice to cancer patients

In 1901 Paul Ehrlich, the pioneering German scientist, medical doctor and immunologist introduced in Section 4.3, received, as the director of the Royal Institute for Experimental Therapy in Frankfurt am Main, an unusual personal request from the German Kaiser Wilhelm II. The royal patron of the Institute asked Ehrlich to focus all his effort on curing cancer. The reason for the Kaiser's request is easy to guess: His mother, Kaiserin Victoria, died of breast cancer in 1901, while his father, Kaiser Friedrich III, died of laryngeal cancer in 1888. In response, Ehrlich established the Department for Cancer Research within the Institute. He also informed the institute's sponsors that studying cancer meant doing basic research and that a cure could not be expected soon. Ehrlich's assessment of cancer cure is still relevant today. Despite many breakthroughs in the study of cancer, partially outlined in Section 6.6, and substantial progress in prevention, treatment and management of a few particular types of cancer, the incidence of many other major types of cancer accounting for the vast majority of cancer-related deaths continues to stubbornly rise or shows only moderate decline and, even worse, the same is also true for mortality from some of these malignancies (see Section 2.1).

So why is winning the War on Cancer declared by President Richard Nixon in 1971 still elusive? Why have many areas of cancer research lost site of the cancer patient and have become insulated academic disciplines? Why are some modes of cancer treatment designed and administered in blind pursuit of short-term benefits without even asking if this might exacerbate the disease in the long term and shorten the lives of cancer patients? I viewed shining some light on these questions as an overarching goal of this book.

14.1 The essence of the book

In a nutshell, the content of this book can be summarized as follows:

1. The book calls the attention of cancer patients, their families, caregivers, treating physicians, cancer researchers and healthcare specialists to various conscious and unwitting misconceptions described in Chapter 4, that have spread far and wide in theoretical and practical oncology. One of them is a common belief in, and dogmatic adherence to, the linear cancer progression theory and its numerous theoretical offshoots such as: (a) rigid separation between local and systemic cancer; (b) conventional staging systems; (c) insistence on early cancer detection including mass cancer screening programs; and (d) the idea that cancer should universally be treated as soon as possible with the maximum dose of anticancer agents a patient can tolerate (the front loading and MTD principles). Another misconception is that, once established, various primary and secondary tumors within the same host

https://doi.org/10.1515/9783111334035-018

develop largely independently. The book presented numerous arguments against these notions and described many ways in which they could harm cancer patients.

2. An important upshot of the book is that conservative approaches to treatment of invasive solid cancers deserve much greater attention and can often be expected to be superior to the aggressive ones. Most such cancers are by and large incurable by contemporary means. However, the vast arsenal of anticancer interventions can be deployed to control the growth of both primary and secondary tumors over long periods of time. Probably the best outcome many patients can hope for is to push cancer into dormancy—a stable, frequently occurring state of equilibrium between cancer cell proliferation and death in the dominant presence of angiogenesis inhibitors (see Section 3.6). Once maintaining the state of dormancy of primary and secondary tumors by therapeutic means becomes achievable, the urgency to employ other treatments and perhaps even the necessity of some of them would be diminished. One way to maintain the dormant state of metastases is to use the Ehrlich effect—the ability of primary tumor to suppress the growth and vascularization of metastases, as discussed in Section 4.3. Equally important is avoiding any perturbations to cancer dormancy (see Section 14.3). Conversely, I demonstrated that aggressive interventions, including the use of surgery and radiation therapy as first-line cancer treatments, are likely to cause explosive metastatic recurrence of the disease in a considerable fraction of patients (see Sections 5.2–5.4). Additionally, it was shown in Chapter 11 that aggressive systemic treatments can lead to the emergence and clonal expansion of increasingly faster proliferating cancer cells and thus reduce overall survival of cancer patients.
3. The book enlisted mathematics to aid cancer research and treatment in a fundamentally new way. While traditional mathematical models provide detailed mechanistic description of particular biomedical processes and are solved for a particular set of observations, the new method, outlined in Section 6.6, employs very general mathematical models and enables the discovery of general principles under minimal mathematical and biomedical assumptions in a data-free fashion. However, any such model must satisfy a crucial requirement—the existence of universal, i. e., data-independent, maximum likelihood estimates of some model parameters. Fortunately, a very general model of metastatic cancer progression described in Chapter 8 meets this requirement. This led to the discovery in Chapter 9 of the following general principle, or a natural law: *The most likely scenario of metastatic cancer progression in an individual patient whose primary tumor was resected or ablated by radiation is invariably the same—suppression of metastatic growth while primary tumor is in place followed by an abrupt growth acceleration after primary tumor removal.* Although these two related effects were first discovered experimentally 110–120 years ago and since then have enjoyed innumerable experimental and clinical confirmations, the concurrent experimental and clinical observations of the opposite effects prevented empirical discovery of the stated natural law.

4. In this book, I identified a number of methodological barriers to winning the War on Cancer. This includes serious methodological and practical problems with clinical trials and especially with statistical analysis of trial data explicated in Chapter 13. The book also exposed in Chapter 12 a credibility crisis across the entire realm of quantitative biomedical and social sciences caused by cavalier and ritualistic use of inferential statistics, which has led to accumulation of false knowledge and irreplicable research findings on an appalling scale. A few measures that could rein in statistical orthodoxy and put applied statistics back on track were proposed in Chapter 12. Finally, the book made a case for a more rigorous use of the scientific method including careful formulation of assumptions and being more fastidious about mathematical modeling and computation.

14.2 The double-edged sword of aggressive cancer treatment

The dominant paradigm of aggressive cancer treatment stems from the ostensibly self-evident idea that cancer cells should be eliminated as soon as possible lest they proliferate and exacerbate the disease. This idea is embodied in the front loading principle and, for interventions that have treatment dose, in the MTD approach to cancer therapy (see Section 5.6). Many of the arguments and results presented in this book point to a distinct possibility that for many categories of patients, such a frontal assault on cancer may actually be counterproductive. Here is a précis of points made to this effect throughout the book:

1. Radical interventions such as extirpation of primary tumor by surgery or radiation are likely to cause dormant solitary metastatic cells and indolent or slowly growing micrometastases lodged at various sites in the body to escape their dormant state and start to actively proliferate, vascularize and aggressively grow. This is due to four disparate but synergistic mechanisms: (a) abrogation of the Ehrlich effect; (b) boost to metastasis caused by spillover of cancer cells into the bloodstream during surgery for primary tumor; (c) elimination of a significant source of antigens expressed by an immunogenic primary tumor as a result of its removal by surgery or radiation, which may cause metastases to escape immune surveillance; and (d) acceleration of metastasis stemming from the medical procedure itself due to wounding, associated inflammation and transient immunosuppression resulting from both surgery and radiotherapy. Of note is that item (d) applies to *any* surgery, including the one unrelated to the cancer.
2. Apart from toxicity and harmful side effects, the main danger of systemic cancer treatments comes from the emergence of resistance. The presence of preexisting or emerging resistant cancer cells in a treated tumor is a universal phenomenon rooted in the heterogeneity of tumor cell population, genomic instability of cancer cells and selection processes causing resistant cells to survive, evolve, adapt and gradually take over as sensitive cancer cells are being progressively eliminated.

When a high-dose treatment is paused or terminated, which inevitably occurs due to mounting toxicity, the surviving residual tumor will mostly consist of resistant cells. Tackling them would require new, more potent agents or their combinations, whose administration will produce new side effects and will likely lead to the emergence of an even more resistant lineages. Resistance can also develop in the course of radiation therapy due to heritable differences in cancer cell radiosensitivity, selection processes, accelerated repopulation of cancer cells between fractions of radiation, and the presence of hypoxic and quiescent cancer cells refractory to radiation.

3. As I argued in Chapter 11, every treatment that does not eliminate a tumor completely or induce a stable disease may encounter another setback—progressive enrichment of the residual tumor with increasingly faster proliferating cells. The enrichment process will make subsequent treatments even less likely to succeed.

Thus, aggressive cancer therapy faces a number of roadblocks rooted in the basic biology of cancer and its response to treatment, and in selection processes triggered by the anticancer intervention. Cancer is a living and evolving entity with complex interactions with its environment and a tendency to *homeorhesis* (dynamic stability; in other words, return to the previous developmental trajectory after a perturbation). This causes rigid, predetermined treatment strategies such as the front loading and MTD principles to eventually fail.

What are the alternatives to aggressive cancer treatment? The idea is to abandon the universal goal of vanquishing cancer and instead trying to force it, when feasible, into a naturally occurring dormant or indolent state, or, in the words of Judah Folkman and Raghu Kalluri, "cancer without disease" [73].

How to achieve cancer dormancy? It could come about as a result of a "smart" approach to cancer treatment that avoids an all-out attack on the "enemy", but rather capitalizes on its inherent vulnerabilities and natural competitors. This approach could utilize: (a) homeostatic influence of a primary tumor on metastases (the Ehrlich effect); (b) critical dependence of the growth of primary and secondary tumors on angiogenesis; and (c) competition between sensitive and resistant as well as slower and faster proliferating cancer cells, and between cancer and normal cells. The emergence of resistant cells is often due to acquisition by these cells of new biological functions. Because maintaining them requires extra energy and material resources, resistant cells are likely to be less fit than sensitive cells. This makes it theoretically possible to reduce the overall size of the tumor to the point of dormancy while preventing runaway expansion of the populations of resistant and/or rapidly proliferating cancer cells.

Thus, the state of cancer dormancy can be achieved using an armamentarium of interventions at the disposal of modern oncology. The fact that they often fail to tackle a full-blown, aggressively growing, invading and metastasizing cancer, doesn't mean that smaller doses of the same agents or their combinations cannot be used to maintain and fine-tune the state of equilibrium between cancer cell proliferation, quiescence and death.

14.3 Oncology: a path forward

The arguments and results presented in the book suggest several directions of research, described next, that may potentially bring about breakthroughs in understanding and treating cancer, reduction in cancer-related mortality and improvement in the length and quality of the lives of cancer patients. A recurrent theme in these avenues of research is metastatic dormancy including its detection and designing therapies to maintain it. I believe that mastering metastatic dormancy represents the Holy Grail of the oncology of solid cancers.

1. As was described in Section 4.1, Bernard Fisher discovered that invasive breast cancer typically metastasizes long before primary tumor is discovered. What other solid cancers and to what extent fall under the umbrella of the Fisher effect?
2. The Ehrlich effect is the phenomenon of suppression of metastatic progression by primary tumor, which oftentimes results in metastatic dormancy (see Section 4.3). As was explained there, the putative mechanism involves local and systemic generation of growth and angiogenesis inhibitors and their spread through blood circulation. Although the Ehrlich effect was studied on animal models for more than a century, its mechanisms are still poorly understood, and so are qualitative and quantitative differences in its manifestation between various types of metastasizing tumors. Uncovering these mechanisms could be critical to the design of therapies aimed at maintaining metastatic dormancy.
3. As a logical consequence of the Ehrlich effect, resection of a primary tumor or its ablation by radiation could cause metastases to escape from dormancy and start aggressive vascularization and growth, which has been confirmed empirically in scores of experimental studies and myriad of clinical observations, and even proven mathematically using a very general model of cancer progression in Chapter 9. Other known causes of accelerated metastatic progression are traumatic, inflammation-inducing and immunity-suppressing effects of surgery and radiation, outlined in Sections 5.3 and 5.4. Beyond that, very little is, but a lot should be, known about metastasis-promoting effects of surgery, radiotherapy and other treatments. In particular, what cancer types are most prone to manifesting these effects, and what countermeasures could thwart or mitigate them and induce metastatic dormancy? Apparently, biomedical chivalry has not shown much zeal to pursue the Holy Grail.
4. Answering the following two questions about cancer diagnosis and prognosis would likely have the greatest impact on survival and well-being of cancer patients: (1) *How to detect dormant micrometastases?* and (2) *What is the likelihood that such metastases will remain dormant, and for how long, if the primary tumor is left intact vs. eradicated by surgery or radiation?* Designing definitive assays and image-processing algorithms providing answers to these questions would go a long way in guiding cancer treatment (or determining that leaving cancer untreated is the best

option). Because neural networks can be trained on millions of images and clinical histories of cancer patients, AI systems employing such neural networks could prove valuable aids in cancer diagnosis and prognosis.

5. The idea of converting aggressive cancer into a manageable chronic condition seems to be a very promising future direction of oncology. Implementing it would require a creative, adaptive, personalized approach to cancer treatment. Mounting evidence suggests that the standard one-size-fits-all MTD-based aggressive treatment is not in the best interest of many categories of cancer patients.
6. A tantalizing line of research, although perhaps with a taste of a pie in the sky, is deciphering the causes of miraculous cancer regression, be it spontaneous or unexpectedly brought about by supercharging of the immune system triggered by an intercurrent infectious disease or a medical intervention. Unlike other directions of oncological research already mentioned, this one could potentially lead to genuine cancer cure.
7. In the grand scheme of things, the inability of molecular biology and genomics to develop a lucid, universal understanding of cancer that would naturally lead to effective treatments is probably rooted in their reductionist nature. This approach knows no limit to the levels of complexity and detail it seeks to uncover and therefore is unlikely to converge to some final truth about cancer expressible as a comprehensive yet manageable catechism. This calls for devising a more macroscopic, systemic and holistic approach to cancer (and biological phenomena more broadly) that would view living organisms and their organs in health and disease as self-organizing dynamical entities governed by first principles, an alternative ardently advocated in [272], [273, Chapter 1] and [35]. This book can be viewed as a step in this direction.

14.4 Advice to cancer patients

This book offered many arguments, observations and specific recommendations, to be considered by cancer patients and those standing by their side when weighing treatment options, thinking about the questions to ask treating physicians, and pondering whether to seek a second or third opinion. The following pieces of general advice are parts of a mindset that, in my opinion, could be helpful in these deliberations. This advice is informed by the findings of this book, my 30 years of studying literature on cancer, and communicating with cancer patients and examining the course of their disease.

Attitude and philosophy

Have you noticed that all things cancer are routinely characterized in military terms? Ever since the US embarked on the War on Cancer in 1971, oncologists, cancer researchers and patient advocates are dubbed cancer warriors, patients who were cured or are in a state of remission are called cancer survivors and those who succumbed to the disease "have lost their battle with cancer." Implicit in these familiar labels are the ideas that cancer is an external enemy that should be vanquished and that, like in a mortal combat, there are only two outcomes in a patient's fight against cancer—victory or death.

These dualistic ideas, especially when pushed to the extreme, are a serious distortion of truth. When internalized by patients, they become a false, limiting belief. Medical events such as infectious diseases and traumas may indeed just happen to us due to forces beyond our control, with a caveat that even they can often be traced back to our failure to take preventative or safety measures. By contrast, spontaneous cancer is typically the end result of a long, intricate chain of internal events and processes that have more to do with our genetic make-up, family history of cancer, strength of our immune system and frequently with our lifestyle, dietary and other choices. And even the emergence of cancer induced by carcinogenic chemicals or radiation is mediated by internal factors, for it only affects a fraction of exposed individuals. Thus, perhaps a more productive idea would be to view cancer not just as an existential external enemy that has nothing to do with us but also as a manifestation of a weaker, imperfect side of our biological self. From this perspective, waging an all-out war on cancer is tantamount to doing so upon oneself.

The belligerent attitude to cancer shared by many oncologists goes hand in hand with the practice of radical cancer treatment including the "slash, burn and poison" triad (i. e., surgery, radiation therapy and cytotoxic chemotherapy) and other aggressive cancer interventions. Cancer patients, naturally, have a passionate desire to "just obliterate it." Thus, supply meets the demand, and this creates a powerful pressure to achieve short-term success in the long game of cancer, often at the expense of overall survival and the quality of life.

Find the right doctor

Finding the "right" doctor should always be the first priority for the patient and his/her family. Trust in the physician is, among many other things, a powerful magnifier of the placebo effect of treatment. Such a doctor would respect and follow the patient's preferences (see the following), commit to treating the patient and not the disease and would not benefit in any way, shape or form from the biomedical industry. The "right" doctor would carefully analyze outcomes of previous treatment cycles and adjust or, when necessary, even radically change the course of treatment, constantly learn and be unafraid to venture into unchartered clinical territory including off-label use of approved medications and tapping into the vast arsenal of alternative medicine. Such a personalized, inventive approach to treatment is hard, time consuming, may put pressure on the physician's financial bottom line and carry certain risks. But for those doctors who truly aim to forge a sacred bond with their patients and alleviate their suffering, treating patients at the cutting edge of scientific knowledge and clinical practice, and doing so in pursuit of the highest benefit for the patient, is honorable, exciting and morally rewarding.

Communicate your existential priorities

If you have a clear preference regarding length versus quality of life, you should state it to your treating physician unequivocally, for this may give your doctor an important clue regarding treatment strategy, e. g., more aggressive vs. more conservative. Cancer patients should also be aware that the quality and length of life are not necessarily mutually exclusive. Better quality of life is achieved through a delicate balance between cancer control and the severity of the side effects of treatment. This affords the patient the ability to maintain, to a certain degree, regular lifestyle and activities and spares immune defenses and other self-healing resources of the organism, which leads to greater overall vitality and zest and, therefore, likely, to longer life. The patient should also ask the treating physician directly if he or she would be better off by going with palliative care or watchful waiting alone. Because nowadays leaving cancer untreated is generally considered unethical, rigorous large-scale clinical trials of cancer interventions with a no-treatment arm as control are scarce. Equally meager is historical survival data on untreated cancers. Therefore, it is possible that the opposition to not treating certain cancers is not so much evidence-based but rather a reflection of the fear by sponsors of clinical trials that their agents might, in the end, fare not much better than the "leave cancer alone and live with it" approach.

What to avoid

The leading factors that can exacerbate cancer progression are *surgery*, related or unrelated to cancer (see Sections 5.2 and 5.3); significant doses of *radiation* received in the course of cancer radiotherapy (see Section 5.4), for other medical or diagnostic purposes, or due to a professional hazard; exposure to *carcinogenic chemicals*; *chronic bacterial or viral infection*; and *injury* (see Section 3.8). As was stated in Section 14.1, for many patients with invasive solid cancer, the best thing to realistically pin one's hope on is that treatment will convert cancer into a slowly progressing or, still better, dormant disease. If this is achieved, the patient is advised to avoid the just-listed perturbing factors at all costs because they are well-known for their ability to cause primary tumor recurrence and explosive outgrowth of metastases. Evidence from animal studies, reviewed in [129], also suggests that cancer including metastases can be stimulated by many seemingly innocuous drugs and other medical interventions with systemic effects on the body such as certain analgesics, steroids, antidepressants, antioxidants, some vitamin supplements, hypo- and hyperthermia and hypo- and hyperoxia.

Beware of harmful medications and medical errors

I urge cancer patients to heed a passionate plea by Peter Gøetzsche, introduced to the reader in Subsections 13.4.2 and 13.4.4, regarding ineffective and outright harmful drugs that are marketed to patients by pharmaceutical industry using its corrupt relationships with regulatory agencies, lawmakers, medical doctors and patient advocacy groups [7, 253]. As a reminder from Subsection 13.4.2, many among even the most highly prescribed medicines on the US market have very low efficacy [1]. As yet another stark reminder, the harmful effects of properly used prescription medications is the *fourth* leading cause of death in the US [252]. This does not include the considerable death toll from overdoses, self-prescribing and other unauthorized deviations from approved treatment protocols that patients or their caregivers may be responsible for.

Patients are also advised to gain as much knowledge as possible about drugs and other prescribed treatments, their side effects and deleterious interactions. Read carefully and understand the provided package insert. Because your doctor is simultaneously treating many patients and has limited time, chances are that if you do your homework well, you will know more about potential harms of your medicines than your doctor. Equally important is to use the acquired knowledge to carefully check the details of your medication's label and how your medicine is actually administrated. This is not a trivial matter or a vain exercise in control but rather a matter of life and death because, as was already mentioned in Subsection 13.4.2, medical errors constitute the appalling *third* leading cause of death in the US [252].

Practice medical self-knowledge

Nobody knows your body, the course of your past maladies and your responses to medications and other treatments better than you. Likewise, only you possess a unique knowledge of the family history of illnesses including cancer and which treatments worked or didn't work. This information may prove indispensable in selecting the best options for your cancer therapy. No doctor can predict your response to treatment and the toxic side effects it may cause with certainty, and your knowledge and intuition developed through observation, talking to relatives and journaling may provide the much needed insight.

Ignore survival statistics

The lethality of a particular type and stage of cancer is quantified by the survival rate over a given period of time counted from the occurrence of some event, e. g., reaching a certain age, detection of primary tumor, discovery of metastases, completion of treatment, etc. For example, a 5-year postdiagnosis survival rate of 60 % for patients with a particular type and stage of cancer means that according to historical data, 60 % of such patients were alive five years after their diagnosis. This survival statistic may be useful to a cancer epidemiologist or drug developer who deals with populations of patients. But for an individual cancer patient, it is largely meaningless, and here is why.

Among patients forming a certain population, their survival times vary widely and cannot be predicted in advance at the start of the 5-year, or any other, period. The survival time depends on many individual attributes of the patient and his/her disease including the aggressiveness of the particular phenotype of cancer cells, the degree of their differentiation (called *histological grade*), the presence of particular mutations, the strength of the immune system, age and overall health. Even more importantly, the duration of the residual lifetime may depend on other characteristics of the disease that are unobservable at the start of the 5-year period (see Subsection 13.6.3 for an example). Additionally, the individual 5-year survival probability depends heavily on the choice of treatment.

Thus, the observed 5-year historical survival rate is the *average survival rate* over a large unknown number of relatively homogeneous patient subpopulations weighted by their unknown fractional sizes within the relevant notional population. Neither the patient nor the physician knows with certainty to which subpopulation the patient belongs at the beginning of the 5-year period. If the entire population were homogeneous in all respects relevant to survival time, which never really happens in practice, only then would the population survival rate be roughly applicable to an individual patient.

Most significantly, fixation on the population survival rate sows gloom and discourages patients from increasing their individual survival probability by choosing the right doctor, aiming for the best treatment tailored to their individual needs and characteristics of the disease, avoiding exposure to factors that could exacerbate the disease and by pursuing alternative anticancer countermeasures. And if many cancer patients adopt such a proactive approach, the population survival rate would improve as well!

Never lose hope

The fact that cancer still remains a somewhat mysterious illness that stubbornly resists curative efforts has somewhat of a silver lining—unpredictability of the course of the disease and treatment outcomes. Sometimes, for reasons unknown to science, cancer undergoes spontaneous regression and disappears for good (see Section 5.6). Occasionally, the results of treatment by far exceed expectations. For instance, treatment may induce a stable disease that does not progress for an extended period of time due to reaching an equilibrium between the proliferation and death of surviving cancer cells. The medical literature comprises many case reports where resection of the primary tumor alone led to inexplicable disappearance of metastases. For example, a well-documented case of a clear cell renal cell carcinoma patient whose multiple lung metastases vanished altogether after removal of the primary kidney tumor was reported in [274].

Another source of hope is the so-called *abscopal effect* whereby radiation treatment triggers such a strong activation of the immune system that it starts to recognize cancer cells and wipes off all cancer deposits throughout the body [275, 276]. Furthermore, it has been known for centuries that the same can result from a spontaneous intercurrent bacterial infection causing high fever [277]. Bacteria, their toxins and other microorganisms have been deliberately used to inhibit or cure cancer [277]. For example, the antituberculosis Bacillus Calmette–Guérin (BCG) vaccine (a live attenuated *Mycobacterium*) is a standard treatment employed with considerable success as immunotherapy to cure early stage localized bladder cancer. Finally, scientists are working around the clock to discover new anticancer agents, so that despite methodological and other problems with cancer research and testing new treatments exposed in this book, a cancer incurable today may become curable or manageable tomorrow.

Appendix: Poisson process

This Appendix provides a background on Poisson processes as well as rigorous and largely self-contained proofs for some of their properties essential for Chapter 8. The Appendix also contains a detailed proof of Theorem 8.1, one of the major results in Chapter 8. The material of the Appendix forms a mathematical underpinning for the findings of Chapters 9 and 10. The appendix presupposes some knowledge of basic probability and calculus. Relevant prerequisite material in probability can be found in [148, 178].

A.1 The Poisson distribution

The Poisson distribution holds a special place among discrete probability distributions due to its remarkable properties and the ability to provide accurate quantitative description of various real-world events and processes.

Definition A.1. Let $\lambda > 0$. A nonnegative integer-valued random variable X has Poisson distribution (notation: $X \sim P(\lambda)$) if

$$\Pr(X = n) = e^{-\lambda}\frac{\lambda^n}{n!}, \quad n \geq 0. \tag{A.1}$$

In particular, $\Pr(X = 0) = e^{-\lambda}$. Together with (A.1), this makes it natural to set $P(0) = \delta_0$, the unit point mass (or Dirac measure) at 0. This imputation leads to a convenient extension of various properties of the Poisson distribution to the limiting case $\lambda = 0$.

A simple computation based on the well-known power series representation of the exponential function shows that $P(\lambda)$ is a proper probability distribution:

$$\sum_{n=0}^{\infty} \Pr(X = n) = \sum_{n=0}^{\infty} e^{-\lambda}\frac{\lambda^n}{n!} = e^{-\lambda}\sum_{n=0}^{\infty}\frac{\lambda^n}{n!} = e^{-\lambda}e^{\lambda} = 1.$$

A similar elementary computation establishes a formula for the expected value of the Poisson distribution (i. e., the expected value of any random variable $X \sim P(\lambda)$):

$$\mathbb{E}X = \sum_{n=0}^{\infty} n\Pr(X = n) = e^{-\lambda}\sum_{n=1}^{\infty} n\frac{\lambda^n}{n!} = e^{-\lambda}\lambda\sum_{n=1}^{\infty}\frac{\lambda^{n-1}}{(n-1)!} = \lambda e^{-\lambda}e^{\lambda} = \lambda.$$

Also, for the moment generating function $M_X(t)$, $t \in \mathbb{R}$, of a random variable $X \sim P(\lambda)$ we have:

$$M_X(t) = \exp\{\lambda(e^t - 1)\}. \tag{A.2}$$

In fact,

https://doi.org/10.1515/9783111334035-019

$$M_X(t) = \mathbb{E}e^{tX} = \sum_{n=0}^{\infty} e^{nt} e^{-\lambda} \frac{\lambda^n}{n!} = e^{-\lambda} \sum_{n=0}^{\infty} \frac{(\lambda e^t)^n}{n!} = e^{-\lambda} e^{\lambda e^t} = e^{\lambda(e^t-1)}.$$

In a typical application, random variable $X \sim P(\lambda)$ is interpreted as the number of events of a specific kind occurring over a fixed interval of time.

One of the remarkable properties of the Poisson distribution deals with the distribution of a *marked* (or filtered) Poisson random variable arising in the following setting. Suppose the occurrence of a certain kind of events is counted by a Poisson random variable X. Imagine that events are marked (or filtered out) independently of each other and of X with the same probability p, $0 \le p \le 1$. Let random variable Y represent the number of marked events. The following statement specifies the distribution of random variable Y.

Proposition A.1. $Y \sim P(p\lambda)$.

Proof. The description of the process of "marking" implies that, for any $n \ge 1$, the distribution of random variable Y, conditional on the event $\{X = n\}$, is binomial $\mathrm{Bin}(n, p)$:

$$\Pr(Y = m|X = n) = \binom{n}{m} p^m (1-p)^{n-m}, \quad 0 \le m \le n, \tag{A.3}$$

where the binomial coefficient

$$\binom{n}{m} = \frac{n!}{m!(n-m)!} \tag{A.4}$$

represents the number of ways to select a subset of m elements out of a set of n elements. Using the formula of total probability and formulas (A.1), (A.3) and (A.4), we obtain for $m \ge 0$:

$$\begin{aligned}\Pr(Y = m) &= \sum_{n=m}^{\infty} \Pr(Y = m|X = n) \Pr(X = n) = e^{-\lambda} \sum_{n=m}^{\infty} \frac{\lambda^n}{m!(n-m)!} p^m (1-p)^{n-m} \\ &= e^{-\lambda} \frac{(p\lambda)^m}{m!} \sum_{n=m}^{\infty} \frac{[(1-p)\lambda]^{n-m}}{(n-m)!} = e^{-\lambda} \frac{(p\lambda)^m}{m!} \sum_{j=0}^{\infty} \frac{[(1-p)\lambda]^j}{j!} = e^{-\lambda} \frac{(p\lambda)^m}{m!} e^{(1-p)\lambda} \\ &= e^{-p\lambda} \frac{(p\lambda)^m}{m!},\end{aligned}$$

where we set $j = n - m$. Therefore, $Y \sim P(p\lambda)$. □

Remark A.1. Proposition A.1 can be interpreted in terms of *compounding*. Let $X \sim P(\lambda)$. Suppose that, for every $n \ge 0$, random variable $Y_n \sim \mathrm{Bin}(n, p)$, conditional on $X = n$ (with $B(0, p)$ set by definition to be δ_0). If random variables X and Y_n are defined on the same sample space S, then we define the compounded random variable Z by $Z(s) = Y_{X(s)}(s)$, $s \in S$. Then the claim of Proposition A.1 is that $Z \sim P(p\lambda)$, or symbolically $\mathrm{Bin}[P(\lambda), p] = P(p\lambda)$.

Another important feature of the Poisson distribution is the following "additivity" property of (stochastically) independent Poisson random variables.

Proposition A.2. *Suppose random variables* $X \sim P(\lambda)$ *and* $Y \sim P(\mu)$ *are independent. Then* $X + Y \sim P(\lambda + \mu)$.

Proof. Using independence of random variables X and Y, formula (A.1) and the binomial formula, we have for $n \geq 0$:

$$\Pr(X + Y = n) = \sum_{k=0}^{n} \Pr(X = k,\ Y = n - k) = \sum_{k=0}^{n} \Pr(X = k)\Pr(Y = n - k)$$

$$= e^{-(\lambda+\mu)} \sum_{k=0}^{n} \frac{\lambda^k \mu^{n-k}}{k!(n-k)!} = \frac{e^{-(\lambda+\mu)}}{n!} \sum_{k=0}^{n} \frac{n!}{k!(n-k)!} \lambda^k \mu^{n-k} = e^{-(\lambda+\mu)} \frac{(\lambda + \mu)^n}{n!}.$$

□

Finally, the following proposition, which represents a converse to Proposition A.2, will be instrumental for interpretation of Poisson processes in the next section.

Proposition A.3. *Let* $\lambda \geq \mu \geq 0$. *Suppose random variables* $X \sim P(\lambda)$ *and* $Y \sim P(\mu)$ *have the property that* Y *and* $X - Y$ *are independent. Then* $X - Y \sim P(\lambda - \mu)$.

Proof. Denote $Z = X - Y$, then $X = Y + Z$. Since random variables Y and Z are independent, $M_X(t) = M_Y(t)\, M_Z(t)$ for all $t \in \mathbb{R}$. Therefore, in view of formula (A.2),

$$M_Z(t) = \frac{M_X(t)}{M_Y(t)} = \frac{\exp\{\lambda(e^t - 1)\}}{\exp\{\mu(e^t - 1)\}} = \exp\{(\lambda - \mu)(e^t - 1)\}, \quad t \in \mathbb{R}.$$

Because the distribution of a random variable is determined by its moment generating function uniquely, we again refer to (A.2) to conclude that $Z \sim P(\lambda - \mu)$. □

Remark A.2. Proposition A.3 implies that random variable Z is nonnegative with probability 1, a fact not immediately evident from the definition of Z.

A.2 Definition of the Poisson process

A *Poisson process* is a collection of random variables $X(t)$ parameterized by $t \geq 0$ with the properties codified in the following definition. In a typical real-world application, $X(t)$ represents the number of events of a certain kind that have occurred over the time interval $[0, t]$.

Definition A.2. Let $\lambda(t)$ be a nonnegative locally integrable function on $[0, \infty)$, called the rate (or intensity) function. Let $\Lambda(t) = \int_0^t \lambda(u)du$ be the corresponding cumulative (or integrated) rate function. A collection of random variables $\{X(t) : t \geq 0\}$ is called a Poisson process with rate $\lambda(t)$ if it satisfies the following three conditions:

(1) $X(0) = 0$ with probability 1;
(2) $X(t) \sim P[\Lambda(t)]$ for all $t > 0$;
(3) For any $n \geq 2$ and any time moments $0 \leq t_0 < t_1 < \cdots < t_n$, random variables $X(t_k) - X(t_{k-1})$, $1 \leq k \leq n$, termed increments of the process $\{X(t) : t \geq 0\}$, are jointly independent.

For $0 \leq s < t$, denote $X = X(t)$ and $Y = X(s)$. In view of properties 1 and 3 of the Poisson process with $n = 1$, random variables Y and $X - Y$ are independent. Then, according to Proposition A.3,

(2′) $X - Y \in P[\Lambda(t) - \Lambda(s)]$, where $\Lambda(t) - \Lambda(s) = \int_s^t \lambda(u)du$.

In particular, $X \geq Y$ with probability 1. Therefore, Poisson processes always describe *accumulation* of events, which is not obvious from properties 1–3. Also, it follows from Proposition A.3 that properties 1–3 in Definition A.2 of the Poisson process can equivalently be replaced with the more general set of properties 1, 2′ and 3.

A.3 Marked Poisson process

The goal of this section is to prove the following result, which was essential in Chapter 8.

Theorem A.1. *Suppose that events in a Poisson process $X(t)$ with rate $\lambda(t)$ are marked independently of each other and of the Poisson process itself with the same probability p, $0 \leq p \leq 1$. Denote by $Y(t)$ the number of marked events that have occurred by time t. Then $Y(t)$ is a Poisson process with the rate $p\lambda(t)$.*

Proof. We have to show that stochastic process $Y(t)$ has properties 1–3 from the definition of the Poisson process. That property 1 holds is obvious. Next, it follows from Proposition A.1 that $Y(t) \sim P[p\Lambda(t)]$, which establishes property 2. Thus, only property 3 on the independence of increments remains to be shown.

Let $n \geq 2$ and $0 \leq t_0 < t_1 < \cdots < t_n$ be any time points. Denote $W_i = X(t_i) - X(t_{i-1})$ and $Z_i = Y(t_i) - Y(t_{i-1})$, $1 \leq i \leq n$. Thus, W_i is the number of events in the Poisson process $X(t)$ that have occurred on the interval $(t_{i-1}, t_i]$, while Z_i is the number of marked events on the same interval. Clearly, $Z_i \leq W_i$, $1 \leq i \leq n$.

We have to demonstrate that random variables $Z_1, Z_2, \ldots, Z_n$ representing increments of the process $Y(t)$ are jointly independent, i. e.,

$$\Pr(Z_1 = k_1, Z_2 = k_2, \ldots, Z_n = k_n) = \Pr(Z_1 = k_1)\Pr(Z_2 = k_2) \cdot \cdots \cdot \Pr(Z_n = k_n) \quad \text{(A.5)}$$

for any integers $k_1, k_2, \ldots, k_n \geq 0$.

In the rest of the proof, we use a shorthand notation $W = (W_1, W_2, \ldots, W_n)$ and $Z = (Z_1, Z_2, \ldots, Z_n)$ for random vectors and a similar notation $m = (m_1, m_2, \ldots, m_n)$,

$k = (k_1, k_2, \ldots, k_n)$ for vectors with nonnegative integer components. Define $m \geq k$ to mean that $m_i \geq k_i$ for $1 \leq i \leq n$. Finally, set $\mu_i = \Lambda(t_i) - \Lambda(t_{i-1})$, then $W_i \sim P(\mu_i), 1 \leq i \leq n$.

If m is any vector as before, then, in accordance with the assumptions of "marking," conditional on $W = m$ random variables $Z_1, Z_2, \ldots, Z_n$ are independent and have binomial distributions $Z_i \sim \text{Bin}(m_i, p), 1 \leq i \leq n$. Therefore,

$$\Pr(Z = k|W = m) = \prod_{i=1}^{n} \frac{m_i!}{k_i!(m_i - k_i)!} p^{k_i}(1-p)^{m_i - k_i}. \tag{A.6}$$

The formula of total probability, formula (A.6) and independence of the increments $W_1, W_2, \ldots, W_n$ yield

$$\begin{aligned}\Pr(Z = k) &= \sum_{m \geq k} \Pr(Z = k|W = m)\Pr(W = m) \\ &= \sum_{m \geq k} \prod_{i=1}^{n} \left[\frac{m_i!}{k_i!(m_i - k_i)!} p^{k_i}(1-p)^{m_i - k_i} e^{-\mu_i} \frac{\mu_i^{m_i}}{m_i!} \right] \\ &= \left[\prod_{i=1}^{n} e^{-\mu_i} \frac{(p\mu_i)^{k_i}}{k_i!} \right] \sum_{m \geq k} \prod_{i=1}^{n} \frac{[(1-p)\mu_i]^{m_i - k_i}}{(m_i - k_i)!}.\end{aligned}$$

Setting $j = m - k$ in the last sum, we find that

$$\Pr(Z = k) = \left[\prod_{i=1}^{n} e^{-\mu_i} \frac{(p\mu_i)^{k_i}}{k_i!} \right] \sum_{j \geq 0} \prod_{i=1}^{n} \frac{[(1-p)\mu_i]^{j_i}}{j_i!}. \tag{A.7}$$

For an infinite matrix $[a_{ir}]$, $1 \leq i \leq n, r \geq 0$, with nonnegative entries, we have by an extension of the elementary "product of sums" rule in algebra that

$$\sum_{j_1, j_2, \ldots, j_n \geq 0} a_{1j_1} a_{2j_2} \ldots a_{nj_n} = \sum_{r=0}^{\infty} a_{1r} \cdot \sum_{r=0}^{\infty} a_{2r} \cdot \cdots \cdot \sum_{r=0}^{\infty} a_{nr}.$$

Applying this to the sum in (A.7) and using the power series expansion for the exponential function, we obtain

$$\sum_{j \geq 0} \prod_{i=1}^{n} \frac{[(1-p)\mu_i]^{j_i}}{j_i!} = \prod_{i=1}^{n} \sum_{r=0}^{\infty} \frac{[(1-p)\mu_i]^r}{r!} = \prod_{i=1}^{n} e^{(1-p)\mu_i}.$$

Finally, we continue (A.7) to get, in view of Proposition A.1, that

$$\Pr(Z = k) = \prod_{i=1}^{n} e^{-\mu_i} \frac{(p\mu_i)^{k_i}}{k_i!} \cdot \prod_{i=1}^{n} e^{(1-p)\mu_i} = \prod_{i=1}^{n} e^{-p\mu_i} \frac{(p\mu_i)^{k_i}}{k_i!} = \prod_{i=1}^{n} \Pr(Z_i = k_i),$$

which coincides with (A.5). □

A.4 Proof of Theorem 8.1

In this section, I aim to prove the following result, which is Theorem 8.1 from Section 8.2.

Theorem A.2. *Let $t > 0$, λ be a continuous nonnegative function on $[0, \infty)$ such that $\Lambda(t) = \int_0^t \lambda(u)du > 0$, and $X(s)$ be a Poisson process with rate $\lambda(s)$. Suppose random variables $T_1, T_2, \ldots, T_n$ with $0 \le T_1 < T_2 < \cdots < T_n \le t$ represent the times of occurrence of the first $n \ge 1$ events in the Poisson process $X(s)$. Then the joint distribution of random variables $T_1, T_2, \ldots, T_n$, conditional on $X(t) = n$, is absolutely continuous with pdf*

$$f_{T_1,T_2,\ldots,T_n|X(t)=n}(t_1, t_2, \ldots, t_n) = n!\,\frac{\prod_{j=1}^n \lambda(t_j)}{\Lambda^n(t)} \quad \text{for } 0 \le t_1 < t_2 < \cdots < t_n \le t, \tag{A.8}$$

and 0 otherwise.

Remark A.3. A useful interpretation of Theorem A.2 is that, under the assumptions of this theorem, random vector $(T_1, T_2, \ldots, T_n)$ is equidistributed, conditional on $X(t) = n$, with the vector of order statistics based on a random sample of size n drawn from the distribution with pdf $\lambda(s)/\Lambda(t)$ for $s \in [0, t]$ and 0 otherwise (see [148, Section 10.3]).

A.4.1 Preliminaries

I would like to start with reminding the reader about some basic definitions and properties related to the cumulative distribution function (cdf) of a random variable.

Cdf of a random variable X is defined by the formula $F(x) = \Pr(X \le x)$, $x \in \mathbb{R}$. It follows from this definition that F is an increasing function such that $\lim_{x\to-\infty} F(x) = 0$, $\lim_{x\to\infty} F(x) = 1$ and $\Pr(X \in (a, b]) = F(b) - F(a)$ for all intervals $(a, b]$. Also, $F'(x)$ exists and is finite and nonnegative for almost all $x \in \mathbb{R}$ with respect to Lebesgue measure. However, in general one can only conclude that $\int_{-\infty}^{\infty} F'(x)dx \le 1$.

The condition $\int_{-\infty}^{\infty} F'(x)dx = 1$ defines the class of *absolutely continuous* random variables X. In this case, the function $f = F'$ is called the *probability density function* (pdf) of random variable X. For such random variables,

$$\Pr(X \in (a, b]) = \int_a^b f(x)dx \quad \text{for all intervals } (a, b] \subset \mathbb{R}. \tag{A.9}$$

The existence of a measurable function f on $\mathbb{R}$ with the property (A.9) serves as an equivalent definition of an absolutely continuous random variable X. Clearly, the values of pdf f can be changed arbitrarily on a set of Lebesgue measure 0. Also, cdf F can be computed from the pdf f by the formula $F(x) = \int_{-\infty}^{x} f(t)dt$.

The relationship between the cdf and pdf, $f = F'$, implies that, for almost all $x \in \mathbb{R}$,

$$f(x) = \lim_{h \to 0+} \frac{\Pr(X \in (x, x+h])}{h}. \tag{A.10}$$

In other words, f is the "physical" density of the probability distribution of random variable X viewed as a distribution of the unit mass on $\mathbb{R}$.

My principal goal in the next subsection is to extend the "physical" definition of pdf given by (A.10) to multivariate absolutely continuous random vectors. The latter are defined along the lines of (A.9), but instead of intervals $(a, b]$, I will use cubes

$$Q = (a_1, a_1 + h] \times (a_2, a_2 + h] \times \cdots \times (a_n, a_n + h] \tag{A.11}$$

in $\mathbb{R}^n$, assume $h > 0$ and set $r(Q) = h$. Specifically, a random vector $X = (X_1, X_2, \ldots, X_n)$ is called *absolutely continuous* if there exists a measurable function $f : \mathbb{R}^n \to \mathbb{R}$ such that, for every cube Q of the form (A.11),

$$\Pr(X \in Q) = \int_Q f(x)dx.$$

This implies that $f \geq 0$ almost everywhere (a. e.) with respect to Lebesgue measure m_n on $\mathbb{R}^n$ and $\int_{\mathbb{R}^n} f(x)dx = 1$.

The extension of formula (A.10) to the multivariate case will make use of the concept of *Vitali covering* and its important property, called the *Vitali covering theorem*. Recall that a collection $\mathcal{F}$ of subsets in $\mathbb{R}^n$ is called a *covering* of a subset A in $\mathbb{R}^n$ if the union of all sets in $\mathcal{F}$ contains A. A covering $\mathcal{F}$ of A composed of *cubes* in $\mathbb{R}^n$ is termed a Vitali covering if, for every point $x \in A$ and every $\delta > 0$, there is a cube $F \in \mathcal{F}$ such that $x \in F$ and $r(F) < \delta$. The following important technical result constitutes the Vitali covering theorem:

Theorem A.3. *If $\mathcal{F}$ is a Vitali covering of a measurable subset A in $\mathbb{R}^n$, then there exists a finite or countable subcollection $\{F_1, F_2, \ldots\}$ of disjoint cubes in $\mathcal{F}$ with the property that $m_n[A \setminus (\cup_k F_k)] = 0$.*

For a proof of the Vitali covering theorem, the reader is referred to any standard textbook in real analysis or measure theory (see, e. g., [278]).

A.4.2 A description of the pdf of a multivariate distribution

The purpose of this subsection is to present a proof of the following statement:

Lemma A.1. *Let $X = (X_1, X_2, \ldots, X_n)$ be a random vector in $\mathbb{R}^n$ supported on an open set $G \subset \mathbb{R}^n$ in the sense that $\Pr(X \in G) = 1$. Suppose there exists a measurable nonnegative function f on G with $\int_G f(u)du = 1$ that has the following property: For almost all $x \in G$*

with respect to Lebesgue measure and for every $\varepsilon > 0$, there exists $\delta = \delta(x) > 0$ such that for every cube Q containing x with $r(Q) < \delta$,

$$\left|\frac{\Pr(X \in Q)}{m_n(Q)} - f(y)\right| \le \varepsilon \quad \textit{for all } y \in Q. \tag{A.12}$$

Then random vector X is absolutely continuous, and f is the pdf of X.

Proof. Denote by E the set of all points $x \in G$ for which the property stated in Lemma A.1 does not hold; then $m_n(E) = 0$.

We have to show that, for every cube $B \subset G$,

$$\Pr(X \in B) = \int_B f(x)dx. \tag{A.13}$$

To this end, fix any such B and $\varepsilon > 0$. By the assumptions of Lemma A.1, for every $x \in B\backslash E$, there is $\delta = \delta(x) > 0$ with the following property: for all cubes $Q \subset B$ such that $x \in Q$ and $r(Q) < \delta$, relation (A.12) holds. The collection, $\mathcal{F}$, of all such cubes selected for all $x \in B\backslash E$, forms a Vitali covering of $B\backslash E$. By the Vitali covering theorem (see Theorem A.3), there is a finite or countable *disjoint* subcollection $\{F_1, F_2, \ldots\}$ of cubes from $\mathcal{F}$ such that $m_n[(B \setminus E) \setminus (\cup_k F_k)] = 0$. Denote $F = \cup_k F_k$, and observe that $F \subset B$. Due to the inclusion $B \setminus F \subset [(B \setminus E) \setminus F] \cup E$, we also have $m_n(B \setminus F) = 0$. In view of disjointness of the sets in $\{F_1, F_2, \ldots\}$ and (A.12),

$$\begin{aligned}\left|\Pr(X \in F) - \int_F f(u)du\right| &= \left|\sum_k \Pr(X \in F_k) - \sum_k \int_{F_k} f(u)du\right| \\ &= \left|\sum_k \int_{F_k} \left[\frac{\Pr(X \in F_k)}{m_n(F_k)} - f(u)\right] du\right| \le \sum_k \int_{F_k} \left|\frac{\Pr(X \in F_k)}{m_n(F_k)} - f(u)\right| du \\ &\le \varepsilon \sum_k m_n(F_k) = \varepsilon m_n(F) = \varepsilon m_n(B).\end{aligned}$$

Therefore,

$$\int_B f(u)du = \int_F f(u)du \le \Pr(X \in F) + \varepsilon m_n(B) \le \Pr(X \in B) + \varepsilon m_n(B),$$

which implies, due to arbitrariness of ε, that for every cube $B \subset G$,

$$\Pr(X \in B) \ge \int_B f(u)du. \tag{A.14}$$

In order to show the reverse inequality, suppose that

$$\Pr(X \in B_0) > \int_{B_0} f(u)du \tag{A.15}$$

for some cube $B_0 \subset G$. The open set $G \setminus \bar{B}_0$, where $\bar{B}_0$, the closure of B_0, is a closed cube, can be represented as a finite or countable disjoint union of cubes, $G \setminus \bar{B}_0 = \cup_k Q_k$. Then G can also be represented as a disjoint union: $G = (\bar{B}_0 \cap G) \cup (\cup_k Q_k)$. In view of our assumption (A.15), inequality (A.14) and the fact that $m_n[(\bar{B}_0 \cap G) \setminus B_0] \le m_n(\bar{B}_0 \setminus B_0) = 0$, we have

$$
\begin{aligned}
1 &= \Pr(X \in G) = \Pr(X \in \bar{B}_0 \cap G) + \Pr(X \in \cup_k Q_k) = \Pr(X \in \bar{B}_0) + \sum_k \Pr(X \in Q_k) \\
&\ge \Pr(X \in B_0) + \sum_k \Pr(X \in Q_k) > \int_{B_0} f(u)du + \sum_k \int_{Q_k} f(u)du \\
&= \int_{\bar{B}_0 \cap G} f(u)du + \int_{\cup_k Q_k} f(u)du = \int_{(\bar{B}_0 \cap G) \cup (\cup_k Q_k)} f(u)du = \int_G f(u)du = 1.
\end{aligned}
$$

This contradiction proves (A.13). □

A.4.3 Proof of Theorem A.2

The proof follows the notation used in the formulation of Theorem A.2. Additionally, set

$$
G = \{u = (t_1, t_2, \ldots, t_n) \in \mathbb{R}^n : 0 < t_1 < t_2 < \cdots < t_n < t\}. \tag{A.16}
$$

Clearly, G is an open subset in $\mathbb{R}^n$. Recall that $T = (T_1, T_2, \ldots, T_n)$ is the random vector of the occurrence times for the first n events in a Poisson process $X(s)$. Finally, denote by f the function on the right-hand side (RHS) of formula (A.8).

Owing to Lemma A.1, we only have to show that

1. $\Pr[T \in G | X(t) = n] = 1$;
2. Function f satisfies condition (A.12); and
3. $\int_G f(u)du = 1$.

To prove statement 1, we need to verify that $\Pr[T_1 = 0 | X(t) = n] = 0$ and $\Pr[T_n = t | X(t) = n] = 0$. The first equality follows from property 1 of the Poisson process. To demonstrate the second equality, denote by Φ_n the cdf of T_n, conditional on $X(t) = n$. Observe that $\{T_n \le t\} = \{X(t) \ge n\}$. Then, for $0 \le s \le t$, we have using properties 2 and 3 of the Poisson process:

$$
\begin{aligned}
\Phi_n(s) &= \Pr[T_n \le s | X(t) = n] = \frac{\Pr[T_n \le s, X(t) = n]}{\Pr[X(t) = n]} = \frac{\Pr[X(s) \ge n, X(t) = n]}{\Pr[X(t) = n]} \\
&= \frac{\Pr[X(s) = n, X(t) = n]}{\Pr[X(t) = n]} = \frac{\Pr[X(s) = n, X(t) - X(s) = 0]}{\Pr[X(t) = n]} \\
&= \Pr[X(t) - X(s) = 0] \frac{\Pr[X(s) = n]}{\Pr[X(t) = n]} = e^{-[\Lambda(t) - \Lambda(s)]} \frac{e^{-\Lambda(s)} \Lambda^n(s)}{e^{-\Lambda(t)} \Lambda^n(t)} = \left[\frac{\Lambda(s)}{\Lambda(t)}\right]^n,
\end{aligned}
$$

while for $s > t$ we have $\Phi_n(s) = 1$. Thus, function Φ_n is continuous at point t, which implies that $\Pr[T_n = t|X(t) = n] = \Phi_n(t) - \Phi_n(t-) = 0$.

To prove statement 2, fix $u = (t_1, t_2, \dots, t_n) \in G$ and $\varepsilon > 0$. Consider a cube Q of the type (A.11) such that $u \in Q$, and set for convenience $t_0 = 0$ and $t_{n+1} = a_{n+1} = t$. Define

$$\delta_0 = \frac{1}{2}\min\{t_k - t_{k-1} : 1 \le k \le n+1\}.$$

Clearly, $\delta_0 > 0$. We need to establish the following technical result:

Claim. *If $r(Q) < \delta_0$, then $Q \subset G$.*

To prove this claim, in accordance with the definition of the set G in (A.16), we only have to show that (a) $a_1 > 0$; (b) $a_k + h < a_{k+1}$ for $1 \le k \le n-1$, and (c) $a_n + h < t$.

To verify inequality (a), note that due to the fact that $u = (t_1, t_2, \dots, t_n) \in Q$,

$$a_1 \ge t_1 - h > t_1 - \delta_0 > t_1 - (t_1 - t_0) = t_0 = 0.$$

As for (b),

$$a_{k+1} - (a_k + h) > (t_{k+1} - h) - (t_k + h) > (t_{k+1} - t_k) - 2\delta_0 \ge (t_{k+1} - t_k) - (t_{k+1} - t_k) = 0.$$

Finally, we demonstrate (c) by noting that

$$t - (a_n + h) > t - (t_n + h) > t_{n+1} - t_n - \delta_0 > (t_{n+1} - t_n) - (t_{n+1} - t_n) = 0,$$

which concludes the proof of the claim.

To verify condition (A.12), we first compute, assuming $r(Q) < \delta_0$,

$$\Pr[T \in Q|X(t) = n] = \frac{\Pr[T \in Q, X(t) = n]}{\Pr[X(t) = n]}, \tag{A.17}$$

where

$$\Pr[X(t) = n] = e^{-\Lambda(t)}\frac{\Lambda^n(t)}{n!}. \tag{A.18}$$

The event $\{T \in Q, X(t) = n\}$ can be represented as follows:

$$\begin{aligned}
&\{T \in Q, X(t) = n\}\\
&= \prod_{k=1}^{n}\{T_k \in (a_k, a_k + h], 1 \le k \le n\} \cap \{X(t) = n\}\\
&= \{0 < a_1 < T_1 \le a_1 + h < a_2 < T_2 \le a_2 + h < \cdots < a_n < T_n \le a_n + h < t\} \cap \{X(t) = n\}\\
&= \{X(a_1) = 0, X(a_1 + h) = X(a_2) = 1, \dots, X(a_{n-1} + h) = X(a_n) = n-1, X(a_n + h) = X(t) = n\}\\
&= \{X(a_1) = 0\} \cap [\cap_{k=1}^{n}\{X(a_k + h) - X(a_k) = 1\}] \cap [\cap_{k=1}^{n}\{X(a_{k+1}) - X(a_k + h) = 0\}].
\end{aligned}$$

Observe that in the last representation, all intersected events are independent. Therefore,

$$\Pr[T \in Q, X(t) = n] = e^{-\Lambda(a_1)} \cdot \prod_{k=1}^{n} e^{\Lambda(a_k)-\Lambda(a_k+h)} [\Lambda(a_k + h) - \Lambda(a_k)] \cdot \prod_{k=1}^{n} e^{\Lambda(a_k+h)-\Lambda(a_{k+1})}$$
$$= e^{-\Lambda(t)} \prod_{k=1}^{n} [\Lambda(a_k + h) - \Lambda(a_k)].$$

Taking (A.17) and (A.18) into account, we find that

$$\frac{\Pr[T \in Q|X(t) = n]}{m_n(Q)} = \frac{n!}{\Lambda^n(t)} \prod_{k=1}^{n} \frac{\Lambda(a_k + h) - \Lambda(a_k)}{h}. \tag{A.19}$$

For every $y = (y_1, y_2, \ldots, y_n) \in Q$, we have $a_k < y_k \le a_k + h, 1 \le k \le n$. Then

$$\left| \frac{\Lambda(a_k + h) - \Lambda(a_k)}{h} - \lambda(y_k) \right| = \left| \frac{1}{h} \int_{a_k}^{a_k+h} [\lambda(x) - \lambda(y_k)]dx \right| \le \frac{1}{h} \int_{a_k}^{a_k+h} |\lambda(x) - \lambda(y_k)|dx.$$

Since function λ was assumed continuous on $[0, t]$, it is also uniformly continuous on $[0, t]$. Therefore, for any $\eta > 0$, there exists $\delta > 0$ such that, for each k, $1 \le k \le n$, and for any pair of points $v, w \in (a_k, a_k + h]$, inequality $h < \delta$ implies $|\lambda(v) - \lambda(w)| \le \eta$. Therefore, if $r(Q) < \delta \le \delta_0$, then

$$\sup_{y_k \in (a_k, a_k+h]} \left| \frac{\Lambda(a_k + h) - \Lambda(a_k)}{h} - \lambda(y_k) \right| \le \eta, \quad 1 \le k \le n.$$

From (A.19) we now conclude that, for the number $\varepsilon > 0$ preselected, there exists $\delta > 0$ with $\delta \le \delta_0$ such that

$$\sup_{y \in Q} \left| \frac{\Pr[T \in Q|X(t) = n]}{m_n(Q)} - f(y) \right| \le \varepsilon$$

for every cube $Q \subset G$ with $r(Q) < \delta$, where

$$f(y) = n! \, \frac{\prod_{k=1}^{n} \lambda(y_k)}{\Lambda^n(t)}, \quad y \in G,$$

compare with the RHS of (A8). This finalizes the proof of statement 2.

We now turn to statement 3. We have to verify that this function f satisfies the normalization condition $\int_G f(u)du = 1$, i. e.,

$$I_n(t) = \int_0^t \int_0^{u_n} \cdots \int_0^{u_2} \lambda(u_1)\lambda(u_2) \ldots \lambda(u_{n-1})\lambda(u_n) du_1 du_2 \ldots du_n = \frac{\Lambda^n(t)}{n!}, \quad t \ge 0. \tag{A.20}$$

To show this, we use the method of mathematical induction. For $n = 1$,

$$I_1(t) = \int_0^t \lambda(u_1)du_1 = \Lambda(t),$$

so that (A.20) is trivially satisfied. Suppose that for some $n \geq 2$ and all $t \geq 0$,

$$I_{n-1}(t) = \int_0^t \int_0^{u_{n-1}} \cdots \int_0^{u_2} \lambda(u_1)\lambda(u_2)\ldots\lambda(u_{n-1})du_1du_2\ldots du_{n-1} = \frac{\Lambda^{n-1}(t)}{(n-1)!}.$$

Then, using the induction hypothesis and making a change of variable $v = \Lambda(u_n)$, we find that

$$I_n(t) = \int_0^t I_{n-1}(u_n)\lambda(u_n)du_n = \int_0^t \frac{\Lambda^{n-1}(u_n)}{(n-1)!}\lambda(u_n)du_n = \int_0^{\Lambda(t)} \frac{v^{n-1}}{(n-1)!}\,dv = \frac{\Lambda^n(t)}{n!},$$

which completes the proof of Theorem A.2.

A.5 Delayed Poisson process

The purpose of this section is to show that, under the conditions stated in Section 8.1, a delayed Poisson process is again a Poisson process and to compute its rate function. Essential components of the argument are developed within the following proof of Theorem A.4. This theorem represents an extension of Theorem A.1 on marked Poisson processes to the setting where the marking probability is time-dependent. This result is also of independent interest.

Suppose that an event in a Poisson process $X(t)$ with rate function $\lambda(t)$ occurring at time s is marked with probability $p(s)$ independently of other events and of the process itself. It is assumed that $p(s)$ is a measurable function on $[0, \infty)$.

Theorem A.4. *Under these assumptions, the marked Poisson process $Y(t)$ is a Poisson process with the rate function $p(t)\lambda(t)$.*

Proof. Demonstrating that $Y(t)$ is a Poisson process requires verification of conditions 1–3 that define the Poisson process (see Section A.2). Condition 1 is trivially satisfied. As to condition 2, we have to compute the distribution of random variable $Y(t)$. Fix $t > 0$ and the number, $n \geq 1$, of events in the original process $X(s)$ on the interval $(0, t]$. Denote by $T_1, T_2, \ldots, T_n$, where $0 < T_1 < T_2 < \cdots < T_n \leq t$, the successive occurrence times for the first n events. We have to evaluate

$$\pi_{kn}(t) = \Pr[Y(t) = k|X(t) = n] = \mathbb{E} \sum_{\xi_1+\xi_2+\cdots+\xi_n=k} \prod_{i=1}^{n} [p(T_i)]^{\xi_i} [1 - p(T_i)]^{1-\xi_i}, \quad 0 \le k \le n, \tag{A.21}$$

where $\xi_i = 0$ or 1 is the marking indicator for i-th event, $1 \le i \le n$, with 1 assigned to a marked event. Observe also that in the case $n = 0$, we have $\pi_{00}(t) = 1$.

Direct computation of probabilities $\pi_{kn}(t)$ is difficult due to the fact that random variables $T_1, T_2, \ldots, T_n$ are stochastically dependent, and this is where Theorem A.2 lends critical help. According to Remark A.3 after Theorem A.2, the event occurrence times in the Poisson process $X(s)$ are equidistributed, conditional on $X(t) = n$, with the vector of order statistics for a random sample $U_1, U_2, \ldots, U_n$ drawn from the pdf $\omega(s) = \lambda(s)/\Lambda(t)$ for $0 \le s \le t$ and 0 elsewhere. Observe that the sum in (A.21) is a symmetric (rearrangement-invariant) function of $T_1, T_2, \ldots, T_n$. This implies that random variables $T_1, T_2, \ldots, T_n$ in (A.21) can be replaced with the iid random variables $U_1, U_2, \ldots, U_n$. Thus, the probabilities $\pi_{kn}(t)$ in (A.21) form the binomial distribution $\mathrm{Bin}(n, p(t))$, where $p(t)$, the overall probability, conditional on $X(t) = n$, that an event that has occurred by time t has been marked, is given by

$$p(t) = \int_0^t p(s)\omega(s)ds = \frac{\int_0^t p(s)\lambda(s)ds}{\Lambda(t)}. \tag{A.22}$$

As expected, $p(t)$ is independent of n. Using Proposition A.1, we conclude that the overall (compounded) distribution of $Y(t)$ is Poisson $P[p(t)\Lambda(t)] = P[\int_0^t p(s)\lambda(s)ds]$.

Finally, we have to make sure that condition 3 on the independence of increments of the process $Y(t)$ is satisfied. This argument represents an extension of the proof of increment independence for the case of constant marking probability (see Theorem A.1).

Let $n \ge 2$ and $0 \le t_0 < t_1 < \cdots < t_n$ be any time points. We retain from the proof of Theorem A.1 the notation $W_k = X(t_k) - X(t_{k-1})$ and $Z_k = Y(t_k) - Y(t_{k-1})$, $1 \le k \le n$. Fix a vector $m = (m_1, m_2, \ldots, m_n)$ of event counts for the random vector of increments $W = (W_1, W_2, \ldots, W_n)$. Observe that for any $k = 1, 2, \ldots, n$, stochastic process defined by the formula $V_k(t) = X(t_{k-1}+t) - X(t_{k-1})$, $t \ge 0$, is a Poisson process with the rate function $\lambda(t_{k-1} + t)$. Note also that $W_k = V_k(t_k - t_{k-1})$, $1 \le k \le n$.

Similar to (A.22), we find that, for any $k = 1, 2, \ldots, n$ and any original event occurring on the interval $(t_{k-1}, t_k]$, the probability that this event has been marked, conditional on $W_k = m_k$, is

$$p_k = \int_{t_{k-1}}^{t_k} p(s)\nu_k(s - t_{k-1})ds = \frac{\int_{t_{k-1}}^{t_k} p(s)\lambda(s)ds}{\Lambda(t_k) - \Lambda(t_{k-1})},$$

where

$$\nu_k(s) = \frac{\lambda(t_{k-1} + s)}{\Lambda(t_k) - \Lambda(t_{k-1})}, \quad 0 \le s \le t_k - t_{k-1},$$

and 0 otherwise is the pdf underlying the occurrence of events in the process $V_k(t)$, conditional on the event $V(t_k - t_{k-1}) = m_k$. Therefore, the conditional distribution of the number, Z_k, of marked events given $W_m = m_k$ is $\mathrm{Bin}(m_k, p_k)$, $1 \le k \le n$. Additionally, independence assumptions built into the marking process imply that random variables $Z_1, Z_2, \ldots, Z_n$ are independent, conditional on $W = m$. Observe that the argument within the proof of Theorem A.1 that established unconditional independence of these random variables, expressed by formula (A.5), holds in the more general case of arbitrary probabilities $p_1, p_2, \ldots, p_n$. Therefore, the process $Y(t)$ has independent increments.

Thus, $Y(t)$ is a Poisson process with the rate function $p(t)\lambda(t)$. This completes the proof of Theorem A.4. □

We are now ready to handle delayed Poisson processes. Suppose that every event in a Poisson process $X(t)$ with rate $\lambda(t)$ is delayed, independently of other events and of the Poisson process, by a random amount of time. It is also assumed that the delay times are iid random variables with pdf f and the corresponding cdf F. Denote by $Y(t)$ the number of events whose delay was completed by time t and call it the *delayed Poisson process*.

Theorem A.5. *Under these assumptions, the delayed Poisson process $Y(t)$ is a Poisson process with the rate function $\mu(t) = \int_0^t f(t-s)\lambda(s)ds$.*

Proof. We have to verify that conditions 1–3 in the definition of Poisson process are satisfied. That condition 1 holds is clear.

As to condition 2, fix $t > 0$. Consider an event in the original Poisson process that has occurred at time $s \in (0, t]$. Let τ be its random delay time. Then, the probability, $q_t(s)$, that the delay will be completed by time t is

$$q_t(s) = \Pr(s + \tau \le t) = \Pr(\tau \le t - s) = F(t - s).$$

To show that $Y(t)$ is a Poisson random variable, pick $n \ge 1$, and consider n original events that happened by time t. As was argued in the proof of Theorem A.4, their occurrence times, conditional on $X(t) = n$, can be thought of as a random sample from the probability distribution with pdf $\omega(s) = \lambda(s)/\Lambda(t)$, $0 \le s \le t$, and 0 otherwise. Then, the overall probability, conditional on the occurrence of n original events by time t, is given by the formula

$$p(t) = \int_0^t q_t(s)\omega(s)ds = \frac{\int_0^t F(t-s)\lambda(s)ds}{\Lambda(t)}.$$

Observe that this probability is independent of n. The distribution of the number of original events, whose delay was completed by time t, conditional on $X(t) = n$, is $\mathrm{Bin}(n, p(t))$. Applying Proposition A.1 we conclude that the distribution of random variable $Y(t)$ is Poisson $P[p(t)\Lambda(t)] = P[\int_0^t F(t-s)\lambda(s)ds]$.

A proof for the independence of increments of the process $Y(t)$ follows verbatim its counterpart in the proof of Theorem A.4.

Thus, $Y(t)$ is a Poisson process with integrated rate $M(t) = \int_0^t F(t-s)\lambda(s)ds$. Then, for its rate we have due to $F(0) = 0$:

$$\mu(t) = M'(t) = F(0)\lambda(t) + \int_0^t F'(t-s)\lambda(s)ds = \int_0^t f(t-s)\lambda(s)ds.$$

This finalizes the proof of Theorem A.5. □

Acknowledgment

On March 29, 2023, destiny knocked at my door in the form of an email from Dr. Scott Bentley, a consulting editor at DeGruyter. He wrote to me asking if I would be interested in writing a book on mathematical biology for this esteemed publishing house founded in 1749. I had been having vague thoughts for quite some time about writing a book summarizing what I had learned about cancer and its treatment over 30 years of work in the field, mostly on the mathematical modeling side. In the past, these thoughts used to be accompanied by doubts and excuses and were quickly washed away by the flow of busy life. But Scott Bentley's request affected me very differently, and a quiet voice inside told me in no uncertain terms that the time had come. I agreed, and Scott Bentley gently carried me through the process of book proposal preparation and its internal review. For this, and for his subsequent support for the book project, I am forever grateful to him. Without him, this book would likely never have seen the light.

I would also like to extend my appreciation to other DeGruyter (and more recently, DeGruyter Brill) editors who have generously shared with me their time and expertise. I am especially thankful to Steven Elliot, who deftly steered the book project through external review and the inking of the contract, and helped on the stage of manuscript submission. My special thanks also go to Dr. Bettina Noto, a senior manager for Science, Technology and Medicine, for her decisive help and guidance at critical junctions on the road leading to a published monograph. I am also obliged to Nadja Schedensack and Ute Skambraks, the former content editors of books, who guided me through manuscript preparation, and to Kristina Grigorjeva who assisted me on the production stage. Finally, I am grateful to Dr. Ranis Ibragimov, the former acquisition editor for Mathematics & Computer Science, for his warm welcome.

Another person without whom this book would have never been written is Andrei Yakovlev, my dear friend and collaborator whom I met back in Russia in 1986. He rekindled my interest in biology and medicine, which figured prominently in my life until 1973, the year I entered Leningrad (St.Petersburg) State University to study mathematics, and helped me put it on a more professional footing. Our friendship and joint work had spanned 22 years until his untimely death in 2008. Andrei was a universal scientist of the highest caliber with expertise in medicine, biology, mathematics and statistics. Unsurprisingly, his innovative ideas about cancer and his insights into radiation biology had a great influence on my views on these subjects. His profound thoughts about mathematical modeling in biomedical sciences have continued to guide my work ever since the time he left this world. I cannot thank him enough for his presence in my life.

Three other notable scientists left an indelible mark on my vision of cancer and the effects of its treatment. Coincidentally, or perhaps not at all, all of them were physicists by training. My interaction with them accelerated germination of the ideas that form the core of this book. They helped and supported me in more ways than can be listed here, and for that I am eternally grateful to them.

https://doi.org/10.1515/9783111334035-020

The first among them is my friend and long-time collaborator Marco Zaider, a renowned expert in radiation biology and, until his retirement, one of the leading radiation oncologists at the Memorial Sloan Kettering Cancer Center in New York City. He not only helped me hone my theoretical understanding of the mechanisms and effects of radiation but also to bring the clinical reality of cancer to the forefront of my thinking about the disease and its mitigation.

The second colleague and friend is Michael Retsky, a maverick cancer researcher whose pioneering ideas about accelerating effects of surgery on metastasis were one of those transformative “aha!” moments that gave new dimension to my cancer-related research. Although I have never met him in person, Michael Retsky has never failed to share with me his novel ideas, bold plans and latest publications.

And the third scientist is Ray Sachs, who worked most of his life in the Physics and Mathematics Departments at the University of California, Berkeley. In his younger years, Sachs made a number of fundamental discoveries in theoretical astrophysics and cosmology. But later, for reasons apparently known to him alone, he switched to radiation biology and mathematical oncology. I have learned tremendously from reading, and occasionally refereeing, his papers in these two fields. I never had an opportunity to meet him face-to-face, but our correspondence over the last 15 years and, more recently, our collaborative work, convinced me that in him I met both a profound scholar and a caring friend. His death in 2024 has left a void in my heart.

Last but not least, I want to thank my family for their keen interest in my work and unwavering support. My elder son Mark gave much thought to the book’s content vis-a-vis potential readership and went with his sharp editorial eye through some parts of the book, which greatly improved their style. My younger son Boris gave me a lot of inspiration and never failed to ask me about the progress with the book. His incisive, erudite mathematical and scientific mind was an invaluable resource for me. But above anything else, I am filled with gratitude to my wife Marina. Her profound knowledge of biology made her a natural target for my incessant inquiries about this subject, and for each question I received a thorough and thoughtful answer. I cannot thank her enough for her encouragement, appreciation of my work, patience and for being the main driving force behind so many things that are good, caring and creative in my life and that of our family.

Bibliography

[1] Schork N. Time for one-patient trials. Nature 2015, 520, 609–11.
[2] Poincaré H. Science and hypothesis. New York, NY, USA, Dover Publications, 1952.
[3] https://paulingblog.wordpress.com/2008/10/28/clarifying-three-widespread-quotes/ (Accessed March 14, 2026.)
[4] Angell M. Drug companies & doctors: A story of corruption. The New York review of books, January 15, 2009.
[5] Leaf C. The truth in small doses. Why we're losing the war on cancer – and how to win it. New York, NY, USA, Simon & Schuster, 2013.
[6] Servan-Schreiber D. Anticancer: A new way of life. New York, NY, USA, Penguine Group, 2008.
[7] Gøetzsche PC. Deadly medicines and organised crime: How Big Pharma has corrupted healthcare. London, UK, Radcliffe Publishing, 2013.
[8] Penston J. Stats.con. How we've been fooled by statistics-based research in medicine. London, UK, London Press, 2010.
[9] Hanin L. Why statistical inference from clinical trials is likely to generate false and irreproducible results. BMC Med Res Methodol 2017, 17, 127.
[10] Kolitz D. 'Evidence-based medicine' and the expulsion of Peter Gøetzsche. Undark, December 30, 2019. (Accessed March 14, 2026 at https://undark.org/2019/12/30/peter-gotzsche-cochrane/.)
[11] Hanin L. Cavalier use of inferential statistics is a major source of false and irreproducible scientific findings. Mathematics 2021, 9(6), 603.
[12] https://www.pewresearch.org/science/2023/11/14/confidence-in-scientists-medical-scientists-and-other-groups-and-institutions-in-society/ (Accessed March 14, 2026).
[13] Greenhalgh T, Howick J, Maskrey N. Evidence based medicine: A movement in crisis? BMJ 2014, 348, g3725.
[14] Fall K, Fang F, Mucci LA et al. Immediate risk for cardiovascular events and suicide following a prostate cancer diagnosis: Prospective cohort study. PLoS Med 2009, 6(12), e1000197.
[15] Geffen J. The journey through cancer. Healing and transforming the whole person. New York, NY, USA, Three Rivers Press, 2006.
[16] Cooke R. Dr. Folkman's war. Angiogenesis and the struggle to defeat cancer. New York, NY, USA, Random House, 2001.
[17] Atlas S. A plague upon our house: My fight at the Trump White House to stop COVID from destroying America. New York, NY and Nashville, TN, USA, Liberatio Protocol. 2021.
[18] Gusev Y, Hanin L, Klebanov L, Tsodikov A, Yanev N, Zorin A. Dr. Andrei Yakovlev: Visionary, leader, iconoclast. Biol Direct 2008, 3, 10.
[19] Hanin LG. Principles of mathematical modeling in biomedical sciences: An unwritten gospel of Andrei Yakovlev. In: Almudevar A, Oakes D, Hall J, ed. Statistical modeling for biological systems: In memory of Andrei Yakovlev. Cham, Switzerland, Springer Nature Switzerland AG, 2020, 321–31.
[20] Force LM, Kocarnik JM, May ML et al. The global, regional, and national burden of cancer, 1990–2023, with forecasts to 2050: A systematic analysis for the Global Burden of Disease Study 2023. The Lancet, 24 September 2025.
[21] American Cancer Society. Global cancer facts and figures. 5th ed. Atlanta, GA, USA, American Cancer Society, 2024.
[22] American Cancer Society. Cancer facts and figures. Atlanta, GA, USA, American Cancer Society, 2025.
[23] Zheng R, Wang S, Zhang S et al. Global, regional, and national lifetime probabilities of developing cancer in 2020. Sci Bull 2023, 68(21), 2620–8.
[24] Elmadani M, Mokaya PO, Omer AAA, Kiptulon EK, Klara S, Orsolya M. Cancer burden in Europe: A systematic analysis of the GLOBOCAN database (2022). BMC Cancer 2025, 25(1), 447.
[25] https://www.who.int/news/item/01-02-2024-global-cancer-burden-growing--amidst-mounting-need-for-services (Accessed March 14, 2026.)

https://doi.org/10.1515/9783111334035-021

[26] Sultan I, Ahmad S, Alfaar AS, Sultan Y, Salman Z, Qaddoumi I. Trends in childhood cancer: Incidence and survival analysis over 45 years of SEER data. PLoS ONE 2025, 20(1), e0314592.
[27] Zhao J, Xu L, Sun J et al. Global trends in incidence, death, burden and risk factors of early-onset cancer from 1990 to 2019. BMJ Oncology 2023, 2, e000049.
[28] Siegel RL, Kratzer TB, Giaquinto AN, Sung H, Jemal A. Cancer statistics, 2025 CA Cancer J Clin 2025, 75(1), 10–45.
[29] Mukherjee S. The Emperor of all maladies. A biography of cancer. New York, NY, USA, Scribner, 2025.
[30] Rous FP. The challenge to man of the neoplastic cell. Nobel Lecture, December 13, 1966.
[31] Hayflick L, Moorhead PS. The serial cultivation of human diploid cell strains. Exp Cell Res 1961, 25(3), 585–621.
[32] Sonnenschein C, Soto AM. Somatic mutation theory of carcinogenesis: Why it should be dropped and replaced. Mol Carcinog 2000, 29, 205–11.
[33] Soto AM, Sonnenschein C. The somatic mutation theory of cancer: Growing problems with the paradigm? BioEssays 2004, 26, 1097–107.
[34] Sonnenschein C, Soto AM. Theories of carcinogenesis: An emerging perspective. Semin Cancer Biol 2008, 18, 372–7.
[35] Demicheli R, Hrushesky WJM, Saenger E, Biganzoli E. Medical and scientific evidence for the cancer attractor. Acad Oncol 2024, 1(2), https://doi.org/10.20935/AcadOnco7445.
[36] Smithers DW. Cancer, an attack on cytologism. Lancet 1962, 1, 493–9.
[37] Mintz B, Illmensee K. Normal genetically mosaic mice produced from malignant teratocarcinoma cells. Proc Natl Acad Sci USA 1975, 72, 3585–9.
[38] Kenny PA, Bissell M. Tumor reversion: Correction of malignant behavior by microenvironmental cues. Int J Cancer 2003, 107(5), 688–95.
[39] Brand KG, Buoen LC, Brand I. Foreign-body tumorigenesis induced by glass and smooth and rough plastic. Comparative study of preneoplastic events. J Natl Cancer Inst 1975, 55(2), 319–22.
[40] Tarin D. Clinical and biological implications of the tumor microenvironment. Cancer Microenviron 2012, 5, 95–112.
[41] Kenny PA, Nelson CM, Bissell MJ. The ecology of tumors: By perturbing the microenvironment, wounds and infection may be key to tumor development. Scientist 2006, 20(4), 30–5.
[42] Folkman J. Tumor angiogenesis factor. Cancer Res 1974, 34, 2109–13.
[43] Moiseenko VM. "Natural history" of breast cancer growth. Pract Oncol 2002, 3(1), 6–14 (in Russian).
[44] O'Reilly MS, Holmgren L, Shing Y et al. Angiostatin: A novel angiogenesis inhibitor that mediates the suppression of metastases by a Lewis lung carcinoma. Cell 1994, 79, 315–28.
[45] O'Reilly MS, Boehm T, Shing Y et al. Endostatin: An endogenous inhibitor of angiogenesis and tumor growth. Cell 1997, 88(2), 277–85.
[46] Folkman J. Role of angiogenesis in tumor growth and metastasis. Semin Oncol 2002, 29(6), Suppl 16, 15–8.
[47] Tirino V, Desiderio V, Paino F et al. Cancer stem cells in solid tumors: An overview and new approaches for their isolation and characterization. FACEB J 2013, 27, 13–24.
[48] Bonnet D, Dick JE. Human acute myeloid leukemia is organized as a hierarchy that originates from a primitive hematopoietic cell. Nat Med 1997, 3, 730–7.
[49] Al-Hajj M, Wicha MS, Benito-Hernandez A, Morrison SJ, Clarke MF. Prospective identification of tumorigenic breast cancer cells. Proc Natl Acad Sci USA 2003, 100(7), 3983–8.
[50] Collins AT, Berry PA, Hyde C, Stower MJ, Maitland NJ. Prospective identification of tumorigenic prostate cancer stem cells. Cancer Res 2005, 65, 10946–51.
[51] Fidler IJ. Critical factors in the biology of human cancer metastasis: Twenty-eighth G. H. A. Clowes memorial award lecture. Cancer Res 1990, 50, 6130–8.
[52] Friberg S, Nyström A. Cancer metastases: Early dissemination and late recurrences. Cancer Growth Metastasis 2015, 8, 43–9.

[53] Fidler IJ, Ellis LM. The implications of angiogenesis for the biology and therapy of cancer metastasis. Cell 1994, 79, 185–8.

[54] Pantel K, Otte M. Occult micrometastases: Enrichment, identification and characterization of single disseminated tumour cells. Semin Cancer Biol 2001, 11, 327–37.

[55] Paget S. The distribution of secondary growths in cancer of the breast. Lancet 1889, 133(3421), 571–3.

[56] Obenauf AC, Massagué J. Surviving at a distance: Organ specific metastasis. Trends Cancer 2015, 1(1), 76–91.

[57] Tarin D, Price JE, Kettlewell MG, Souter RG, Vass AC, Crossley B. Mechanisms of human tumor metastasis studied in patients with peritoneovenous shunts. Cancer Res 1984, 44(8), 3584–92.

[58] Ashworth TR. A case of cancer in which cells similar to those in the tumour were seen in the blood after death. Med J Aust 1869, 14, 146–7.

[59] Yu M, Stott S, Toner M, Maheswaran S, Haber DA. Circulating tumor cells: Approaches to isolation and characterization. J Cell Biol 2011, 192(3), 373–82.

[60] Marches R, Scheuermann R, Uhr J. Cancer dormancy. From mice to man. Cell Cycle 2006, 5(16), 1772–8.

[61] Okumura Y, Tanaka F, Yoneda K et al. Circulating tumor cells in pulmonary venous blood of primary lung cancer patients. Ann Thorac Surg 2009, 87(6), 1669–75.

[62] Miller MC, Doyle GV, Terstappen LW. Significance of circulating tumor cells detected by the CellSearch system in patients with metastatic breast, colorectal and prostate cancer. J Oncol 2010, 617421, 1–8.

[63] Moore GE, Sandberg AA, Watne AL. The comparative size and structure of tumor cells and clumps in the blood, bone marrow, and tumor imprints. Cancer 1960, 13, 111–7.

[64] Zeidman I. The fate of circulating tumor cells I. Passage of cells through capillaries. Cancer Res 1961, 21, 38–9.

[65] Hanin LG. The circulation stage of the metastatic cascade: A mathematical description and its clinical implications. J Theor Biol 2023, 572, 111582.

[66] Dujon AM, Capp J-P, Brown JS et al. Is there one key step in the metastatic cascade? Cancers 2021, 13, 3693.

[67] Hadfield G. The dormant cancer cell. Br Med J 1954, 2, 607–10.

[68] Demicheli R, Biganzoli E. Clinical tumor dormancy. In: Montagner M, ed. Cancer cell dormancy. Methods and protocols. Totowa, NJ, USA, Humana Press, 2024, 1–26.

[69] Holmgren K, O'Reilly MS, Folkman J. Dormancy of micrometastases: Balanced proliferation and apoptosis in the presence of angiogenesis suppression. Nat Med 1995, 1, 149–53.

[70] Sanders ME, Schuyler PA, Dupont WD, Page DL. The natural history of low-grade ductal carcinoma in situ of the breast in women treated by biopsy only revealed over 30 years of long-term follow-up. Cancer 2005, 103(12), 2481–4.

[71] Mamby CC, Love RR, Heaney E. Metastatic breast cancer 39 years after primary treatment. Wisc Med J 1993, 92(10), 567–9.

[72] Loh E, Couch FG, Hendricksen C et al. Development of donor-derived prostate cancer in a recipient following orthotopic heart transplantation. JAMA 1997, 277, 133–7.

[73] Folkman J, Kalluri R. Cancer without disease. Nature 2004, 427, 787.

[74] Andersen J, Nielsen M, Jensen J. Essential histological findings in the female breast at autopsy. In: Zander J, Baltzer J, ed. Early breast cancer. Berlin, Heidelberg, New York, Tokyo, Springer Verlag, 1985, 52–63.

[75] Bell KJL, Del Mar C, Wright G, Dickinson J, Glasziou P. Prevalence of incidental prostate cancer: A systematic review of autopsy studies. Int J Cancer 2015, 137, 1749–57.

[76] Sandhu GS, Andriole GL. Overdiagnosis of prostate cancer. J Natl Cancer Inst Monogr 2012, 45, 146–51.

[77] Alexander P. Dormant metastases: Studies in experimental animals. J Pathol 1983, 141, 379–83.

[78] Lança T, Silva-Santos B. The split nature of tumor-infiltrating leukocytes. Implications for cancer surveillance and immunotherapy. OncoImmunology 2012, 1(5), 717–25.

[79] Cussens LM, Werb Z. Inflammation and cancer. Nature 2002, 420(6917), 860–7.

[80] Murthy SM, Goldschmidt RA, Rao LN, Ammirati M, Buchmann T, Scanlon EF. The influence of surgical trauma on experimental metastasis. Cancer 1989, 64(10), 2035–44.

[81] Hoover HC, Ketcham AS. Techniques for inhibiting tumor metastases. Cancer 1975, 35, 5–14.

[82] Bogden AE, Moreau J-P, Eden PA. Proliferative response of human and animal tumours to surgical wounding of normal tissues: Onset, duration and inhibition. Br J Cancer 1997, 75(7), 1021–7.

[83] El Saghir NS, Elhajj II, Geara FB, Hourani MH. Trauma-associated growth of suspected dormant micrometastasis. BMC Cancer 2005, 5, 94.

[84] De Giorgi V, Maida P, Salvati L et al. Trauma and foreign bodies may favour the onset of melanoma metastases. Clin Exp Dermatol 2020, 45(5), 619–21.

[85] Hanin L. Do breast cancer patients benefit from surgery? Hypotheses, mathematical models and false beliefs. In: Retsky M, Demicheli R, ed. Perioperative inflammation as a triggering origin of metastasis development. Cham, Switzerland, Springer Nature, 2017, 161–82.

[86] Virchow R. Die krankhaften Geschwülste. Berlin, Germany, A. Hirschwald, 1863 (in German).

[87] Fisher B. Laboratory and clinical research in breast cancer: A personal adventure. The David A. Karnofsky memorial lecture. Cancer Res 1980, 40, 3863–74.

[88] Fisher B. From Halsted to prevention and beyond: Advances in the management of breast cancer during the twentieth century. Eur J Cancer 1999, 35, 1963–73.

[89] Douglas JRS. Significance of the size distribution of bloodborne metastases. Cancer 1971, 27, 379–90.

[90] Chantrain CF, Feron O, Marbaix E, DeClerck YA. Bone marrow microenvironment and tumor progression. Cancer Microenviron 2008, 1(1), 23–35.

[91] Demicheli R. Cancer: Nurture and Nature. In: Retsky M, Demicheli R, ed. Perioperative inflammation as a triggering origin of metastasis development. Cham, Switzerland, Springer Nature, 2017, 209–25.

[92] Scott JG, Gerlee P, Basanta D, Fletcher AG, Maini PK, Anderson ARA. Mathematical modeling of the metastatic process. In: Experimental metastasis: Modeling and analysis. Dordrecht, the Netherlands, Springer, 2013, 189–208.

[93] Gøetzsche P. Mammography screening: Truth, lies and controversy. London, UK, Radcliffe Publishing, 2012.

[94] Baines CJ. Rational and irrational issues in breast cancer screening. Cancers 2011, 3, 252–66.

[95] Cox B. Variation in the effectiveness of breast screening by year of follow-up. J Natl Cancer Inst Monogr 1997, 22, 69–72.

[96] Retsky M, Demicheli R, Hrushesky W. Breast cancer screening: Controversies and future directions. Curr Opin Obstet Gynecol 2003, 15(1), 1–8.

[97] Welch HG, Black WC. Overdiagnosis in cancer. J Natl Cancer Inst 2010, 102(9), 605–13.

[98] Ablin RJ. The great prostate mistake. The New York Times, March 10, 2010.

[99] Ehrlich P. Experimentelle Karzinomstudien an Mäusen. Arch Königlichen Inst Exp Ther Frankfurt am Main 1906, 1, 65–103 (in German).

[100] Bashford E, Murray J, Cramer W. The natural and induced resistance of mice to the growth of cancer. Proc R Soc Lond 1907, 79, 164–87.

[101] Gorelik E. Concomitant tumor immunity and resistance to a second tumor challenge. Adv Cancer Res 1983, 39, 71–120.

[102] Chiarella P, Bruzzo J, Meiss RP, Ruggiero RA. Concomitant tumor resistance. Cancer Lett 2012, 324, 133–41.

[103] Prehn RT. Two competing influences that may explain concomitant tumor resistance. Cancer Res 1993, 53, 3266–9.

[104] Tohme S, Simmons RL, Tsung A. Surgery for cancer: A trigger for metastases. Cancer Res 2017, 77(7), 1548–52.

[105] Hanin L. Paradoxical effects of tumor shrinkage on long-term survival of cancer patients. Front Appl Math Stat – Systems Biology 2020, 6, 27.
[106] Gatenby RA. A change of strategy in the war on cancer. Nature 2009, 459, 508–9.
[107] Enriquez-Navas PM, Wojtkowiak JW, Gatenby RA. Application of evolutionary principles to cancer therapy. Cancer Res 2015, 75(22), 4675–80.
[108] Nikolaou M, Nikolaou G, Digklia A et al. Immunotherapy of cancer: Developments and reference points, an unorthodox approach. Integr Cancer Ther 2019, 18(1), 1–10.
[109] Esfahani K, Roudaia L, Buhlaiga N, Del Rincon SV, Papneja N, Miller Jr WH. A review of cancer immunotherapy: From the past, to the present, to the future. Curr Oncol 2020, 27(S2), 87–97.
[110] Min H-Y, Lee H-Y. Molecular targeted therapy for anticancer treatment. Exp Mol Med 2022, 54, 1670–94.
[111] Coleman RE, Rubens RD, Fogelman I. Reappraisal of the baseline bone scan in breast cancer. J Nucl Med 1988, 29, 1045–9.
[112] Marie P, Clunet J. Fréquences des métastases viscérales chez les souris cancéreuses après ablation chirurgicale de leur tumeur. Bull Assoc Fr Étude Cancer 1910, 3, 19–23 (in French).
[113] Demicheli R, Retsky M, Hrushesky WJM, Baum M, Gukas ID. The effects of surgery on tumor growth: A century of investigations. Ann Oncol 2008, 19, 1821–8.
[114] Retsky M, Demicheli R, Hrushesky W, Baum M, Gukas I. Surgery triggers outgrowth of latent distant disease in breast cancer: An inconvenient truth? Cancers 2010, 2(2), 305–37.
[115] Deylgat B, Van Rooy F, Vansteenkiste F, Devriendt D, George C. Postsurgery activation of dormant liver micrometastasis: A case report and review of literature. J Gastrointest Cancer 2011, 42(1), 1–4.
[116] Tseng WW, Doyle JA, Maguiness S, Horvai AE, Kashani-Sabet M, Leong SPL. Giant cutaneous melanomas: Evidence for primary tumour induced dormancy in metastatic sites? Br Med J Case Reports, October 5, 2009.
[117] Okada K, Makihara K, Okada M et al. A case of primary squamous cell carcinoma of the breast with rapid progression. Breast Cancer 2000, 7(2), 160–4.
[118] Hanin L, Rose J. Suppression of metastasis by primary tumor and acceleration of metastasis following primary tumor resection: A natural law? Bull Math Biol 2018, 80(3), 519–39.
[119] Pachmann K. Die Bedeutung der im Blut zirkulierenden Tumorzellen in der Metastasierungskaskade. Dtsch Z Onkol 2012, 42, 11–6 (in German).
[120] Sandler HM, Hanks GE. Analysis of the possibility that transurethral resection promotes metastasis in prostate cancer. Cancer 1988, 62, 2622–7.
[121] Tyzzer EE. Factors in the production and growth of tumor metastases. J Med Res 1913, 28, 309–32.
[122] Hogan BV, Peter MB, Shenoy HG, Horgan K, Hughes TA. Surgery induced immunosuppression. Surgeon 2011, 9(1), 38–43.
[123] Krall JA, Reinhardt F, Mercury OA et al. The systemic response to surgery triggers the outgrowth of distant immune-controlled tumors in mouse models of dormancy. Sci Transl Med 2018, 10, eaan3464.
[124] Maida V, Ennis M, Kuziemsky C, Corban J. Wounds and survival in cancer patients. Eur J Cancer 2009, 45, 3237–44.
[125] Isern AE, Manjer J, Malina J et al. Risk of recurrence following delayed large flap reconstruction after mastectomy for breast cancer. Br J Surg 2011, 98, 659–66.
[126] Sugarbaker E, Thornthwaite J, Ketcham A. Inhibitory effect of a primary tumor on metastasis. In: Day SB, Myers WPL, Stanley P, Garattini S, Lewis MG, ed. Progress in cancer research and therapy. New York, NY, USA, Raven, 1977, 227–40.
[127] Camphausen K, Moses MA, Beecken W-D, Khan MK, Folkman J, O'Reilly MS. Radiation therapy to a primary tumor accelerates metastatic growth in mice. Cancer Res 2001, 61, 2207–11.
[128] Sundahl N, Duprez F, Ost P, De Neve W, Mareel M. Effects of radiation on the metastatic process. Mol Med 2018, 24, 16.

[129] Ebos JM. Prodding the beast: Assessing the impact of treatment-induced metastasis. Cancer Res 2015, 75, 3427–35.

[130] Housman G, Byler S, Heerboth S et al. Drug resistance in cancer: An overview. Cancers 2014, 6, 1769–92.

[131] Boyd W. The spontaneous regression of cancer. Springfield, IL, USA, Thomas, 1966.

[132] Everson TC, Cole WH. Spontaneous regression of cancer. Philadelphia, PA, USA, Saunders, 1966.

[133] Smithers DW. Spontaneous regression of cancer. Ann R Coll Surg Engl 1967, 41(Suppl), 160–2.

[134] Zahl P-H, Mæhlen J, Welch HG. The natural history of invasive breast cancer detected by screening mammography. Arch Intern Med 2008, 168, 2311–6.

[135] Hanin L, Korosteleva O. Does extirpation of the primary breast tumor give boost to growth of metastases? Evidence revealed by mathematical modeling. Math Biosci 2010, 223, 133–41.

[136] Hanin L, Zaider M. Effects of surgery and chemotherapy on metastatic progression of prostate cancer: Evidence from the natural history of the disease reconstructed through mathematical modeling. Cancers 2011, 3, 3632–60.

[137] Hanin L, Bunimovich-Mendrazitsky S. Reconstruction of the natural history of metastatic cancer and assessment of the effects of surgery: Gompertzian growth of the primary tumor. Math Biosci 2014, 247, 47–58.

[138] Hanin L, Rose J. Uncovering the natural history of cancer from post mortem cross-sectional diameters of hepatic metastases. Math Med Biol 2015, 33(4), 397–416.

[139] Hanin L, Seidel K, Stoevesandt D. A "universal" model of metastatic cancer, its parametric forms and their identification: What can be learned from site-specific volumes of metastases. J Math Biol 2016, 72(6), 1633–62.

[140] Sachs RK, Heidenreich WF, Brenner DJ. Dose timing in tumor radiotherapy: Considerations of cell number stochasticity. Math Biosci 1996, 138, 131–46.

[141] Fakir H, Hlatky L, Li H, Sachs R. Repopulation of interacting tumor cells during fractionated radiotherapy: Stochastic modeling of the tumor control probability. Med Phys 2013, 40(12), 121716.

[142] Hanin L, Zaider M. Optimal schedules of fractionated radiation therapy by way of the greedy principle: Biologically-based adaptive boosting. Phys Med Biol 2014, 59, 4085–98.

[143] Retsky MW. Metronomic chemotherapy was originally designed and first used in 1994 for early stage cancer-why is it taking so long to proceed? J Bioequivalence & Bioavailability 2011, 3(4), i–iv.

[144] Retsky MW. An argument for discovery-driven research: From physicist to cancer researcher ecancer 2014, 8, ed38.

[145] Bernstein J. MIA in the war in cancer: Where are the low-cost treatments? ProPublica, April 23, 2014. (Accessed March 14, 2026, at https://www.propublica.org/article/where-are-the-low-cost-cancer-treatments.)

[146] Bhattacharya A. The man from the future. The visionary ideas of John von Neumann. New York, NY, USA, W. W. Norton & Company, 2021.

[147] Sachs RK, Hahnfeld P, Brenner DJ. The link between low-LET dose-response relations and the underlying kinetics of damage production/repair/misrepair. Int J Radiat Biol 1997, 72(4), 351–74.

[148] Bartoczyński R, Niewiadomska-Bugaj M. Probability and statistical inference. 2nd ed. Hoboken, NJ, USA, Wiley & Sons, 2008.

[149] Moolgavkar SH, Venzon DJ. Two-event models for carcinogenesis: Incidence curves for childhood and adult tumors. Math Biosci 1979, 47, 55–77.

[150] Moolgavkar SH, Knudson AG. Mutation and cancer: A model for human carcinogenesis. J Natl Cancer Inst 1981, 66, 1037–52.

[151] Kopp-Schneider A, Portier CJ, Sherman CD. The exact formula for tumor incidence in the two-stage model. Risk Anal 1994, 14, 1079–80.

[152] Zheng Q. On the exact hazard and survival functions of the MVK stochastic carcinogenesis model. Risk Anal 1994, 14, 1081–4.

[153] Hanin LG, Yakovlev AY. A nonidentifiability aspect of the two-stage model of carcinogenesis. Risk Anal 1996, 16, 711–5.
[154] Heidenreich WF. On the parameters of the clonal expansion model. Radiat Environ Biophys 1996, 35, 127–9.
[155] Hanin LG. Identification problem for stochastic models with application to carcinogenesis, cancer detection and radiation biology. Discrete Dyn Nat Soc 2002, 7, 177–89.
[156] Wigner EP. The unreasonable effectiveness of mathematics in the natural sciences. Commun Pure Appl Math 1960, 13, 1–14.
[157] Hill AB. The environment and disease: Association or causation? Proc R Soc Med 1965, 58(5), 295–300.
[158] Hanin LG. Seeing the invisible: How mathematical models uncover tumor dormancy, reconstruct the natural history of cancer and assess the effects of treatment. In: Almog N, Enderling H, Hlatky L, ed. Systems biology of tumor dormancy. Advances in Experimental Medicine and Biology, v. 734. New York, NY, USA, Springer, 2013, 261–82.
[159] Stigler SM. The epic story of maximum likelihood. Stat Sci 2007, 22(4), 598–620.
[160] Karr AF. Probability. New York, NY, USA, Springer, 1993.
[161] Benzekry S, Lamont C, Beheshti A et al. Classical mathematical models for description and prediction of experimental tumor growth. PLoS Comput Biol 2014, 10(8), e1003800.
[162] Talkington A, Durett R. Estimating tumor growth rates in vivo. Bull Math Biol 2015, 77(10), 1934–54.
[163] Speer JF, Petrosky VE, Retsky MW, Wardwell RH. A stochastic numerical model of breast cancer growth that simulates clinical data. Cancer Res 1984, 44, 4124–30.
[164] Retsky M, Swartzendruber DE, Wardwell RH, Bame PD. Is Gompertzian kinetics a valid description of individual tumor growth? Med Hypotheses 1990, 33(2), 95–106.
[165] Bedford JS, Dewey WC. Historical and current highlights in radiation biology: Has anything important been learned by irradiating cells? Radiat Res 2002, 158, 251–91.
[166] Skipper H, Schabel Jr F. Quantitative and cytokinetic studies in experimental tumor systems. In: Holland JF, Frei III E, ed. Cancer medicine. 2nd ed. Philadelphia, PA, USA, Lea and Febiger, 1982, 636–48.
[167] Klein M, Bartoszyński R. Estimation of growth and metastatic rates of primary breast cancer. In: Arino O, Axelrod DE, Kimmel M, ed. Mathematical population dynamics. New York, NY, USA, Marcel Dekker, 1991, 397–412.
[168] Cauchy A-L. Cours d'analyse de l'École Polytechnique, 1: L'analyse algébrique. Paris, 1821 (in French).
[169] Gompertz B. On the nature of the function expressive of the law of human mortality, and on a new mode of determining the value of life contingencies. Philos Trans R Soc Lond 1825, 115, 513–85.
[170] Laird AK. Dynamics of tumour growth. Br J Cancer 1964, 18, 490–502.
[171] Norton L, Simon R. Growth curve of an experimental solid tumor following radiotherapy. J Natl Cancer Inst 1977, 58, 1735–41.
[172] Norton L. A Gompertzian model of human breast cancer growth. Cancer Res 1988, 48, 7067–71.
[173] Hanin LG, Rose J, Zaider M. A stochastic model for the sizes of detectable metastases. J Theor Biol 2006, 243, 407–17.
[174] Hanin LG. Distribution of the sizes of metastases: Mathematical and biomedical considerations. In: Tan W-Y, Hanin LG, ed. Handbook of cancer models with applications. Series in Mathematical Biology and Medicine, v. 9. Singapore, World Scientific, 2008, 149–72.
[175] Hanin L, Jandrig B, Pavlova L, Seidel K. The natural history of renal cell carcinoma with pulmonary metastases illuminated through mathematical modeling. Math Biosci 2019, 309, 118–30.
[176] Kendal WS. Chance mechanisms affecting the burden of metastases. BMC Cancer 2006, 5, 138.
[177] Folkman J. Tumor angiogenesis: Therapeutic implications. N Engl J Med 1971, 285, 1182–6.
[178] Taylor HM, Karlin S. An introduction to stochastic modeling. 3rd ed. San Diego, CA, USA, Academic Press, 1998.
[179] Tait CR, Dodwell D, Horgan K. Do metastases metastasize? J Pathol 2004, 203, 515–8.

[180] Price JE, Carr D, Jones LD, Messer P, Tarin D. Experimental analysis of factors affecting metastatic spread using naturally occurring tumours. Invasion Metastasis 1982, 2(2), 77–112.
[181] Hölzel D, Eckel R, Emeny RT, Engel J. Distant metastases do not metastasize. Cancer Metastasis Rev 2010, 29, 737–50.
[182] Kleffel S, Schatton T. Tumor dormancy and cancer stem cells: Two sides of the same coin? In: Almog N, Enderling H, Hlatky L, ed. Systems biology of tumor dormancy. Advances in Experimental Medicine and Biology. v. 734. New York, NY, USA, Springer, 2013, 145–79.
[183] Bartoszyński R, Edler L, Hanin LG et al. Modeling cancer detection: Tumor size as a source of information on unobservable stages of carcinogenesis. Math Biosci 2001, 171, 113–42.
[184] Dick JE. Breast cancer stem cells revealed. Proc Natl Acad Sci USA 2003, 100(7), 3547–9.
[185] Hanin L, Pavlova L. A quantitative insight into metastatic relapse of breast cancer. J Theor Biol 2016, 394, 172–81.
[186] Zastrow S, Phuong A, von Bar I, Novotny V, Hakenberg OW, Wirth MP. Primary tumor size in renal cell cancer in relation to the occurrence of synchronous metastatic disease. Urol Int 2014, 92, 462–7.
[187] Thorstenson A, Bergman M, Scherman-Plogell AH et al. Tumour characteristics and surgical treatment of renal cell carcinoma in Sweden 2005-2010: A population-based study from the national Swedish kidney cancer register. Scand J Urol 2014, 48(3), 231–8.
[188] Dabestani S, Thorstenson A, Lindblad P, Harmenberg U, Ljungberg B, Lundstam S. Renal cell carcinoma recurrences and metastases in primary non-metastatic patients: A population-based study. World J Urol 2016, 34, 1081–6.
[189] Daugherty M, Sedaghatpour D, Shapiro O, Vourganti S, Kutikov A, Bratslavsky G. The metastatic potential of renal tumors: Influence of histologic subtypes on definition of small renal masses, risk stratification, and future active surveillance protocols. Urol Oncol 2017, 35, 153.e15–153.e20.
[190] Bianchi M, Sun M, Jeldres C et al. Distribution of metastatic sites in renal cell carcinoma: A population-based analysis. Ann Oncol 2012, 23(4), 973–80.
[191] Hock LM, Lynch J, Balaji KC. Increasing incidence of all stages of kidney cancer in the last two decades in the United States: An analysis of surveillance, epidemiology and end results program data. J Urol 2002, 167, 57–60.
[192] MacMahon H, Austin JHM, Gamsu G et al. Guidelines for management of small pulmonary nodules detected on CT scans: A statement from the Fleischner Society. Radiology 2005, 237, 395–400.
[193] Vallander SS. Calculation of the Wasserstein distance between probability distributions on the line. Theory Probab Appl 1974, 18(4), 784–6.
[194] Kai K, Arima Y, Kamiya T, Saya H. Breast cancer stem cells. Breast Cancer 2010, 17, 80–5.
[195] Bussolati B, Dekel B, Azzarone B, Camussi G. Human renal cancer stem cells. Cancer Lett 2013, 338(1), 141–6.
[196] Corrò C, Moch H. Biomarker discovery for renal cancer stem cells. J Pathol Clin Res 2018, 4(1), 3–18.
[197] Ang KK, Thames HD, Jones SD, Jiang G-L, Milas L, Peters LJ. Proliferation kinetics of a murine fibrosarcoma during fractionated irradiation. Radiat Res 1988, 116, 327–36.
[198] Jones B, Dale RG. Cell loss factors and the linear-quadratic model. Radiother Oncol 1995, 37, 136–9.
[199] Tucker SL, Taylor JM. Improved models of tumour cure. Int J Radiat Biol 1996, 70(5), 539–53.
[200] Eisenhauer EA, Therasse P, Bogaerts J et al. New response evaluation criteria in solid tumours: Revised RECIST guideline (version 1.1). Eur J Cancer 2009, 45, 228–47.
[201] Johnson JR, Ning Y-M, Farrell A, Justice R, Keegan P, Pazdur R. Accelerated approval of oncology products: The Food and Drug Administration experience. J Natl Cancer Inst 2011, 103(8), 636–44.
[202] Johnson JR, Williams G, Pazdur R. End points and United States Food and Drug Administration approval of oncology drugs. J Clin Oncol 2003, 21(7), 1404–11.
[203] Dethlefsen LA, Prewitt JMS, Mendelsohn ML. Analysis of tumor growth curves. J Natl Cancer Inst 1968, 40(2), 389–405.
[204] Humphries A, Wright NA. Colonic crypt organization and tumorigenesis. Nat Rev Cancer 2008, 8, 415–24.

[205] Piessevaux H, Buyse M, Schlichting M et al. Use of early tumor shrinkage to predict long-term outcome in metastatic colorectal cancer treated with cetuximab. J Clin Oncol 2013, 31(30), 3764–75.
[206] Douillard JY, Siena S, Peeters M, Koukakis R, Terwey JH, Tabernero J. Impact of early tumour shrinkage and resection on outcomes in patients with wild-type RAS metastatic colorectal cancer. Eur J Cancer 2015, 51(10), 1231–42.
[207] Sakamaki K, Kito Y, Yamazaki K et al. Exploration of time points and cut-off values for early tumour shrinkage to predict survival outcomes of patients with metastatic colorectal cancer treated with first-line chemotherapy using a biexponential model for change in tumour size. ESMO Open 2017, 2, e000275.
[208] Advanced Colorectal Cancer Meta-Analysis Project. Modulation of fluorouracil by leucovorin in patients with advanced colorectal cancer: Evidence in terms of response rate. J Clin Oncol 1992, 10(6), 896–903.
[209] Grothey A, Hedrick EE, Mass RD et al. Response-independent survival benefit in metastatic colorectal cancer: A comparative analysis of N9741 and AVF2107. J Clin Oncol 2008, 26(2), 183–9.
[210] Colloca GA, Venturino A, Guarneri D. Early tumor shrinkage after first-line medical treatment of metastatic colorectal cancer: A meta-analysis. Int J Clin Oncol 2019, 24(3), 231–40.
[211] Basanta D, Scott JG, Fishman MN, Ayala G, Hayward SW, Anderson ARA. Investigating prostate cancer tumour-stroma interactions: Clinical and biological insights from an evolutionary game. Br J Cancer 2012, 106, 174–81.
[212] Staňková K, Brown JS, Dalton WS, Gatenby RA. Optimizing cancer treatment using game theory: A review. JAMA Oncol 2019, 5(1), 96–103.
[213] Enriquez-Navas PM, Wojtkowiak JW, Gatenby RA. Application of evolutionary principles to cancer therapy. Cancer Res 2015, 75(22), 4675–80.
[214] Doll R, Hill AB. Smoking and carcinoma of the lung; preliminary report. Br Med J 1950, 2(4682), 739–48.
[215] Altman DG. The scandal of poor medical research. Br Med J 1994, 308, 283–4.
[216] Romero F. Philosophy of science and the replicability crisis. Philos Compass 2019, 14, e12633.
[217] National Academies of Sciences, Engineering, and Medicine. Reproducibility and replicability in science. Washington, DC, USA, The National Academies Press, 2019.
[218] Ioannidis JPA. Contradicted and initially stronger effects in highly cited clinical research. JAMA 2005, 294(2), 218–28.
[219] Open Science Collaboration. Estimating the reproducibility of psychological science. Science 2015, 349, aac4726.
[220] Goodman SN. Toward evidence-based medical statistics, 1: The *P* value fallacy. Ann Intern Med 1999, 130, 995–1004.
[221] Goodman SN. A dirty dozen: Twelve *p*-value misconceptions. Semin Hematol 2008, 45, 135–40.
[222] Ziliak S, McCloskey D. The cult of statistical significance: How the standard error costs us jobs, justice, and lives. Ann Arbor, MI, USA, University of Michigan Press, 2008.
[223] Gelman A. *P*-values and statistical practice. Epidemiology 2013, 24, 69–72.
[224] Greenland S, Senn SJ, Rothman KJ et al. Statistical tests, *P*-values, confidence intervals, and power: A guide to misinterpretations. Am Stat 2016, 70, 1–12.
[225] Wasserstein RL, Lazar NA. The ASA's statement on *p*-values: Context, process, and purpose. Am Stat 2016, 70(2), 129–33.
[226] Wasserstein RL, Schirm AL, Lazar NA. Moving to a world beyond "$p < 0.05$". Am Stat 2019, 73(sup1), 1–19.
[227] Ioannidis JPA. Why most published research findings are false. PLoS Med 2005, 2, e124.
[228] Tvesky A, Kahneman D. Judgement under uncertainty: Heuristics and biases. Science 1974, 185(4157), 1124–31.
[229] Goodman SN. Why is getting rid of *p*-values so hard? Musings on science and statistics. Am Stat 2019, 73(sup1), 26–30.

[230] Rachev ST, Klebanov L, Stoyanov SV, Fabozzi F. The methods of distances in the theory of probability and statistics. New York, NY, USA, Springer, 2013.
[231] Rényi A. On the central limit theorem for the sum of a random number of independent random variables. Acta Math Acad Sci Hung 1960, 11, 97–102.
[232] Hanin L, Zaider M. Cell-survival probability at large doses: An alternative to the linear-quadratic model. Phys Med Biol 2010, 55, 4687–702.
[233] Berry AC. The accuracy of the Gaussian approximation to the sum of independent variates. Trans Am Math Soc 1941, 49, 122–36.
[234] Esseen C-G. A moment inequality with an application to the central limit theorem. Scand Actuar J 1956, 39, 160–70.
[235] Tyurin IS. An improvement of upper estimates of the constants in the Lyapunov theorem. Russ Math Surv 2010, 65, 201–2.
[236] Shiryaev AN. Probability. Graduate Texts in Mathematics. New York, NY, USA, Springer, 1996.
[237] Benjamin DJ, Berger JO, Johannesson M et al. Redefine statistical significance. Nat Hum Behav 2017, 2, 6–10.
[238] Chavalarias D, Wallach JD, Li AHT, Ioannidis JPA. Evolution of reporting *P* values in the biomedical literature. JAMA 2016, 315, 1141–8.
[239] Kennedy-Shaffer L. Before $p < 0.05$ to beyond $p < 0.05$: Using history to contextualize *p*-values and significance testing. Am Stat 2019, 73, 82–90.
[240] Bernard C. An introduction to the study of experimental medicine. New York, NY, USA, Dover Publications, 1957.
[241] Butler D, Callaway E. Scientists in the dark after French clinical trial proves fatal. Nature 2016, 529, 263–4.
[242] Wadman M. London's disastrous drug trial has serious side effects for research. Nature 2006, 440, 388–9.
[243] Honkoop P, Scholte HR, de Man RA, Schalm SW. Mitochondrial injury. Lessons from the fialuridine trial. Drug Saf 1997, 17, 1–7.
[244] Attarwala H. TGN1412: From discovery to disaster. J Young Pharm 2010, 2(3), 332–6.
[245] Lind J. Treatise of the scurvy. Edinburgh, Scotland, Sands, Murray and Cochran, 1753.
[246] Bartholomew M. James Lind's *Treatise of the Scurvy* (1753). Postgrad Med J 2002, 78, 695–6.
[247] https://www.nuffieldtrust.org.uk/resource/cancer-survival-rates (Accessed March 14, 2026.)
[248] Barnett A. Patients used as drug 'guinea pigs'. The Observer, February 9, 2003.
[249] Emanuel EJ. The solution to drug prices. The New York Times, September 9, 2015.
[250] Light DW, Lexchin J, Darrow JJ. Institutional corruption of pharmaceuticals and the myth of safe and effective drugs. J Law Med Ethics 2013, 41(3), 590–600.
[251] Hutchins LF, Unger JM, Crowley JJ, Coltman Jr CA, Albain KS. Underrepresentation of patient 65 years of age or older in cancer-treatment trials. N Engl J Med 1999, 341(27), 2061–7.
[252] Makary MA Daniel M. Medical error – the third leading cause of death in the US. BMJ 2016, 353, i2139.
[253] Gøeztsche PC. Our prescription drugs kill us in large numbers. Pol Arch Intern Med 2014, 124(11), 628–33.
[254] Angell M. The truth about the drug companies. New York Review of Books, vol. 51 July 15, 2004.
[255] Heres S, Davis J, Maino K, Jetzinger E, Kissling W, Leucht S. Why olanzapine beats risperidone, risperidone beats quetiapine, and quetiapine beats olanzapine: An exploratory analysis of head-to-head comparison studies of second-generation antipsychotics. Am J Psychiatry 2006, 163, 185–94.
[256] Mayor S. Rofecoxib caused excess heart disease. BMJ 2005, 330(7485), 212.
[257] Singer N. Medical papers by ghostwriters pushed therapy. The New York Times 4 August 2009.
[258] Fugh-Berman AJ. The haunting of medical journals: How ghostwriting sold "HRT". PLoS Med 2010, 7(9), e1000335.

[259] Collaborative Group on Hormonal Factors in Breast Cancer. Type and timing of menopausal hormone therapy and breast cancer risk: Individual participant meta-analysis of the worldwide epidemiological evidence. Lancet 2019, 394(10204), 1159–68.
[260] Chlebowski RT, Hendrix SL, Langer RD et al. Influence of estrogen plus progestin on breast cancer and mammography in healthy postmenopausal women: The women's health initiative randomized trial. JAMA 2003, 289(24), 3243–53.
[261] Razavi P, Pike MC, Horn-Ross PL et al. Long-term postmenopausal hormone therapy and endometrial cancer. Cancer Epidemiol Biomark Prev 2010, 19(2), 475–83.
[262] Sachdev A, Sharpe I, Bowman M, Booth CM, Gyawali B. Objective response rate of placebo in randomized controlled trials of anticancer medicines. EClinicalMedicine 2023, 55, 101753.
[263] Cherny NI. An appraisal of FDA approvals for adult solid tumours in 2017–2021: has the eagle landed? Nat Rev, Clin Oncol 2022, 19, 486–92.
[264] Chvetzoff G, Tannock IF. Placebo effects in oncology. J Natl Cancer Inst 2003, 95(1), 19–29.
[265] Howick J, Friedemann C, Tsakok M et al. Are treatments more effective than placebo? A systematic review and meta-analysis. PLoS ONE 2013, 8(5), e62599.
[266] Dien Ho. New theory of placebos reframes mind-body problem. IAI news, December 10, 2024. (Accessed March 14, 2026 at https://iai.tv/articles/new-theory-of-placebos-reframes-mind-body-problem-auid-3022?_auid=2020.)
[267] Berger VW. Pros and cons of permutation tests in clinical trials. Stat Med 2000, 19, 1319–28.
[268] Berger VW. Conflicts of interest, selective inertia, and research malpractice in randomized clinical trials: An unholy trinity. Sci Eng Ethics 2015, 21(4), 857–74.
[269] Soares JF, Wu CFJ. Some restricted randomization rules in sequential designs. Commun Stat, Theory Methods 1982, 12, 2017–34.
[270] Berger VW, Ivanova A, Deloria-Knoll M. Minimizing predictability while retaining balance through the use of less restrictive randomization procedures. Stat Med 2003, 22(19), 3017–28.
[271] Collins R, Bowman L, Landray M, Peto R. The magic of randomization versus the myth of real-world evidence. N Engl J Med 2020, 382(7), 674–8.
[272] Woese CR. A new biology for a new century. Microbiol Mol Biol Rev 2004, 68(2), 173–86.
[273] Dyson FJ. A many-colored glass. Charlottesville, VA, USA and London, UK, University of Virginia Press, 2007.
[274] Lekanidi K, Vlachou PA, Morgan B, Vasanthan S. Spontaneous regression of metastatic renal cell carcinoma: case report. J Med Case Rep 2007, 1, 89.
[275] https://www.cancer.gov/news-events/cancer-currents-blog/2020/cancer-abscopal-effect-radiation-immunotherapy (Accessed March 14, 2026.)
[276] Mitsou JD, Tseveleki V. Abscopal effect in melanoma: Effective treatment in situ may unlock systemic antitumor immunity. Academia Oncology 2025, 2, 1–12.
[277] Kucerova P, Cervinkova M. Spontaneous regression of tumour and the role of microbial infection – possibilities for cancer treatment. Anti-Cancer Drugs 2016, 27, 269–77.
[278] Burkill JC. The Lebesgue integral. Cambridge Tracts in Mathematics, vol. 40. Cambridge, UK, Cambridge University Press, 2004.

Index

https://doi.org/10.1515/9783111334035-022

De Gruyter Series in Mathematics and Life Sciences

Volume 10
Fateh Mebarek-Oudina (Ed.)
CFD Simulation. Thermo-Fluids and Nanofluids in Engineering and Biomedicine, 2025
ISBN 978-3-11-140454-7, ISBN (PDF) 978-3-11-140509-4, ISBN (EPUB) 978-3-11-140523-0

Volume 9
Jochen Mau, Sergey Mukhin, Guanyu Wang, Shuhua Xu (Eds.)
BIOKYBERNETIKA. Mathematics for Theory and Control in the Human and in Society, 2025
ISBN 978-3-11-134197-2, ISBN (PDF) 978-3-11-134199-6, ISBN (EPUB) 978-3-11-134204-7

Volume 8/2
Igor M. Rouzine
Mathematical Modeling of Evolution. Volume 2: Fitness Landscape, Red Queen, Evolutionary Enigmas, and Applications to Virology, 2023
ISBN 978-3-11-069731-5, ISBN (PDF) 978-3-11-069738-4, ISBN (EPUB) 978-3-11-069746-9

Volume 8/1
Igor M. Rouzine
Mathematical Modeling of Evolution. Volume 1: One-Locus and Multi-Locus Theory and Recombination, 2020
ISBN 978-3-11-060789-5, ISBN (PDF) 978-3-11-061545-6, ISBN (EPUB) 978-3-11-060819-9

Volume 7
George Dassios, Athanassios S. Fokas
Electroencephalography and Magnetoencephalography, 2020
ISBN 978-3-11-054583-8, ISBN (PDF) 978-3-11-054753-5, ISBN (EPUB) 978-3-11-054578-4

Volume 6
Piotr Biler
Singularities of Solutions to Chemotaxis Systems, 2019
ISBN 978-3-11-059789-9, ISBN (PDF) 978-3-11-059953-4, ISBN (EPUB) 978-3-11-059862-9

Volume 5
S. V. Masiuk, A. G. Kukush, S. V. Shklyar, M. I. Chepurny, I. A. Likhtarov
Radiation Risk Estimation. Based on Measurement Error Models, 2016
ISBN 978-3-11-044180-2, ISBN (PDF) 978-3-11-043366-1, ISBN (EPUB) 978-3-11-043347-0

Volume 4
Sergey Vakulenko
Complexity and Evolution of Dissipative Systems: An Analytical Approach, 2013
ISBN 978-3-11-026648-1, e-ISBN 978-3-11-026828-7

www.degruyterbrill.com

